Social Work and Minorities

Migration and multiculturality are not phenomena new to Europe but recent periods of unprecedented human movement have established new and evolving diasporic configurations. The problems of migration and settlement are many and complex, with different countries presenting their own issues for the minorities within them. In addition, there is a growing awareness of the specific needs of refugees and asylum seekers and particular concerns continue to echo across Europe given the rise in overt racisms and xenophobia. Social work cannot be indifferent to these often turbulent circumstances and the profession needs to accept the responsibility of taking a role in the social integration of Europe.

Social Work and Minorities critically examines key concepts such as assimilation, multiculturalism, racism, marginalisation and social exclusion. It will be an essential resource for social work practitioners and educators working with migrant communities throughout Europe.

Charlotte Williams is a Lecturer in Social Work at the University of Wales, Bangor. **Haluk Soydan** is Research Director of the Centre for Evaluation of Social Services, National Board of Health and Welfare and Professor of Social Work at Gothenburg University, Sweden. **Mark R. D. Johnson** is Reader in Primary Care and Associate Director at the Mary Seacole Research Centre, De Montfort University, Leicester.

Social Work and Minorities

European perspectives

Edited by Charlotte Williams,
Haluk Soydan and
Mark R. D. Johnson

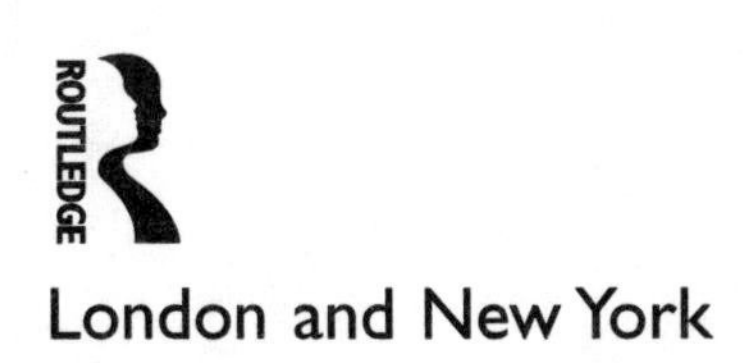

London and New York

First published 1998
by Routledge
11 New Fetter Lane, London EC4P 4EE

Simultaneously published in the USA and Canada
by Routledge
29 West 35th Street, New York, NY 10001

Typeset in Garamond by Keystroke, Jacaranda Lodge, Wolverhampton
Printed and bound in Great Britain by Creative Print and Design
(Wales), Ebbw Vale

British Library Cataloguing in Publication Data
A catalogue record for this book is available from the British Library

Library of Congress Cataloging in Publication Data
Social work and minorities: European perspectives / edited by
Charlotte Williams, Haluk Soydan and Mark R.D. Johnson.
Includes bibliographical references and index.
1. Social work with minorities–Europe. 2. Marginality, Social–
Europe. 3. Assimilation (Sociology) 4. Europe–Social policy.
5. Europe–Race relations. I. Williams, Charlotte, 1954– .
II. Soydan, Haluk, 1946– . III. Johnson, Mark, 1948 Mar. 16–
HV3177.E85S63 1998
362.84'0094–dc21 98–17041
CIP

ISBN 0–415–16962–3 (hbk)
ISBN 0–415–16963–1 (pbk)

Contents

Contributors

Karl-Olov Arnstberg is Professor at the Department of Human Geography, Stockholm University, and Leader of the Institute of Urban Studies, a group conducting qualitative research studies on urban planning.

Martin Baldwin-Edwards is Co-Director of the Mediterranean Migration Observatory in Athens, and joint editor of the journal *South European Society and Politics*.

Lena Dominelli is Director of the Centre for International Social and Community Development at the University of Southampton, and President of the International Association of Schools of Social Work.

Mark Drakeford is Lecturer in Social Policy and Social Work at the University of Wales, Cardiff.

Marie Hessle is a chartered psychologist and Director of the specialised counselling unit serving refugee children and their families in Stockholm.

Sven Hessle is Professor of Social Work at Stockholm University and editor-in-chief of the *Scandinavian Journal of Social Welfare*. Since 1996 he has been directing and participating in UNICEF-funded projects aimed at the reconstruction of social services in Bosnia and Hercegovina.

Maureen Hirsch is Senior Lecturer in Social Policy at Coventry University, following many years' experience in practice settings and higher education, specialising in equalities issues.

Beth Humphries is Research Degrees Co-ordinator in Applied Social Studies at Manchester Metropolitan University, and recently edited a book on *Critical Perspectives on Empowerment*.

Mark R.D. Johnson was Senior Research Fellow at the Centre for Ethnic Relations in the University of Warwick and has been studying issues of ethnic diversity in service delivery for nearly twenty years. He is now a Reader in Primary Care, Mary Seacole Research Centre, De Montfort University, Leicester.

Walter Lorenz holds a Jean Monnet Chair in European Integration Studies at University College, Cork, and is co-editor of the *European Journal of Social Work*. He co-ordinates several European networks concerned with a critical approach to European dimensions in the training of social professions.

Claude Moraes is Director of the Joint Council for the Welfare of Immigrants based in London.

Steve Morris is Lecturer in Continuing Education (Welsh Language) at the University of Wales, Swansea.

Don Naik has worked with the United Nations in Cambodia and South Africa, has taught at the University of North London, and is now an independent consultant in social work.

Naina Patel leads a trans-national project at Bradford University Management Centre, and is Projects Manager in Equal Opportunities and Europe at the UK Central Council for Education and Training in Social Work.

Diana Powell is an Associate Fellow of the Centre for Research in Ethnic Relations at the University of Warwick. Following on from early community work practice, she has been involved in the development of anti-racist social work education for twenty-five years.

Eva Segerström is a social work counsellor in Sweden and has worked with *Rädda Barnen* (Save the Children) on refugee programmes for the past eight years.

Gurnam Singh is a Senior Lecturer in Social Work at Coventry University and currently researching a Ph.D. in Postmodernity and Anti-Racist Social Work.

Haluk Soydan is research director at the Centre for Evaluation of Social Services, Swedish National Board of Health and Welfare. He is also Professor of Social Work and Migration Research at Gothenburg University. He has considerable experience in teaching and research in social work.

Charlotte Williams is a Lecturer in Social Work at the University of Wales, Bangor. She has been writing, researching, practising and training in the field of anti-oppressive practice and work with minority groups for many years.

Foreword

This book has grown out of many years' collaboration and conversation between the editors, and between us and our contributors. Two of the editors (Soydan and Williams) first met within the frame of an ERASMUS programme, designed to bring together social work teachers across Europe. Both have a long background in schools of social work, in Wales and Sweden, and had long felt the need for a textbook of this kind to advance the training of students and practitioners of social work. Previous European textbooks in this field were either totally country-specific or written in another era. The third editor (Johnson) brought to the team a long experience of research into questions of 'ethnic relations' and the delivery of welfare-related services in societies of diversity. We hope that this work will meet all of our professional needs for an up-to-date text which will contribute to the requirements of a curriculum designed to equip social work students for practice in environments of multicultural diversity.

Acknowledgements

The editors would like to express their gratitude and thanks to all those who have contributed to the text and to their respective centres for their ongoing support: The Centre for Applied Community Studies, University of Wales, Bangor; The Centre for Evaluation of Social Services, National Board of Health and Welfare, Stockholm; and the Centre for Research in Ethnic Relations, University of Warwick.

Charlotte Williams, *Bangor*
Haluk Soydan, *Stockholm*
Mark Johnson, *Leicester*

Editors' introduction

> Rather than recycling the illusions of imperial Europe, we should address and welcome the multicultural realities and opportunities of post imperial Europe.
>
> (Nederveen Pieterse 1991:7)

Migration and multiculturality are not new phenomena to Europe. Population movement has long characterised a Europe whose presence was felt across the world and in turn was shaped by a permeation of influences and peoples from beyond its borders. Nederveen Pieterse (1991) pertinently questions the origins and ancestry of contemporary citizens of Europe, asking: 'how many of you hail from non-European worlds?' Yet what is so often part of the 'forgotten memory' of Europe is a recognition of this wide-ranging diversity of cultures as part of its inheritance. Dominant imaginings of Europe emerge, and are defended, that venerate a homogeneity of European culture to which diversity is seen as a threat, or certainly a problem. And so the 'problem of minorities' is constructed. That is, their difference to the supposed 'oneness' of the society rather than that 'oneness' itself is seen as the problem. Such visions of Europe are, of course, fictions, misinterpretations of a history that had been decontextualised from an acknowledgement of the decolonisation that produced the Europe we know, from the history of migrations imperial and post-imperial and from the impact of globalisation.

In the contemporary landscape of Europe there are many good reasons to refocus our attention on the issues of migration and settlement. Economic union implies some form of social union and the European Union has seen as a priority the promotion of social cohesion. Yet we are living in times of rapid change and uncertainty in realising the goals of 'a European society'. The aspirations of social integration, social solidarity, citizenship, mutual respect and tolerance are proposed within a context of increasing contradictions in relation to multiculturalism. This territory is a site of struggle and conflict as well as negotiation. European societies face choices about whether to opt to embrace multiculturalism or to embrace the idea of a 'Fortress Europe' in which they eschew internal differences between member states in order to promote a Union designed to fend off encroachments from outside (Gordon 1989).

Globalisation as a significant feature of the post-industrial era is the key process that has guaranteed renewed focus on the issue of cultural diversity. Our world is getting smaller as events happening many miles away are brought in touch with our local contexts. Beyond the radical reshaping of economic activities, globalisation brings in its wake new and complicated demographic distributions, the diversification of our life-styles as cultural forms interact and also the worldwide spread of commonalities and uniformities between different nation states. This is not, however, just a matter of 'there's a McDonald's in every town': contemporary societies are increasingly marked by a new configuration in the distribution of wealth between the haves and the have-nots and new diasporic conditions are appearing with attendant issues and problems.

Such a process has far-reaching effects on various arenas of social life, such as family, recreation, culture, diet and the nature of work. Migration flows between countries have substantially increased and during the last decade included new countries of origin and destination within Europe as well as across its borders. Italians in Belgium, Turks in Sweden and Germany and Britons in Berlin are evidence of this. It is estimated that approximately 30 million people have entered Western Europe as workers or their dependants in the post-war period (Cannan *et al.* 1992) and there are now some 18 million people settled in Europe who derive from non-EC countries (Eurostat 1996). International migration has never before been so pervasive nor so socially, politically and economically significant. The consequences of this massive social upheaval are immense.

The responses of European states and European political bodies have been piecemeal and *ad hoc*, and lacked any long-term, coherent strategies (Castles 1993:24). What is clear is that national policies have been attempting to realise a number of irreconcilable goals. For example, at one and the same time they seek the integration of minorities into social and political institutions whilst developing policies and practices that promote the differentiation and control of migrants. Castles (1993) argues that the overlap of such divergent policy goals generates serious contradictions with particular ramifications. We may summarise these as follows:

- Exclusionary policies, aimed at controlling migration, create potential for public disorder by denying citizenship rights to full political representation.
- Immigration controls criminalise later migrants and cast suspicion on earlier settlers.
- Cheap labour policies utilising undocumented workers destabilise labour markets and create tensions between ethnic groups within the workforce.

- Crisis management based on 'moral panics' and political appeals to intolerance create racial violence and threaten public order.
- Appeals to national unity based on nationalism invoke separatism (*repli-sur-soi*) and fundamentalism (*intégrisme*) among religious and cultural groups.

These contradictory forces prescribe the position of minorities in Europe and underscore a certain ambivalence of Europe to its minorities and in turn a potential for ambivalence from minorities to the project of Europe.

Minorities themselves are not silent partners in this dynamic. The growing conscientisation amongst minority groups themselves must be a factor in arousing increased attention and focus on issues of multiculturalism. The establishment of the Migrants' Forum, the Black Caucus and the representation of minorities in the European Parliament provide important fora for resistance, self-empowerment and autonomous action. From this arena an awareness is growing of the formulation and articulation of new and changing identities, both individual and collective; of the range of needs and demands voiced by minorities and, of course, of the lived experiences of being one of Europe's many minorities. In some of the nation states such as Great Britain and the Netherlands this trend is complemented by a growing number of people from minority backgrounds in public office, in the welfare bureaucracies and the academy. The sense of presence of minorities has consequently grown.

Alongside the process of globalisation other noticeable trends pattern the current dynamic of minorities and Europe. The restructuring of welfare and a reformulation of the relationship between the nation state and the individual is now advanced in most of the nation states of Western Europe. As the social democratic welfare state comes under attack, not only are the tenuous citizenship rights of many minorities in Europe eroded but a situation is produced which fosters racism and xenophobia, fuelled by social insecurity (Delanty 1996). This crisis of welfare is a significant force in exacerbating the exclusions experienced by migrants and, indeed, by refugees.

Further, the emergence of a body of legislation, policy and proclamations in respect of the protection of minorities at both national and pan-European levels has raised the profile of minorities: the Council Resolution on the Combating of Racism and Xenophobia (90/C 157/01) and Council of Europe Resolutions on migrants' housing (No. R.(88)14) and on equal treatment of national and migrant workers in the sectors of working conditions, remuneration, dismissal, geographical and occupational mobility (No. R.(74)15). The year 1997 is the declared European Year Against Racism, with initiatives being developed with European funding right across Europe. The Council of Europe's Youth Campaign (*all different, all equal*) is introducing a massive educational programme and the ECRI (European Commission on Racism and Intolerance) is also a Council of Europe initiative. These are clear statements of the recognition of the rise of right-wing activism, the development of fascist organisations and the quantitative rise in racism and xenophobia that is characterising all European countries. In every nation state, despite an uneven commitment to anti-racist and anti-discriminatory legislation (Report of the European Parliament 1992), there is an evident and visible rise in overt hostilities, some of which is incurring growing media interest.

This is countered, however, by a growing harmonisation of policies of internal and external control. The Trevi Group (Terrorism, Radicalism, Extremism, Violence International), founded in 1975 in Rome to combat terrorism and drug trafficking, extended their remit to include asylum questions and illegal immigration. The Schengen Accord of June 1985 extended this strategy as countries grouped together (Germany, France, Belgium, Luxembourg, the Netherlands, Denmark, Italy, Spain and Portugal) to co-ordinate their policies on border controls, immigration laws, visa requirements, asylum procedures, sharing of information systems and other stringent controls (Paul 1991). In this way 'the basis of Fortress Europe already exists' (Paul 1991:61) and a segregated system of freedom of movement has emerged for EC and non-EC nationals.

Public concern is also growing in relation to the number of refugees and asylum seekers arriving or already 'here' within European states. European self-identity as the home of tolerance and civilisation is increasingly challenged, and the fragility of civil society brought home by often startling accounts of war or political conflict within Europe's borders. We do not need to detail the current events – every week brings new stories of arrivals on the Italian littoral, or of the experiences of people from the territory formerly known as Yugoslavia, or upheavals and removals somewhere else. For each of these there are a number of human stories, and individuals with their families as well as communities come forward to demand their rights to respect and welfare, and to provoke the conscience of society.

This at times turbulent, dynamic and often conflictual configuration of circumstances creates an encounter with the social professions (to use Lorenz' term, 1994) to which we are obliged to respond. This response is shaped not only by legal requirement and professional concerns but is also fundamentally moral. Herein lie some choices for the profession as social work is implicated both directly and indirectly in the process of change. History attests to the abuse of social work as an arm of internal control either overtly or more subtly through professional practices – assessments, behavioural controls, sectioning under statutes or through indifference, neglect and 'difference blindness'. What is at issue is whether the profession will act to assert and protect minority rights and influence the processes of change that are afoot or whether it will become cowed by political agendas that are oppressive to Europe's minorities (Lorenz 1994). The challenge is to respond appropriately to individual, group and community needs, to contribute to the creation of social solidarity, to resist the oppressive forces of national agendas and pan-national agreements that serve to exacerbate the exclusion of minorities and to contribute towards what Lorenz has called 'negotiated diversity' and the reclaiming of the true meaning of a European citizenship that is non-exclusive.

How equipped are the social professions for the challenges of this new encounter? This book seeks to open debates on the nature of the response that is called for. How is this challenge being perceived and formulated? Are there common themes, perspectives, strategies and conceptual frameworks that can have cross-national relevance? Is there a common value base in relation to the responsibility of social work to protect Europe's visible minorities?

The aim of the book is not to specify particular formulae for 'working with minorities'. Our belief is that there can be no cut and dried methodology for work with minority groups but that the methodology is necessarily an emergent one in which there are many partners and many stories. Our aim is to problematise the issues and to present 'rich descriptions' that may contribute to practice wisdom and prompt the theorising of debates cross-nationally so that new frameworks of action on a pan-European level can be developed.

As with most editorial tasks and particularly those of editing international texts, the selection of material involves difficult decisions about focus and emphasis. One guiding factor was that a substantial number of the contributions should reflect writing by people from minority groups themselves and this has been achieved. This, we would argue, is not only a matter of validating the voice of minority peoples but is in recognition of their role in directing the way knowledge is produced with and on behalf of minority communities. Another consideration was that we should eschew the traditional tendency to bring together contributions around the familiar client groupings: older people, children, people with disabilities and so on, or familiar territory in terms of issues, such as transnational adoption, child protection, interpreting, and the abuse of particular powers or provisions. This may well be a valid exercise in looking at minority experiences which traverse all of these categorisations and practice areas – but we have had to leave them for another time. Our selection is organised to reflect the praxis between theory building, practice wisdom, policy, research and training and the three parts of the book in turn form such a frame, each with a short introduction.

Within the practice area some hard decisions had to be made and we hope we have selected areas that have perhaps had less attention in existing comparative material. One regret is the omission of a chapter on migrant women, as we are of the opinion that the specific issues of gender in this area are often neglected in social work thinking. That said, it is our hope that gender informs all the writings included. In addition, we can but refer you to an excellent book by Gina Buijs (1996) which contains a rich collection of essays, many by migrant women themselves, and leave you to do the work.

The methodology of the book is to construct knowledge through a variety of media: case study and practice accounts, research, theoretical debate, observations and modelling, in an attempt to illustrate that there are different ways of doing things. The text is consequently a product of researchers, teachers and academics, practitioners and administrators drawn from different social science backgrounds. It is hoped that by adopting multiple perspectives we can see things 'in the round'. We have eschewed any didactic approach, and believe in the essential rationality and competence of our readers, to take from the text those lessons which can be best applied to their own situation. There is here no description of ideal types of migrant culture, no 'this is what Sikhs do' or 'how to care for the Muslim family'. Such matters are constantly evolving, and must take account of the personal histories of the participants and local contexts. Instead, we have attempted to portray some of the dilemmas that those entering the field may face, and to show some case studies of possible solutions or lessons that can be learned from the actions of others.

The starting point of the text is that an understanding of issues of migration has to be contextualised against different social, political and economic situations, against the different histories of the nation states and against the different meanings attached to the notion and operation of social work in the nation states. That said, the text has its own history in the collaboration between Sweden and Great Britain and inevitably reflects this. We have tried from the experiences of these two countries to generate possible comparative material rather than bring together a 'many countries' or national studies text.

THEMES AND CONTENT

The text seeks to explore structural issues. It focuses on the importance of looking at *power* relationships, on the positioning of 'being a minority' and in addition on some of the consequent effects of migration.

In summary, we have identified three 'big issues' contributing to disadvantage and inequality which we consider are highlighted within the chapters:

- Exclusion – through the process of minoritisation, marginalisation and racialisation;
- Globalisation – cultural distance and nearness, intolerance, prejudice and discrimination;
- Visibility – does remarking on, or providing for, difference itself discriminate?

In all of these, there are both institutional and personal aspects, but we believe that the essential underlying processes are related, and it is to these processes that we wish to draw attention.

As we explore commonalities from country to country in these thematic terms, and as a consensus builds around the need to practise 'diversity-aware' and 'minority-friendly' social work, so there will be a coming together of solutions in which we hope we can participate. At present, however, we feel that it is necessary to build a common agenda: this is our contribution to the start of that debate.

Part I The dimensions of social work and 'minority' discourse

The structure of this book falls into three related parts. In this introduction and in the first section, we explore the dimensions of social work with minority groups. What is meant by 'minority' – how does a minority emerge, and why does it require special attention? What is the significance of migration and the modern context of Europe for modern (or post-modern) practice of social work? How do changing legal and political definitions affect our consideration of these issues? What are the essential factors or structures which are required in order to address the questions, and begin to meet the social care needs of minorities?

Chapter 1 Soydan and Williams – Exploring concepts

Haluk Soydan and Charlotte Williams here lay out the fundamental concepts of the book, seeking to establish a common vocabulary for our readers, at least for the duration of their perusal of these chapters. The analysis shows that there are a great many perspectives, and that by choosing terms one is taking sides. A critical account of concepts such as minority and ethnicity, race and racism, tolerance and discrimination, citizenship and nation is given within the context of European discourse. The authors argue that it remains crucial that we find ways of going behind the labels, and meet in an understanding of the processes which create tensions and exclusion in our societies. They suggest that the terminology of social work with minorities should be the subject of continual review, reflecting its changing and contextual nature.

Chapter 2 Soydan – Understanding migration

Haluk Soydan's discussion of this fundamental process poses a challenge to conventional views of population mobility, which we intend to pursue throughout the volume. Commonly proposed as a problem, or at least a threat to social institutions, migration is shown to be not merely functional for modern society but an essential component in its formation. It is only because of its intersection with questions of identity – frequently defined by issues of 'what we are not' – that it becomes a political question. He characterises social relations between ethnic minorities and majority populations as power relationships. The social consequences of migration are strongly affected by the gender and age structure of the ethnic minorities. As a backdrop to understanding problems in social work and social policy he presents three fundamental models of diversity: categorical, transactional and universal.

Chapter 3 Dominelli – Multiculturalism, anti-racism and social work in Europe

Lena Dominelli explores some of the ideas informing social work education, and the urgency of addressing issues of diversity in an attempt to evolve a European consciousness. Varieties of discourses can be identified, and a series of histories or traditions needs to be reconciled around such common concerns as social deprivation (or exclusion) and 'need'. Active processes of racialisation interact with these, but it is a mistake to simplify racism or reduce it to a simple set of hierarchies. Social work itself is not a singular entity, although a core set of activities and processes can be discerned. These include processes of 'belonging and othering', which must be addressed in the struggle against racism. Equally, it is important that social workers should not be 'disabled' by racism and ignore the fact that people in minorities also have 'generic' needs like those of the majority. An understanding of when a need is 'specific', and when it is altered by the minority status, is critical.

Chapter 4 Johnson, Baldwin-Edwards and Moraes – Controls, rights and migration

Mark Johnson, Martin Baldwin-Edwards and Claude Moraes review the legislative context affecting migrant and minority entitlement to welfare support. This discussion shows how migration controls and legislation relating to nationality and the rights of refugees can affect minorities. The development of European-wide structures has, while creating a notionally 'common travel area' for free trade, generated barriers and difficulties for minorities and set limits upon the enjoyment of hard-won privileges or rights for those who are seen to be different.

Chapter 5 Johnson – Ethnic monitoring: bureaucratic construction of a 'minority' entity or identity

There are many arguments against making visible the apparent differences in society associated with the concept of 'race'. For very significant proportions of migrants and indeed of 'local' minorities, it is preferable that their differences might pass unnoted. They are, in the model first described in

'Netherlands India' and the plural societies of the Caribbean, and more recently asserted by Rex, content to assert their differences in the private sphere, but to meet on common ground in the 'public' or 'marketplace'. An alternative formulation, however, insists that one cannot respect the identity and welfare needs of minorities unless these are identified, labelled and counted. Johnson writes, from experience of Britain and the USA, about the value and problems of 'ethnic record keeping', or more properly, the use of these data for monitoring the quality of services delivered and received. In the process, the nature of difference, and the appropriate dimensions on which these categories are constructed, must be considered.

Part II Case studies of some common themes

In the second part, we present a series of studies based upon particular situations, which draw out specific issues – dimensions, as it were, of the question. Each can be read in its own right as a case study which illustrates both good and bad practice, and might form the basis of a tutorial, or give insight into the needs of and ways of working with a particular minority group. Clearly it would be impossible to present case studies of every minority in Europe – but the themes, of language and religion, refugee status and travellers, and of community organisation, should be common to most societies and settings.

Chapter 6 Drakeford and Morris – Social work with linguistic minorities

By drawing upon the example of an autochthonous but disadvantaged language, Mark Drakeford and Steve Morris explore the implications of multilingualism for social work. Assertive acquisition of second (or indeed subsequent) languages, rather than the traditional expectation of a 'regression to the mean' of the dominant majority tongue, is shown as presenting another set of challenges to social policy. As the authors observe, choice of language is as much a power-relation activity as more familiar sites of struggle. With growing mobility and the creation of micro-communities which can interact and sustain each other through global communication linkages, such challenges appear set to increase. Equally, speakers of minority languages can be marginalised or minoritised as they seek to reassert their own identity through that medium. Social work, which deals with the excluded and the vulnerable, cannot confine its practice to using the language of the powerful, but must find ways to offer that empowerment in its own services.

Chapter 7 Hirsch and Powell – Non-governmental organisations and the welfare of minority ethnic communities in Britain and Germany

Maureen Hirsch and Di Powell compare and contrast the roles played by 'grassroots' organisations. Migrant and minority communities are not static recipients of services: they are actively involved in their own destinies. Despite divergent histories, there are some significant commonalities between Germany and Britain. In both, a need to form defences against racist attacks and social exclusion stimulates community organisation – generating bodies which provide convenient solutions for service providers faced with demands arising from cultural diversity. Where citizenship rights are withheld or denied, this provision is even more crucial. Even so-called community work may, however, act to marginalise genuine community initiative and the role of the state in providing support is also critical. In both states, minority communities have had to struggle to set up their own agencies and to maintain ownership of these. The emergence of a diversity of community groups reflecting varied interests may also present new problems of policy and legitimacy. There is a need to find more satisfactory ways of working together, and a recognition of mutual interdependence.

Chapter 8 Hessle and Hessle – Child welfare in wartime and under post-war conditions: the Bosnian case as a point of departure for reflections on social work with refugees

Europe has a long history of wars and conflicts creating traumatic movements of population. Refugees are again a growing constituency for the provision of welfare across the continent. Associated with this has been a political debate whose tone has aggravated the isolation and sense of fear which the asylum seekers had sought to escape. Sven and Marie Hessle show that principled approaches towards the welfare of children, based upon ideals which are at least conventionally universally supported, have consequences for social work's encounter with refugee populations. The ability of Centres for Social Work to continue functioning in the territory of former Yugoslavia has been enhanced by the rediscovery of these natural principles, and the recognition that many families are perfectly capable of working on the same basis without formal training. Indeed, some workers in welfare settings create problems by their adherence to professional rather than humanitarian protocols. The authors propose a more suitable model of practice. A recognition that refugees rarely seek to be displaced, and that homeostasis – a return to a form of normality – is the goal of most human beings, is required. The encounter of refugees with care workers at home or abroad will leave both parties changed.

Chapter 9 Segerström – Collective action in a refugee camp: a case study

Eva Segerström's case study of Somali refugees in South Yemen illustrates both the dynamism and potential of communities to reorganise and sustain themselves, and the dynamics of the interface between the 'needy' and 'caring' agencies seeking to help them. A Swedish charity (Save the Children) found that its inputs, which had been carefully planned to mesh with their understanding of the community's structures and traditions, had been used in unexpected ways to create a new form of social organisation. Teachers in the school which they had supported had evolved a variety of techniques to meet the needs of children and their families. In contrast, women had turned their backs on the Women's Union which had been set up to assist them, and were working effectively through a network of informal activities. Commitment and personality appeared to be key variables, rather than any formal or more easily measured attributes. This chapter exemplifies the challenges to Western social work operating in non-European settings.

Chapter 10 Arnstberg – Gypsies and social work in Sweden

Some of Europe's oldest migrant minorities are the Gypsies, known by a variety of sobriquets but almost universally described as 'problematic'. Karl-Olov Arnstberg describes the history of the relationship between groups of these people and social work in Sweden, amid the counter-intuitive outcomes of some of the policies which evolved around their welfare. At the same time, his description insists that simplistic labels must be avoided and that even the smallest minority may have significant subdivisions. Experts, of course, may differ, and one of the greatest problems for social workers is to discern which 'knowledge' is authentic, and which policy approaches are 'right'. As Johnson and Singh argue in Chapter 13, social researchers rarely operate in a policy vacuum but take sides, and yet the most deprived and disenfranchised minorities are also capable of exerting their own autonomy, particularly when it comes to sharing that 'authentic' knowledge about themselves. Too rarely does social work act with the client (or, in the new terminology, user), and in an awareness of the compromises and complexity of their lives. This chapter, like those of Segerström, Powell and Hirsch, and the Hessles, reasserts the role of the client or user as actor in his or her own story.

Chapter 11 Patel, Humphries and Naik – The 3 Rs in social work: religion, 'race' and racism in Europe

Naina Patel, Beth Humphries and Don Naik consider the relevance of religion in social work with minorities, challenging the emergent consensus that we live in a materialistic world where faith in the transcendent is redundant. The classic slick formula of human rights – 'regardless of race religion and culture' – rarely interrogates the complexities of that central category. Islamophobia is as much a form of racism as Anti-Semitism, a term more commonly encountered in Europe as a sibling of Racism, Xenophobia and Intolerance. Yet religion is inherent in culture and has historically been a focus for persecution as well as a vehicle for mobilising social groups. Equally, migration has led to challenges for established religious practices, not least in relation to gender roles. This contradictory relationship with the state, society and individuals requires the careful attention of social workers if they are to be effective, even as humanists.

Part III Issues for the structuring of social work's future practice

Third, the book turns back to more general issues of the infrastructure of social work – education, research and policy formulation and management. Here we discuss how the implications of the previous sections can or should be played out in the individual national arenas where social workers and social policy managers operate.

Chapter 12 Williams – Towards an emancipatory pedagogy? Social work education for a multicultural, multi-ethnic Europe

Charlotte Williams proposes a new perspective for social work education, building on models developed since the 1970s and reviewing the multiplicity of paradigms in use. It is time to face up to the deeply embedded intransigence of national and Europe-wide perspectives on minorities, otherwise known perhaps as prejudice and racism. Part of the problem is the lack of a common terminology for the profession to discuss these issues. Other crucial questions include discussion of the role (or use) of people from minority origins within the process, and the nature of learning and assessment in the profession. A synthesis of different models provides pointers to the development of a more satisfactory curriculum, once the central issue is resolved, of the role of social work in serving its sponsors as well as its clients.

Chapter 13 Johnson and Singh – Research with ethnic minority groups in health and social welfare

Two teachers of social research methods explore the challenges and compromises which must be faced when one is conducting research amongst a society of 'ethnic' diversity in order to inform policy and practice. They too are concerned that the use of categories such as minority, migrant, or Muslim may affect the way in which the members of these groups are seen, in ways which are irrelevant to meeting their needs. Practitioners must attempt to work with the groups who form the subject of their research, and transform this approach so that their own practice becomes the true focus of attention. Those whom the social work profession seeks to serve are also active in determining their own destinies, and must be involved as producers and consumers of the research.

Chapter 14 Lorenz – Social work, social policies and minorities in Europe

Walter Lorenz brings the volume to a close with a challenge to the notions of the homogeneity of European society and the 'threat' of diversity. He shows how both are recent – almost post-modern – inventions. This new way of looking at migration and minorities forces attention on the role of social workers as the 'caretakers of society', whose role is therefore defined by, but also affects, how that society is imagined. The myth of 'client self-determination' in a society simultaneously globalising and reasserting nationalism provides a dilemma for social work. Lorenz spells this out in stark terms. The 'special' skills and forms of knowledge required to come to terms with the human needs of minorities, migrants and refugees have fundamental implications for generic social work practice.

IN CONCLUSION?

Throughout this volume, we explore the meaning of migration and its effects, and the repertoire of resources which individuals draw upon to make sense of themselves and society. We find that transfers of population may create a 'crisis of solidarity', which is the root of the challenge that diversity poses to society. Social work with minorities and refugees, while requiring specific skills and approaches, cannot be divorced from the wider field. Similarly, lessons can be learned from the multiplicity of approaches to diversity in social work across Europe in different situations and traditions. Critical to this is a theme which runs through the whole collection of essays – the interplay between the personal (individual need) and the political (or group). Social workers and social policy have a significant role to play in mediating this exigency.

REFERENCES

Buijs, G. (ed.) (1996) *Migrant Women: Crossing Boundaries and Changing Identities* Oxford: Berg.

Cannan, C., Berry, L. and Lyons, K. (1992) *Social Work and Europe* London: Macmillan.
Castles, S. (1993) 'Migrations and minorities in Europe. Perspectives for the 1990s: eleven hypotheses' in J. Wrench and J. Solomos (eds) *Racism and Migration in Western Europe* Oxford: Berg.
Delanty, G. (1996) 'Beyond the nation-state: national identity and citizenship in a multicultural society – a response to Rex' *Sociological Research Online* 1, 3 <http://www.socresonline.org.uk/socresonline/1/3/1.html>
European Parliament (1992) *Report of the Committee of Enquiry into Racism and Xenophobia* Brussels: Office for Official Publications of the European Communities.
Eurostat (1996) *Statistics in Focus: Population and Social Conditions* Luxemburg, no. 2.
Gordon, P. (1989) *Fortress Europe! The Meaning of 1992* London: Runnymede Trust.
Lorenz, W. (1994) *Social Work in a Changing Europe* London: Routledge.
Nederveen Pieterse, J. (1991) 'Fictions of Europe' *Race and Class* 32, 3:3–10.
Paul, R. (1991) 'Black and Third World people's citizenship and 1992' *Critical Social Policy* 11, 2:52–64.
Race and Class (1991) Special issue 'Europe: variations on a theme of racism' 32, 3.

Part I

The dimensions of social work and 'minority' discourse

Professional work and everyday activities of social workers are conditioned by a web of factors that are functioning on different levels in a society. Some factors are closer to and others are more remote from the professional performance of social workers in their daily work. Nevertheless, these activities are framed by micro- as well as macro-level conditions. Social work with minority clients has generic as well as specific characteristics and it is a field of the social work profession that exists at the interface of social work practice and ethnic encounters.

The aim of Part I of the book is to describe and give an understanding of cardinal factors which we believe strongly impact on social work with minorities. Social work methods, practices and everyday encounters between social workers and minority clients are all in one way or another preconditioned by demographic, economic, political, sociological, legal, professional and educational factors. This part is an attempt to give a structure to this complex and intertwined set of factors dominated by issues of migration, globalisation, minoritisation and power.

First, a number of key concepts are explored and introduced with the purpose of demonstrating the complexity of the issues and concepts faced by many of us, that is as students of social work theory and practice as well as practitioners. The concepts of minority and ethnicity, race and racism, tolerance and discrimination, citizenship and nation are discussed from a European perspective.

Second, migration as a fundamental element of modern society is analysed. It is suggested that migration is a problem-solving as well as a problem-generating mechanism at the heart of the globalised society. The diversity of the peoples have also led to development of intervention 'paradigms'. The problem-solving and problem-generating typology is connected to three prominent models of response to the issues of disadvantage and discrimination: the model of categorical diversity, the model of transactional diversity and the model of universal diversity.

Some of the issues that are described and discussed in the first two chapters are elaborated further in the third chapter, where a critical position is taken in terms of some social work practice with subordinated ethnic minority groups. At the same time there is an air of optimism suggested by the challenging of social workers to play a significant role in working with excluded people and to contribute to the creation of a non-racist society.

This part is concluded by an account of the legal framework within which migration to and within Europe takes place and bureaucracies record identity. The political development during the last two decades in Europe has also changed the legal framework of the member states of the European Union. Thus, the issues of in-migration, settlement, citizenship and political and social participation have been and are being reshaped.

Models of understanding of ethnic diversity are presented. The European context of the issue is spelled out. Legal aspects of migration to and within Europe are presented.

Thus, this part with its five chapters offers a theoretical as well as an empirical frame of reference which contextualises the understanding of social work with minority clients.

Chapter 1

Exploring concepts

Haluk Soydan and Charlotte Williams

INTRODUCTION

One of the key considerations in the development of perspectives on social work with minorities in Europe is the issue of terminology. Identifying a shared language for use in these debates, for literature and research, is notoriously difficult given that specific terms can carry a variety of meanings within and across different contexts. Further, terms in use are constantly changing as ideas change and words which have previously had much currency become the subject of debate and criticism. The language we use to mark out difference between indigenous and immigrant peoples is highly salient and words such as 'foreigner', 'stranger', 'alien', 'immigrant' or 'settler' carry specific connotations in different contexts. Language in use reflects particular theories, values, political ideologies and popular thinking of the day and should therefore properly be the subject of constant review and clarification. It is necessary to analyse the terms in which reality is constructed because the selection of particular concepts reflects what it is we are choosing to take into account and what we are choosing to conceal or omitting to consider.

The purpose of this chapter is to provide a critical introductory analysis of some of the key concepts in use in this book and to consider associated debates about their applications in pubic policy making and practice. The aim is to explore the problematic nature of some of the terminology and point to its complexity and not to provide absolute definitions.

MINORITY

The concept of minority is far more complex than may first appear. On a simple level 'minority' refers to any group which is smaller in number than another group or other groups in a given society. In modern social work literature as well as in everyday descriptions the concept is frequently used to refer to groups such as immigrants, people with disabilities, gay and lesbian people, older people, members of certain political, linguistic or religious groupings and is sometimes even applied to women. However, as Norbert Rouland (1991) suggests:

> There are no minorities as such, they are defined only structurally. Minorities are groups which are in a minority position as a result of the balance of power and of law, which subjects them to other groups within a society as a whole, whose interests are the responsibility of a state which perpetuates discrimination, either by means of unequal legal status (apartheid policies), or by means of civil equality principles (by depriving communities with special social and economic status of specific rights, civil equality can create or perpetuate *de facto* inequalities).
>
> (1991:224)

A crucial dimension, therefore, is *power*, which overshadows the issue of number and focuses attention on the relationships between minority and majority groups. In any society power is the main determinant of relationships of domination and subordination and of oppression and discrimination directed towards the minority group (Noel 1994).

Whilst the concepts 'minority' and 'oppression' often go together, that is, minority groups are assumed to be (or objectively are) oppressed or discriminated against, this is not always the case. There are examples of minorities (as groups numerically smaller than other groups) who are able to oppress and discriminate against majority groups. A contemporary and somewhat (in)famous example of a white minority oppressing a large black majority is South Africa, though there are numerous other examples of political minorities oppressing majorities. Further, Rex (1996) points out that a modern state may be the product of a laterally organised minority group imposing its domination over other groups as in the former Yugoslavia. In other European countries, no single group dominates the nation state but several groups share the privilege of governing, as in Belgium and Switzerland.

The notion of 'minority' is not therefore univocal or static but mediated by power. Power itself is a complex concept, which is dynamic and cannot be permanently owned (Lukes 1986). Power is often mobilised transiently by particular groupings within specific contexts, at specific times (Gaventa 1982; Lukes 1974). Therefore the relationship between minorities and majorities is constantly open to change. Contemporary relationships between minority and majority groups in a given society may be the result of historically generated configurations of interaction between these groups but these are not immutable. Mutual valuing and scoring between groups generate specific contextual positions. A few examples of such relationships are the colonised minorities in Europe such as the Basques in Spain, Bretons in France, Welsh in Great Britain and the Lapps in Sweden. Historically, these ethnic groups were colonised in the sense that they are politically, culturally and economically controlled by another group which penetrated their territories. Thus they are accorded ethnic minority status. They continue to be ethnic minorities as long as the power relationship between them and their respective majority group continues to be asymmetric.

Yet the boundaries between groups are fluid and constantly changing. In turn it is possible for individuals at one and the same time to be members of minority groups and majority groups as factors of class, gender, age, race and ethnicity may be intimately intertwined and overlapping to produce an individual patterning of membership across a variety of groups. Being of one community does not preclude the individual's membership of other groups which may complement or be in conflictual relationships. The minority community is therefore much more fragmented, diversified and internally subject to change than may be generally recognised.

Whilst there are both individual and collective considerations built into the concept of minority, an understanding of minority status as used within social work has most frequently come to be grounded in the objective factors of exposure to discrimination and oppression and the consequent factors of inequality.

ETHNIC MINORITIES AND ETHNICITY

Ethnic minority identifies a minority group by reference to a constellation of factors associated with ethnicity. The notion of ethnicity has been the subject of extensive research and discussion. Lange and Westin (1981), amongst others, offer a comprehensive review of definitions of the concept. In most definitions one or a combination of the following variables are used to denote ethnicity: a common religion, a shared culture or set of cultural attributes, a common national or geographic origin, shared language and common physical or physiological characteristics. Latterly, following the footsteps of Norwegian social scientist Fredrik Barth (1969), many writers have sought more open and constructionist definitions of ethnicity in order to both avoid much of the essentialism associated with specific characteristics and the notion of ethnic boundaries as fixed and static (Rex 1996). At its most general level ethnicity implies some sense or feeling of belonging to a particular group and the sharing of its objective conditions of existence (Anthias and Yuval-Davies 1993). An important dimension of ethnicity is clearly therefore the subjective 'us' feeling that can be mobilised for individual and collective group identity. This denotes some notion of 'community' (*Gemeinschaft*, to paraphrase the German sociologist Ferdinand Tönnies), whether the ethnic group be a majority or a minority, co-extensive with a particular nation, a sub-population within a nation, or transcends national boundaries, as in the case of Gypsies. This community comes to be something set apart from the 'them' that are external to it and this generates a feeling of an internal belongingness amongst its members. It becomes ethnicised. In this vein Anthias and Yuval-Davies argue that '*ethnicity is the active face of ethnic consciousness and always involves a political dimension*' (1993:8).

That is to say the mobilisation of ethnic affiliation is necessarily political in that it implies an in-group and an out-group. The sense of 'us' does not therefore simply relate to a cultural grouping. There is, for example, following the 1992 Single European Act the emergence of the notion of supra-European identity transcending the identity of the nation states based on being white and Christian and mobilised around exclusion of non-white and non-Christian minorities (Rex 1996; Anthias and Yuval-Davies 1993). What this indicates is that ethnicity and culture are not necessarily synonymous, as such a mega-ethnic identity, 'white European', embraces a diversity of language, culture, traditions.

Yet within social work writing considerable attention *is* focused on the definitions of ethnic groupings as cultural entities. The notion of a shared culture or a set of shared cultural attributes is often seen as the demarcating factor for the identification of ethnic group. In this respect *culture* is defined as a system of ideas, norms, values, 'ways of being' shared by members of a given group. It is the acquired perspective by which members of a group interpret their environment, make sense of their world and adopt particular conventions. It provides the prescribing frame through which the individual mediates what is right and what is wrong, good and bad. Normally, people's attitude to their own culture is unuttered and often unquestioning.

Migration, however, confronts these cognitive maps in several ways. Migration produces cultural encounters, conflictual or benign. Members of cultural groups have the opportunity to compare cultures and this acts to endorse or challenge *ethnocentrism*, the belief in the superiority of one's own culture. As cultures interact they continually and of necessity change and therefore must be understood as dynamic and fluid entities. Both the majority and the minority cultures are subject to such change. What is often overlooked is the fact that the cultural traditions within immigrant groups have their own modernising elements and these cultural groupings are very often internally divided (Rex 1996). Culture should not therefore be thought of in essentialist terms as unchanging, clearly bounded and homogeneous. This tendency leads to the danger of reifying culture, making it larger than life and in turn inappropriately ethnicising individuals.

Ethnic mobilisation is much more complex than guarding the frontiers of culture and tradition. For example, migrant labourers from very diverse cultural groups may become ethnicised through state legislation and institutional practice or by the ways in which they are identified by the dominant community. Thus ethnic identity may be constructed reactively to particular sets of circumstances as well as being a determinant of such groupings. Ethnic categorisation also significantly cuts across class and gender divisions as well as national boundaries. Gypsies, discussed in Chapter

10 of this book, form an interesting ethnic grouping based on a mixture of ethnic characteristics and they are clearly transnational. Members of other migrant minority ethnic groups may often see themselves in this way as belonging to transnational communities. Rex (1996) argues that this provides the potential for at least three forms of ethnic mobilisation:

- the maintenance of points of reference and connections with a homeland (imagined or real);
- the collective striving for recognition and against inferiorisation in the land of settlement;
- the possibility of onward migration to new countries of settlement given the existence of ethnic boundary markers (Rex 1996).

The mobilisation of ethnicity is clearly multifaceted on both an individual and a collective level. It also importantly relates to the response of the established society to the presence of its minorities:

> It may seek to keep them out or attack them; it may accept them as temporary residents without political rights; it may accept them but demand that they abandon their own culture and organisations; or it may seek to integrate them in a society which sees itself as multi-cultural.
>
> (Rex 1996:7)

These positionalities will in turn dictate the official language used to denote minority ethnic groups, for example the 'guest workers' of Germany, the avoidance of the term 'ethnic minority' in France and the distancing from the term 'immigrant' to denote minority peoples in Britain.

Nation states have also struggled with terminology to mark the transition from immigrant to *settler* status. In some European countries second- and third-generation offspring of migrant families continue to be called 'immigrants' as a marker of their outsider status or at best 'from an immigrant background'. Perotti (1994) usefully provides a number of indicators of settlement. These include: a considerable expansion of family structures as a result of family reunion; an increased number of mixed marriages/cohabitation; an increased number of births to mixed or immigrant couples; the presence of minority children in the school population; an increasing number of non-active or unemployed people in the immigrant population; the extension of the length of stay and a rising number of immigrants receiving citizenship of the country or having dual nationality. To Perotti's delineation can be added noticeable shifts in the majority culture, if only at the level of cuisine, literature and the arts and popular culture and language. This does not, however, mean changes to the minority status of such groups or to the main institutions of a society in responding to pressure for equality, all of which are dependent on power relationships.

THE CONCEPT 'RACE' AND THE ISSUE OF RACISM

The concept 'race' has no generalisable application in European social work literature. Whilst the terms 'race', racism and anti-racism characterise the debates about ethnic minorities in the British context (Dominelli 1988, 1997), wider European writing holds a distinctly more critical approach to their use. In certain European countries, for example France, Germany, the Netherlands and the Scandinavian countries, the powerful negative connotation of the term 'race' has ensured its omission from popular and official discourse. Most commonly throughout Europe such terminology is associated with the political propaganda of extremist and neo-fascist groups, embracing ideas of biological inferiority and notions of a hierarchy of races.

Arguments about the utility of the concept of 'race' to social work policy making and practice range from the overtly political to the theoretical problems posed by the term. The idea of 'race' as a scientific category has long been discredited even within the scientific tradition itself. The notion of fixed and immutable categories determined biologically has no support within genetic research and was significantly discredited across much of Western Europe by the experiences of Nazism and subsequent fears of its revival. The continued usage of the concept is largely based on sociological ideas which either relate 'race' strongly to cultural and ethnic groups or sustain the ideas as essentially an ideological construct and the product of particular discourses (Miles 1993). In Britain the concept presents something of an anomaly in that it has considerable bureaucratic, academic and political currency and is officially recognised in the legislation (The Race Relations Act 1976).

Within social work in Britain, the language of 'race' has been a powerful locus of political mobilisation for change and for defining and operationalising the anti-racist project within social work. Many have argued that pioneering initiatives in this respect developed within social work education, policy and practice that could inform wider European debate on work with ethnic minorities. This ignores the fact, however, that other European countries do not conceptualise the issues in terms of 'race' or more specifically in terms of skin colour, as in the British context.

In France, as in Spain, there is a noticeable absence of colour consciousness. The French concerns pivot more on fears that immigrant cultures (including the majority English) will undermine French culture and political ideals (Rex 1992). This is paralleled in Germany, where the threat is to the homogeneity of the German '*Volk*' posed by '*Ausländer*' (foreigners). The term 'racism' is eschewed in favour of '*Auslanderfeindlichkeit*' (hostility against foreigners). In Belgium, Switzerland and the Netherlands the long experience of religious and linguistic diversity suggests a very different framework on which to build newer forms of multiculturalism. The focus of the European debate seems to be predicated therefore on notions of 'cultural' rather than colour difference and discrimination appears to be more closely associated not with biological inferiorisation but on the basis of cultural ethnocentricity, or more specifically not belonging to the culturally dominant group.

Several writers (Anthias and Yuval-Davies 1993; Donald and Rattansi 1992) suggest that in analysis, rather than seeking to establish the existence of 'race', it may be more useful to consider the way in which 'racial logics and racial frames of reference are articulated and deployed and with what consequences' (Donald and Rattansi 1992:1) and Anthias and Yuval-Davies accordingly use the term 'racialised boundaries', seeing racism as the discourse and practice of inferiorising ethnic groups whatever its basis. When these ideas are translated into social work, the focus would be on asking how policies, practices, ways of thinking and acting reinforce, maintain or promote exclusions based on conceptualisations of cultural differences as inferior (see Dominelli in Chapter 3).

However, the visibility of particular ethnic groups is not irrelevant to an understanding of processes of inferiorisation and ethnic stratification across Europe. Ethnic groups become visible in the sense that particular facets of their difference are marked out in a negative and stigmatising manner. Skin colour is no small factor in this respect and the positioning and treatment of Third World labour migrants throughout Europe indicates it to be an important determining factor in triggering discrimination and inequalities (Paul 1991). Italy provides a contemporary example of the way in which this trend is being manifested (Aluffi-Pentini and Lorenz 1996).

Denial of the explicit use of the salient language of 'race' in social policy and social work and more generally in public policy making has not served to prevent racism from permeating institutional and professional practice. The tendency to avoid this terminology in favour of ethnicity may serve two further purposes. It may serve to mask gross and systematic inequalities associated with differences based on colour, religion, culture in a celebration of the benign pluralism of multiculturality. It serves to detach debates about migration and immigrants from their global and historical context, from the processes of imperialism and colonialism and the moral obligations such a recognition entails. Further, it can be argued that a focus on ethnicity can produce a social work practice driven by concerns with special needs in relation to diet, custom, tradition, language but neglectful of the basis of inequality associated with these differences. Finally, this sanitising of social work language can lead to a distancing of the profession from any responsibility in relation to anti-racism and the countering of xenophobia.

In as much as notions of 'race' and 'ethnicity' provide the grounds for discrimination, oppression and inferiorisation and exploitation, they are central to social work theory and practice. In as much as such categories can be mobilised to provide the basis of political struggle within social work, that is, the anti-racist project, they are important and useful concepts.

THE DIMENSIONS OF DIFFERENCE AND DIVERSITY

Difference and diversity are the bedrock of discussions of immigrant and minority ethnic groups in all European societies. Popular and official notions of cultural pluralism, cultural diversity, multiculturalism imply some type of conceptualisation of difference. The term 'difference' is, however, variously used in welfare discourses and deserves some closer inspection.

Much discussion of immigrant and minority groups pivots on their 'difference', perceived or real, from the dominant ethnic group. It has long been demonstrated that the undesirability of the perceived differences of certain groups can lead to attempts to assimilate, exterminate or exclude them (Anthias 1992). This particular focus on difference points to the often oversimplified dichotomies us/them, norm/other, insider/outsider, in-group/out-group, indigenous/stranger that require much exploration in the context of social work theory, education and practice. Considerable attention has been given to the processes that give rise to such axes, to the construction of relations of domination and subordination, to the marking out of differences as inferior and the creation of ethnic hierarchies (Noel 1994; Anthias and Yuval-Davies 1993).

However, more recently in welfare discourse the term 'difference' has been used with other connotations: with reference to differences *within* particular groupings as well as across them, and to difference as the basis of identity claims by members of groups themselves. This development of the concept is important to social work in at least two respects. First, it acts as a counter to the homogenising tendencies of much ethnicist discourse. This emphasis on difference within particular ethnic groups highlights a rich diversity of experience historical and contemporary, accommodates differences in class, caste, gender, language, religion and so on that have been subsumed under what are often stereotypical notions of 'common cultural needs'. Second, it allows for the problematising of identity claims which transcend rigid and fixed ethnic boundaries; for example, those of Vietnamese children adopted by Swedish parents, or those of second- and third-generation Asians in Britain. Difference therefore can be mobilised to explain in-group and out-group relations; it can be mobilised to define individual needs; it can be mobilised in a managerialist or professional sense to define administrative categories, and it can be claimed by minority participants themselves as a basis for individual or collective identity and mobilised to political effect (Williams 1996).

The concept of 'difference' variously defined can therefore aid social work practice and policy making. It can be utilised to promote sensitivity in meeting individual needs but also to refine an understanding of how needs are defined and articulated by particular groupings. This acts as an important counter to the tendency towards categorising and stereotyping people and makes more accessible a fine-tuned understanding of identity claims. Further, in the British context Luthra (1997) has shown how attention to such difference indicates considerable variations in 'rates of progression' of particular ethnic groups in terms of periodic and intergenerational factors. For example, it is no longer enough to say, 'ethnic minorities have difficulties in accessing welfare services'; we have to be able to identify differences between, say, Afro-Caribbeans and Bangladeshi peoples or look to differences within these groupings based on generational factors.

However, the elevation of difference is in turn problematic. The increasing ethnicisation of minority groups can lead to a proliferation of studies, a focus of specificities of response and 'special' needs that detracts from an understanding of social structural frameworks that determine needs and that define power relationships between groups. It can divert attention away from seeking out patterns and relationships between phenomena to chasing after the endless possibilities of diversity. Further, the problem of difference is that it is not neutral. Ideas of cultural diversity often imply a level playing field, a sense of tolerance and equality between different groups that is not borne out in reality. Finally, a focus on diversity can fragment and divide where a common position may be more strategically effective in producing lasting change for all oppressed groups. The issue of diversity is further illuminated by presentation of the three models of ethnic diversity that have been established in research and literature (see Chapter 2).

TOLERANCE, PREJUDICE AND DISCRIMINATION

The ideal of multiculturality embraces notions of tolerance between individuals and social groups. Nations such as Denmark, Sweden, Holland and Wales have long prided themselves on liberal ideals that embrace tolerance and on so-called cultural attributes that reflect a tolerant people (*Race and Class* 1991; Williams 1995). However, these liberal principles can too often shelter major inequalities and records of intolerance and lead to a type of 'difference-blindness' that ultimately denies minority rights. The idea of tolerance has therefore been the subject of considerable critique (Essed 1991). Tolerance itself implies that there is something intrinsically objectionable to tolerate and invokes much of the paternalism with which multiculturalism has become associated (Husband 1994). Tolerance is no substitute for rights as it relies on a generosity that can easily be withdrawn. Further, it is important to ask, 'What are the limits of tolerance? How far will tolerance extend to the social customs and traditions of minority groups and minority group demands within the liberal democratic framework?' The notion of tolerance must not simply be problematised for its reliance on the inherent qualities of an individual but questioned within the framework of liberal values and the denial of potential conflicts between value systems.

Considerable attention has also been afforded the concepts of *prejudice* and *discrimination* (Lange and Westin 1981). Brown (1995) argues for the phenomenon of prejudice as essentially a 'social psychological orientation' that is most usually negative in character: 'the wary, fearful, suspicious, derogatory, hostile or ultimately murderous treatment of one group of people by another' (1995:7), often based on a false or irrational set of beliefs. Prejudice is not simply a cognitive construct but finds its expression in discrimination – the action of treating someone differently. Whilst discriminatory acts may occur in isolation, they more usually form patterns of behaviour towards powerless groups, and evidence about discrimination in particular societies is often quantitative, indicating the possibility of some people experiencing systematic discrimination (Banton 1994). However, discrimination is only one possible cause of inequality and disadvantage and the terms are not synonymous. Other factors may well be identified as the prime causes of particular disadvantages.

The patterning of discrimination and consequent inequalities has led to strategies of *positive action* and *positive discrimination*. Positive discrimination operates to provide an individual or group with preferential treatment in order to place them on a more equal footing with the majority. In many states this has been outlawed as illegal and institutions deploy positive action strategies aimed more generally at removing the barriers to access of equality of opportunity in order to right patterns of inequality.

Discrimination as a term with both a moral and a legal basis is fundamentally ensconced in the Covention on Human Rights. The European Convention states in Article 14 that its rights shall be secured 'without discrimination on any ground such as sex, race, colour, language, religion, political or other opinion, national or social origin, association with a national minority, property, birth or other status' (quoted in Banton 1994:37). Whilst protection against discrimination may lie ultimately in the hearts and minds of people, there is a need for protective legislation to enforce national and international obligations.

CITIZENSHIP AND NATION

'Citizenship' is a contested and contradictory term when applied to immigrant minorities. Essentially it is an umbrella term describing various types of rights that members of a nation state enjoy by virtue of being subjects of that state. Thomas Marshall (1950) identifies citizenship as a product of modernity and part of the democratisation processes of Western societies over the last three centuries. Marshall saw the development of a triad of rights which would constitute modern citizenship: legal, political and social. The progression to universal social rights such as the granting of welfare and social security irrespective of the individual's position in the market, would come as a complement to the legal and political rights won through class struggle in the eighteenth and nineteenth centuries. Marshall's delineation has been the subject of considerable criticism, not least because of the contradiction between the presumed neutral processes of democratic citizenship and the inequalities engendered by market competition, gender, race and immigration (Williams 1989). Although legal and political rights may be seen as fundamental elements in modern democratic nation states, the social rights of citizens, or social citizenship, are not self-evident.

Ethnic minorities that are immigrant populations do not automatically become citizens of their countries of migration (see Chapter 4). We lack extensive, comparative European analysis that may reveal the situation of different immigrant groups in terms of citizenship, especially given changes that are due to the European Union (Miles 1993:126). However, analysis of the British context highlights the complexity of what citizenship might mean in relation to immigrant minorities. Husband (1996) points out a conceptual distinction made by Bottomore (1992) between 'formal' and 'substantial' citizenship. Formal citizenship refers to a formal membership in a nation state, while substantial citizenship refers to an 'array of civil, political and especially social rights, involving some participation in the business of government' (Husband 1996:43). Formal state membership does not necessarily confer substantive citizenship, as Husband points out:

> one can possess formal state membership yet be excluded (in law or in fact) from certain political, civil or social rights. . . . That formal citizenship is not a necessary condition of substantive citizenship is perhaps less evident. Often social rights, for example, are accessible to citizens and legally resident non-citizens on virtually identical terms.
>
> (Husband 1996:43)

And he concludes: 'The issue here is that within contemporary Britain the majority of ethnic minority persons in the country enjoy formal citizenship in law; yet . . . they are denied equivalence as members of the nation' (Husband 1996:43).

Cannan *et al.* (1992) suggest that this is not a British phenomenon alone. In the Netherlands, France and Germany, ethnic groups speak of the experience of exclusion by their segregation in poor housing and jobs and the racism that they experience (Cannan *et al.* 1992:39).

What this demonstrates is that the notion of citizenship is dialectically determined by the state and its subjects. It is not simply a question of the demands made by disadvantaged subjects for the recognition of full citizenship and belonging – the idea of an appeal to the liberal principle of universal equality – but that this is crucially mediated by state power and other forms of regulation such as civil institutions and social groups who shape citizenship making. Ong (1996) argues for the term 'cultural citizenship' to denote

> a dual process of self-making and being-made within webs of power linked to the nation-state and civil society. Becoming a citizen depends on how one is constituted as a subject who exercises or submits to power relations . . . in shifting fields of power that include the nation-state and the wider world.
>
> (1996:738)

What Ong (1996) includes here and what is often missed in such discussions is some understanding of how global economic conditions can also construct the citizenship of individuals within nation states. This is particularly pertinent given the number of Third World migrant workers within Europe.

European integration now provides a new cultural space for the construction of citizenship in which the notion of citizenship as belonging is increasingly opposed to ethnicity (Rex 1996) and in which so often incoming workers come to be classed as 'denizens' or second-class residents without political citizenship (Hammar 1990). Rex (1996) suggests that this approach is very evident in the German *Gastarbeider* system whereby the denial of legal and political rights has led to the protection of some social rights through the paternalistic activities of some indigenous religious and trade union organisations (Rex 1996:8).

An understanding of citizenship rights is central to the work of social professionals working with minorities in Europe. The rise of nationalism throughout Europe and the tendency towards the development of an exclusionary Fortress Europe (Gordon 1989) stand in clear opposition to what is implied by citizenship in a multicultural Europe. The challenge of a multicultural Europe is to definitions of citizenship based on birth, blood, ethnic descent or some reified notion of culture. Delanty argues optimistically:

> the kind of citizenship commensurate with the needs of multicultural European society will have to be addressed to the question of residence as a qualification. Only by shifting the focus to residence will it be possible to move beyond national citizenship. . . . It will have to enfranchise immigrants who frequently do not have any citizenship rights. European citizenship, as a supplementary citizenship, can thus compensate for the shortcomings of national citizenship and embrace the universalistic norms of European nationality in a new form.
>
> (Delanty 1996:8)

Lorenz (1994:19) links social workers to the frontline of those microprocesses that determine inclusion or exclusion from social citizenship

(1994:19). Clearly arguments for the extension of the social rights of citizenship, which is the interface the social professions span, must be contextualised against the attack across Europe on the social democratic welfare state. The undermining of welfarism in many European countries feeds social insecurities which lead to a rise in protectionist and exclusionary national agendas (Delanty 1996). Other writers contend that the ideology of nationalism based on the cultural inferiority of immigrant groups to the dominant group provides the basis for a new kind of nationalism based on the anxieties about the national identity of communities perceived to be under threat (Rex 1996).

EUROPE

The question 'What is Europe?' will provoke a variety of responses. The construction of the meaning of Europe is neither fixed nor agreed and is the focus of much debate, economic, political, cultural and sociological. Its geographical boundaries have been subject to constant change; its cultural heritage is diverse and the product of multitude of non-European influences (Nederveen Pieterse 1991) and internally there are deep political and social divisions. Lorenz argues that 'Europe is therefore more of a project, the construction of an object, a vision not yet realised' (1994:1).

Europe embraces many visions, many discourses, often representing conflicting sets of interests and pressures for both unity and divergence, continuity and change, connection and separateness (Bailey 1992). Whilst Europe as an economic entity has dominated debates, the social arena has been much marginalised and an understanding of Europe as a society is still underdeveloped (Bailey 1992). This evolutionary nature of the social project of Europe necessarily engages social work.

The conceptual puzzle becomes therefore to deconstruct the discourses of Europe and to consider the nature of social work in relation to specific visions of Europe. The term 'Fortress Europe' has become popularised to denote the ways in which European countries are increasingly integrating policies of exclusion in relation to minorities (Paul 1991; Gordon 1989).

ON SOCIAL WORK

The term 'social work' is increasingly difficult to pin down both within and across national boundaries. Munday and Ely (1996) suggest that in most European countries, with the exception of Britain, the term 'social work' constitutes a specific title conferred on those holding a recognised professional qualification and whose names are included on a professional register. However, Lorenz (1994) and the Council of Europe (1997) illustrate the considerable complexity surrounding the term Europe-wide, which Lorenz suggests covers a range of tasks, roles and professional territory. He adopts the generic term 'the social professions' to embrace this diversity (Lorenz 1994). Certainly the social pedagogues in Germany and the *educateurs specialisés* and *animateurs* in French-speaking Europe have a distinct professional training but undertake many of the tasks that would be considered traditional social work (Munday and Ely 1996). In Britain the term 'care manager' is now fast replacing 'social worker' and distinguishing a range of activities that are distinct from those of the social care worker. The diverse nature of terminology in this area has been a concern to the IASSW (International Association of Schools of Social Work), who have undertaken a survey to identify terms in use. The European Institute has also endeavoured to gain clarity in this area by producing an extensive dictionary of key social service terms translated into four European languages.

The term 'social services' itself is no less problematic in terms of cross-European comparison. In Britain the specific use of the term 'personal social services' has no generalisable currency. Munday and Ely (1996) have accordingly opted for the term 'social care' to encompass statutory, independent and informal social service delivery. In respect of work with minorities this is an important point, as evidence suggests that in the face of the neglect of provision by the statutory services, ethnic minority communities have historically in many countries evolved independent and informal ways of meeting the welfare needs of their communities. Outstanding examples are the Swedes and the Italians in the United States of America and the black communities of Great Britain. This in turn means the need for recognition of a vast amount of activity, roles and welfare tasks performed by community-appointed individuals who may not have any professional status or formal qualifications. These individuals or autonomous groups often undertake considerable liaison, translation work and advocacy roles on behalf of their communities. In addition the nation state may co-opt without recognised status a range of workers to mediate welfare to these communities, such as youth workers, link workers, interpreters, etc. These individuals may work only sporadically or casually in partnership with the 'official agencies'. In some countries mistrust of government officials leads to an increasing role for voluntary organisations, community workers and a plethora of informal care workers in servicing minority communities.

The professional status of social work is therefore an ambivalent one in relation to minorities. Struggles against co-option and incorporation of workers from minority communities are well documented (Stubbs 1988) and the problem of exclusion and elitism of much professional training is challenged by the nature of work with ethnic minority communities (see Chapter 13).

CONCLUSION

The construction of language and the selection of terminology is necessarily political. Common language in use reflects a world view and in itself can reproduce relations of dominance and subordination (Noel 1994). Language is a key medium through which dominating groups reinforce their superiority and prescribe the inferior status of minority groups. There has, for example, been considerable debate on the use of labels such as 'black' people, 'coloured' people, 'people of colour' in reference to ethnic minority groups and it is clear that the acceptability of labels depends on the speaker and who owns the terminology and the agenda for communication. For example, black people in Britain have claimed the word 'black' as a political term to demarcate a collective position and rejected the term 'coloured' as the language used by the dominating group to describe them.

The issue of terminology highlights the dynamic nature of social reality and the construction of language as ever-changing and historically and contextually determined. The search for a universal language for social work with minorities may therefore be misplaced. What is clear, however, is that it is possible to conceptualise the processes of social exclusion and marginalisation, to identify common characteristics that transgress geographical boundaries of nation states and that mark out relations of dominance and subordination in any society (Noel 1994). The distribution of power in society is central to such an understanding. Focusing on analytical tools and conceptual frameworks to deconstruct these processes makes it possible to tap into this dynamic, to accommodate the constant reconfiguration of minorities and the emergence of new minorities and to track patterns of inequality and exclusion that are associated with membership of certain groups. The search for appropriate conceptual frameworks is vital to the development of public policy making and practice in this area. In Chapter 3 Lena Dominelli explores the response of established societies to the presence of their minorities, reviewing concepts of assimilation, integration, multiculturalism and power as the bases of different social work responses.

Summary points

- This chapter provides a critical introductory analysis of some key concepts.
- It is shown that there is a great amount of diversity in terms and concepts used within the field of social work and ethnicity.
- Language and terminology in use tend to reflect relations of dominance and subordination.
- Prejudice and discrimination permeate the tasks of social work.
- An understanding of citizenship rights is crucial to the work of professionals working with minorities.

- Language and terminology in use should be the subject of continual review since the social reality they reflect is contextual and changing.

REFERENCES

Aluffi-Pentini, A. and Lorenz, W. (1996) *Anti-Racist Work with Young People: European Experiences and Approaches*. Lyme Regis: Russell House Publishing.

Anthias, F. (1992) *Ethnicity, Class and Migration: Greek Cypriots in Britain*. Aldershot: Gower.

Anthias, F. and Yuval-Davies, N. (1993) *Racialised Boundaries*. London: Routledge.

Bailey, J. (ed.) (1992) *Social Europe*. London: Longman.

Banton, M. (1994) *Discrimination*. Milton Keynes: Open University Press.

Barth, F. (1969) 'Introduction' in *Ethnic Groups and Boundaries*. Oslo: Universitetsforlaget.

Bottomore, T. (1992) 'Citizenship and social class, forty years on' in T.H. Marshall and T. Bottomore (eds) *Citizenship and Social Class*. London: Pluto Press.

Brown, R. (1995) *Prejudice – its Social Psychology*. Oxford: Blackwell.

Cannan, C., Berry, L. and Lyons, K. (1992) *Social Work in Europe*. London: Macmillan.

Council of Europe (1997) *The Initial and Further Training of Social Workers Taking into Account their Changing Role*. Strasbourg: The Steering Committee on Social Policy.

Delanty, G. (1996) 'Beyond the nation-state: national identity and citizenship in a multi cultural society – a response to Rex' *Sociological Research Online*, 1, 3. <http: www.socresonline.org.uk/socresonline/1/3/1.html>

Dominelli, L. (1988) *Anti Racist Social Work*. London: Macmillan; 2nd edition (1997).

Donald, J. and Rattansi, A. (eds) (1992) *'Race', Culture and Difference*. London: Sage.

Essed, P. (1991) *Understanding Everyday Racism: An Interdisciplinary Theory*. London: Sage.

Gaventa, J. (1982) *Power and Powerlessness. Quiescence and Rebellion in an Appalachian Valley*. Urbana: University of Illinois Press.

Gordon, P. (1989) *Fortress Europe! The Meaning of 1992*, London: Runnymede Trust.

Hammar, T. (1990) *Democracy and the Nation State. Denizens and Citizens in a World of International Migration*. Aldershot: Avebury.

Husband, C. (1994) *Race and Nation: The British Experience*. Perth, WA: Paradigm Press.

—— (1996) 'Defining and containing diversity: community, ethnicity and citizenship' in W.I.U. Ahmad and K. Atkin (eds) *Race and Community Care*. Buckingham: Open University Press.

Lange, A. and Westin, C. (1981) *Etnisk Diskriminering och Social Identitet*. Stockholm: LiberFörlag.

Lorenz, W. (1994) *Social Work in a Changing Europe*. London: Routledge.

Lukes, S. (1974) *Power – a Radical View*. London: Macmillan.

—— (ed.) (1986) *Power*. Oxford: Blackwell.

Luthra, M. (1997) *Britain's Black Population*. Ashgate: Arena.

Marshall, T. (1950) *Citizenship and Social Class, and Other Essays*. Cambridge: Cambridge University Press.
Miles, R. (1993) *Racism after Race Relations*. London: Routledge.
Munday, B. and Ely, P. (1996) *Social Care in Europe*. London: Prentice Hall.
Nederveen Pieterse, J. (1991) 'Fictions of Europe' *Race and Class* 32, 3:3–11.
Noel, L. (1994) *Intolerance: A General Survey*. London: McGill-Queen's University Press.
Ong, A (1996) 'Cultural citizenship as subject-making' *Current Anthropology* 37, 5: 737–62.
Paul, R. (1991) 'Black and Third World people's citizenship and 1992' *Critical Social Policy* II, 2:52–64.
Perotti, A. (1994) *The Case for Intercultural Education*. Strasburg: Council of Europe Press.
Race and Class Vol. 32, Special Edition. Racism and Europe.
Rex, J. (1992) 'Race and ethnicity in Europe' in J. Bailey (ed.) *Social Europe*. London: Longman.
—— (1996) 'National identity in the democratic multi cultural state' *Sociological Research Online* 50, 2. <http://www.socresonline.org.jk/socresonline/1/2/1,html>
Rouland, N. (1991) *Aux confins du droit. Anthropologie juridique de la modernité*. Paris: Odile Jacob.
Stubbs, P. (1988) 'The employment of black social workers: from ethnic sensitivity to anti-racism' *Critical Social Policy* 12:6–27.
Williams, F. (1989) *Social Policy: A Critical Introduction*. Cambridge: Polity Press.
—— (1995) 'Some reflections on race and racism in the Welsh context' *Contemporary Wales* 8:113–31.
—— (1996) 'Postmodernism, feminism and the question of difference' in N. Parton (ed.) *Social Theory, Social Change and Social Work*. London: Routledge.

Chapter 2

Understanding migration

Haluk Soydan

INTRODUCTION

In this chapter, the impact of modern migration is explored by using a typology that describes migration as a problem-solving and problem-generating phenomenon. Negative impacts of migration at individual as well as at societal levels are understood as social problems within the framework of modern society, more specifically, the welfare state. The problem-solving and problem-generating typology is connected to three prominent models of response to the issues of disadvantage and discrimination: the model of categorical diversity, the model of transactional diversity and the model of universal diversity.

MIGRATION

In general, migration means the flow of people from one settlement place to another. Migration can take place within a national territory as well as across national borders, international migration. The duration of migration might change due to a number of factors. Some people migrate and settle down temporarily, while others do so for generations or for a lifetime. In this book the focus is on international migration as outflows and inflows that can be labelled as 'in-migration' and 'out-migration'. This terminology applies to movements and is not easy to differentiate from concepts such as (im)migration and emigration. Whenever the dynamic character of migration is in focus, the concepts of in-migration and out-migration are used. In a more general sense, 'migration' is used as the key concept.

Migration is seen as a phenomenon which is generated by the mutual interference of push and pull factors. Geographical nearness tends to catalyse push and pull factors. Push factors are forces that push people out of regions, countries or maybe even from large areas of continents. Famine, war, unemployment are typical push factors. Pull factors are identified in the in-migration areas and attract people to these areas. Better living conditions, peace, the image of a country as being a 'paradise' are typical pull factors. Migration flows follow possible combinations of push and pull factors in any given contexts.

Probably, migration is as old as human society and settlement itself. When modern migration is discussed, especially from a European perspective, the character of migration as an ancient phenomenon is neglected or at least underestimated. Even when a remote and peripheral region such as Scandinavia is considered, the importance of migration in this region's history should be recognised. The first colonisation of what today is Swedish territory, for example, was due to migration generated by propitious climatic changes. The oldest archaeological discoveries in the southern part of Sweden are 11 to 12 thousand years old (Svanberg and Tydén 1992).

In modern times, that is, post-1945, migration to Western European countries has taken a special shape. Many European countries, especially the north-western ones, became immigration countries due to heavy in-migration after the Second World War. During the period between 1945 and 1970, the economic boom in countries like Germany, France, the Netherlands and Sweden led to the settlement of some 16 million immigrants. In a classic book, *Immigrant Workers and Class Structure in Western Europe*, Castles and Kosack (1993) argued that most of these immigrants were imported to fill the jobs which indigenous workers were reluctant to take, or for which indigenous manpower was lacking. Castles (1984:23) used the term 'industrial reserve army' to characterise the role played by out-migrating workers in the in-migration countries.

However, as Miles (1993) argues in his book *Racism after Race Relations*, modern migration to Europe as well as to and in other parts of the world is a complex phenomenon and must be contextualised in order to be correctly understood. Miles (1993: 127) states that 'it is not only that many migrations are politically determined (although some are thereafter economically mediated), but also that international migrations determined by labour demand are necessarily mediated by the political institutions of nation and state'. Thus, migration flows include not only labour migration between 'Third' and 'First' Worlds but also refugee migration as well as migration of professional, technical and managerial labour over national boundaries. Miles concludes that there is reason to believe that these migrations will continue on an increased scale. 'Uneven economic development, class conflict and the political instability of many nation states all ensure that a large proportion of the world's population has a good reason to consider migration across national boundaries' (Miles 1993:127).

Publications of Eurostat (see for example *Statistics in Focus*, 1996a, no. 2) show that in January 1993 the European Union had a population of 368 million, of whom almost 18 million persons did not have the citizenship of the country in which they were migrants. Turks were the largest single group of non-nationals, living mainly in Germany. With 2.6 million persons, Turks constitute the largest non-EU contingent. One-third of the non-nationals were nationals of another EU country, the largest groups being Italians and Portuguese. Almost two-thirds of the non-nationals live in Germany, France and the United Kingdom. However, the proportion of non-nationals in the total population is higher in smaller countries (31 per cent in Luxembourg, 9 per cent in Belgium, and almost 6 per cent in Sweden). From outside the European Union, the largest sources of out-migration are Turkey, former Yugoslavia and the Maghrebian countries. The non-national population is made up of more men than women. However, this imbalance, caused by successive waves of in-migration, is diminishing over the course of time. There is a tendency towards feminisation of poverty, and thus increasing female human traffic across countries. Since the beginning of the 1980s, European Union migration has been rather limited, whereas in-migration of non-European Union citizens has been considerable. There are also a large number of unregistered illegal immigrants.

Table 2.1 gives a picture of the constitution of non-nationals, EU migrants and non-EU migrants in the EU countries. It shows that Germany, France, the United Kingdom, Belgium and the Netherlands have been receiving the largest number of migrants. Germany, France and the United Kingdom host the largest number of non-EU migrants, and the largest number of non-nationals.

Table 2.1 Immigrants in European Union countries (in thousands)

Country	*Total citizens January 1993*	*Non-nationals January 1993*	*EU migrants January 1994*	*Non-EU migrants January 1994*
Austria	7,795	517	–	706
Belgium	10,068	909	548	372
Denmark	5,180	180	42	147
Finland	5,055	46	12	43
France	56,652	3,596	1,322	2,275
Germany	80,974	6,495	1,750	5,128
Greece	10,350	200	43	106
Ireland	3,563	89	–	21
Italy	56,960	923	120	504
Luxembourg	395	–	116	12
Netherlands	15,239	757	194	586
Portugal	9,864	121	39	118
Spain	39,048	393	201	230
Sweden	8,692	499	183	325
United Kingdom	57,222	2,020	827	1,207

Source: *Statistics in Focus. Population and Social Conditions*, Eurostat 1996a, no. 2; *Demographic Statistics*, Eurostat 1996b.

MIGRATION AS A PROBLEM-SOLVING AND PROBLEM-GENERATING PHENOMENON

One of the distinguishing marks of modern post-war societies is the globalisation of these societies in various ways. Globalisation can be defined as 'the intensification of world-wide social relations which link distant localities in such a way that local happenings are shaped by events occurring many miles away and vice versa' (Giddens 1990:64). Anthony Giddens argues that globalisation in modern times should be analysed in terms of four dimensions: the nation state system, the world capitalist economy, the world military order, and the international division of labour. Although he does not discuss migration as such, he implicitly includes preconditions of migration in his description of the fourth dimension, which basically concerns industrial development. With industrial development, an expansion of the global division of labour has become a considerable necessity. Thus, differentiation between more and less industrialised areas and regions of the world has taken place at a tremendous pace and on a wide scale. International migration, like international and regional specialisation of industry, skills and the production of raw materials, is thus generated as a natural consequence of globalisation of industrial activities. Daniel Kubat (1979) characterises the same phenomenon as an exchange between poor and well-to-do nations. The globalisation of labour is reflected in the political sphere in terms of migration policies which might be defined as

> short term responses of nations and countries faced with the consequences of steps, taken only shortly before, to meet the needs for economic growth with their own supply of labour, to match their political aims with their population policies, and to accommodate the demographic pressures either from within or from outside the country.
>
> (Kubat 1979:xviii)

Furthermore, migration due to political unrest, violent hostilities and war is to be taken into consideration. Although European Union countries have not been strongly affected by in-migration of people from regions of political unrest and war, as a number of countries in other continents have, in-migration of refugees and asylum seekers is still an important factor in the European context.

The statistics presented in the previous section show the demographic constitution of the European Union countries in terms of their ethnic and cultural mix. The demographic alterations due to in-migration are huge, and most probably irreversible. The impact of migrant groups on the countries of in-migration in terms of structural changes and cultural strains are obvious. Thus, migration appears to be a mechanism which fundamentally influences and alters social, economic and political spheres of emigration and, in particular, in-migration countries. The social and ethnic structure of the labour force, the relative proportion of gender composition, and the age structure of the population are altered. Societies are transformed into new multicultural shapes.

In this perspective, migration is seen as a problem-solving and a problem-generating mechanism. It means that, while migration solves problems in certain instances, it also generates problems in other contexts. This dual character of migration might appear obvious; however, it is seldom spelled out. The problem-solving aspect of migration is an important source of knowledge, in particular for social work practice, which by its nature aims at problem solving. The two aspects of migration have their impact either simultaneously or with various degrees of time lag. Problem-solving and problem-generating mechanisms are differentiated and complex processes, and might be better understood on different analytic levels (Leyder 1993:72). Individual and societal contexts are adequate levels of analysis. In other words, a micro–macro perspective on migration's role in societal and individual development is established.

A cross-tabulation of these two aspects illustrates variations of problem-solving and problem-generating processes as simultaneous, parallel and interacting phenomena. Figure 2.1 displays the interplay between migration as problem-solving and problem-generating mechanisms, and the two levels of analysis, namely individual and societal.

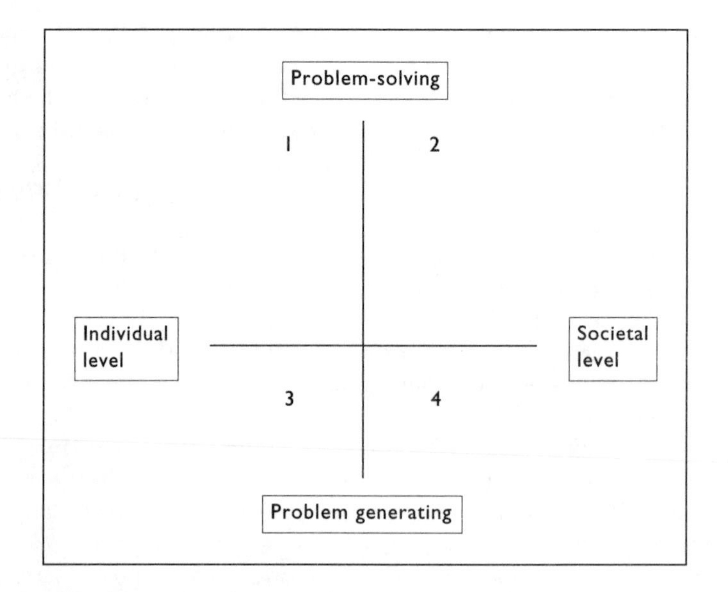

Figure 2.1 Migration as problem-solving/generating mechanisms at individual and societal levels

The figure indicates social processes, each taking place in time and space. What does it mean that migration is a problem-solving mechanism at an individual level? At the individual level, migration becomes problem-solving, for example, when an individual who in the country of out-migration was unemployed may in-migrate to a country, get a job and create a new future for himself or herself and his or her dependants. Or, the same is true for a politically threatened person who in-migrates to another country, is given asylum and can build himself or herself a safe life. In such instances migration is positive and problem-solving for individuals.

At a societal level also, migration may be a problem-solving mechanism. In the post-war period, in particular from the late 1950s to the early 1970s, the economic boom in the north-western European countries stimulated labour migration between central and peripheral countries of Europe. This type of labour inflows and outflows is a natural consequence of globalisation of the world economy. Thus, economically expanding countries have solved their labour force shortage problems by attracting labour reserve armies that were available in other countries. The inflow of experts, especially in trans-national high-technology companies, solves the shortage of highly specialised labour needed in the country of in-migration. It should be emphasised that in-migration countries have through the inflow of migrants also incorporated other types of resources with positive effects for variation and diversity in the country; to mention only a very few, gaining better sportsmen/women, the diversification and supply of cuisines and catering, and the enrichment of the cultural life of the country.

In one sense, the problem-solving effect of this migration was mutual, at least for some periods, by affecting the out-migration countries positively in terms of absorbing labour surplus, the acquisition of skills by migrants and migrant workers' remittances home. The policies of out-migration countries were formed with the assumption that out-migration was a good thing for the country. Nevertheless, this matter is questioned by critical writers such as Castles and Kosack (1993: chapter 9), and it remains a complex phenomenon and an empirical issue to investigate.

What can be said of migration as a problem-generating mechanism? At an individual level, migration may mean strains of various types and adaptation problems that appear as social, psychological and somatic. These stresses may produce disturbances of interpersonal relationships, family and marriage problems, abuse of intoxicants. One of the major problems that face migrants is loss of social status, underemployment and non-recognition of their educational and professional qualifications. A European account of these types of problems is given in the proceedings of workshops organised by the European Science Foundation as early as the beginning of the 1980s (*Human Migration* 1980/1). By the mid-1990s, the immigrants' situation is still characterised by social hierarchy and problematic social landscape (Perotti 1994). The impact of migration at an individual level is mediated by complex mechanisms where class, gender and age certainly play an important role. A growing literature focuses, for instance, on the question of whether migration leads to a loss or gain in the status of women as a result of changes of power within the family. Migrant women who have been able to enter the labour market experience increasing importance within the family. Those women who have been excluded from the labour market and isolated from an extended family network find their role in the family undermined (Buijs 1993:8–9). The family consists of members of different generations. Migrant labour is generally young, but may leave behind children and older relatives who may later rejoin the family. Refugees frequently comprise younger children and older people. Consequently, benefits and problems may be different for different age groups. Thus, the contextuality of the impact of migration is important.

At the societal level, the problem-generating role of migration is obvious. Massive in-migration, especially from poorer economies and remote cultures, tends to create a new social stratification in the in-migration countries in terms of the labour market, housing segregation, cultural and ethnic segregation, and social status hierarchy. Migrant populations as groups often suffer from bad living conditions, and are exposed to exclusion, racism and discrimination (see for example Castles 1984; Castles and Kosack 1993; Lorenz 1994; Rex 1992). Phenomena such as exclusion, discrimination and racism are uncomfortable not only for those who are struck by it but also for those who see it being practised in their native countries. Thus, these types of phenomena create disintegrative and destructive tendencies in immigration countries. Recent strong efforts demonstrated by the European Commission through the European Social Policy Forum clearly show strong concern about disintegrative and anti-democratic tendencies generated by unemployment, segregation and discrimination. The recommendations of a Comité des Sages, published in *For a Europe of Civic and Social Rights* (1996), aim at remedying such tendencies.

The problem-solving and problem-generating model discussed above helps us to locate traditional fields of social work action and social policy measures. Panel 3 in the fourfold table locates the working area of social work, while panel 4 indicates social policy fields.

The focus of social work intervention has been defined and delimited in various ways. Social work researchers and practitioners have very much debated the focus of social work practice, and suggested different definitions of the object of intervention (Soydan 1998). Here it is useful to refer to a widely used definition of social work practice given by Alex Gitterman and Carel Germain (1976:602):

> Social workers focus on problems in living which fall into three areas: (1) problems and needs associated with tasks involved in life transitions; (2) problems and needs associated with tasks in using and influencing

> elements of the environment; and (3) problems and needs associated with interpersonal obstacles which impede the work of a family or a group as it deals with transitional and/or environmental tasks.

Thus, concern about social functioning and focus on both person/group and social situations have profound implications for social work practice. In this book, it is suggested that in social work with minority clients, individual-oriented case-work is not sufficient and the interplay between the individual and his or her environment should be emphasised (see further Chapters 8, 9 and 14). In social work practice a problem is defined, and then planned actions are taken in order to solve that problem. Social work intervention is based on scientific research and tested experience.

Correspondingly, social policy measures focus on social problems located in panel 4, and interact in many ways with social work practice. Thus, there exists a complementary connection between the problem fields of panels 3 and 4, involving social work action and social policy measures. Social policy has been defined and delimited in various ways. A common type of definition is given by Hagenbuch in terms of 'ensuring every member of the community certain minimum standards and certain opportunities' (Titmuss 1974:29). In referring to this definition, Richard Titmuss stresses the following objectives and value judgements of social policy:

> First, they aim to be beneficent – policy is directed to provide welfare for citizens. Second, they include economic as well as non-economic objectives; for example, minimum wages, minimum standards of income maintenance and so on. Third, they involve some measures of progressive redistribution in command-over-resources from rich to poor.
>
> (Titmuss 1974:29)

In sum, social work action and social policy measures have very much to do with disadvantage, powerlessness, inequality and discrimination. In terms of understanding social problems generated within the sphere of migration and ethnic relations, three models of approaching social work action and social policy have been developed. In the next section, these models are presented: categorical diversity, transitional diversity and universal diversity, respectively.

MODELS OF RESPONSE TO ISSUES OF DISADVANTAGE AND DISCRIMINATION

These models are approaches crystallised within the frame of reference of the welfare state and are claimed as responses to social problems generated by migration and ethnic diversity. The models are conceptualisations of what ethnic diversity is, and how it could and should be approached. Thus, each model has empirical, theoretical and normative elements as constituent parts. Empirical elements often refer to implementations of ideas and policies in terms of social work practice or social policy measures. Theoretical elements refer to the theoretical knowledge base of the model. Normative elements prescribe what is good and what is bad in societies with ethnic diversity. These elements often appear in mixed configurations in the self-presentations of these models.

Categorical diversity

First to be discussed is categorical diversity since this model with its variations seems to be the most frequently implemented one in social policy and in social work. Categorical diversity understands ethnicity as a set of markers that persons belonging to the ethnic group possess. Thus, persons categorised in a certain ethnic group are assumed to have all the markers that the ethnic group is supposed to have. All the members share common markers, and the ethnic group is considered to be homogeneous. This model stresses the cultural content of the ethnic group and takes ethnic patterns at face value. Ethnic groups are seen as culturally uniform. Factors such as social class and gender are not taken into consideration when approaching ethnic groups. As Green (1995:25) puts it: 'Categorical thinking is comparative but only in the most simplistic and ethnocentric sense; it presumes a central point of reference that is a standard, myself, and measures all others against that standard.'

The two most frequent manifestations of categorical diversity at a policy level are the 'melting-pot' model and the cultural pluralism model. Both models approach ethnic groups as separate and distinctive cultural communities with specific sets of cultural features. In the melting-pot model, ethnic markers are taken as cultural baggage, a set of cultural markers that are expected to disappear as the ethnic group adopts the culture of the dominant group. The melting-pot model, which was originally launched by the sociologists of the Chicago School with Robert Park as the leading figure, has been debated since then and is still a question of controversy (Steinberg 1989).

Cultural pluralism also underlines the specific content of ethnic groups. As an ideology it stresses the need for ethnic groups to exist autonomously, but side by side and in harmony with the dominant ethnic group. Ethnic differences are seen as a source of richness contributing to a diversification and strengthening of society. Formally, cultural pluralism and cultural relativism seem to harmonise. However, cultural pluralism's acceptance of cultural differences and particularities is limited. Cultural pluralism supports survival of ethnic minorities only to a certain extent; this is due to the fact that relationships between ethnic minorities and the dominant group are power relations. If all groups had equal power, the idea of cultural pluralism could be realised to a certain extent. The relationship between ethnic minorities and the dominant group involves competition in terms of resources whose distribution is also dependent on other factors such as class, age and gender. Furthermore, the dominant group is the one that sets the fundamental standards of the society, including value systems that regulate important life spheres. Green's summary of categorical diversity is rather strong:

> the problem with categorical ways of thinking about ethnicity and cultural differences is that it is ultimately political: the dominant group dictates the categories that help it manage and control uncertain and potentially contentious relationships. The implicit assumption is that cross-cultural relationships are essentially competitive and hostile, competitive for the scarce resources of position, power, rank, authority, goods, time, services, and moral worthiness. Cultural difference is a challenge, even a threat, one that invokes self-protection and personal distancing. In service relationships, that is hardly an effective way of learning about others or of responding to their needs.
>
> (Green 1995:27)

In societies where categorical diversity thinking is the foundation of ethnic relations, social policy measures are taken in order to create 'equal opportunities' for all ethnic groups. Politicisation of cultural pluralism may sometimes lead to positive discrimination of ethnic minorities. Special measures are, then, taken in order to equalise inter-group differences. With this approach it also follows that ethnic groups should be integrated into society, basically on the conditions of the dominant group. By the same token, there are similar approaches in social work. What is basically found is that lack of cultural awareness, sensitivity and competency in dealing with the variety of ethnic groups enforces the use of social work models and tools developed for indigenous groups.

Transactional diversity

The transactional diversity model has its basis in the work of a Norwegian social anthropologist, Fredrik Barth (1969). In encounters between different ethnic groups, boundaries between these groups develop and are defined as ethnic boundaries. The ethnic groups tend to maintain their boundaries. Boundary maintenance comes to the fore and creates the cultural core of the group. Thus, the protection of the ethnic group's boundaries, and not the cultural content in itself, comes into focus. What the members of an ethnic group do in given situations indicates group membership. In interaction with other ethnic groups, one becomes a member of a given ethnic group.

Ethnicity is, then, a situational, or a transactional phenomenon which is generated within the boundaries of ethnic groups. Members of a specific group acquire or refer to their group identity in given situations and under given structures.

The transactional diversity model stresses the complexity of ethnic identities and searches for them in a comparative perspective. While the categorical diversity model stresses the content of the ethnic culture, the transactional diversity model focuses on the interaction. This difference has an important consequence in terms of social policy and social work action. Social policy and social work interventions seek to bring about measures in harmony with the prerequisites of the ethnic group. Thus, any intervention must have as its starting point the group's own definition of social problems.

Universal diversity

The third model that will be presented here has been debated during the last decade, mainly in the United States and to some extent in the United Kingdom, principally in the field of working life research, and is mostly known under the name of 'managing diversity' (Kandola and Fullerton 1994). It could be labelled as universal diversity since the model embraces all individuals, who are seen as different from one another in many ways. The model as a research and action tradition has emerged in controversy with the model of categorical diversity, and especially with the idea of 'equal opportunities'. So, what are the characteristics of this model?

The universal diversity model is based on the assumption that diversity in human societies and social institutions emanates from differences in a number of human aspects such as gender, ethnicity, religious affiliation, age, physical and mental capability, economic class, sexual orientation and many other factors which cause individuals to develop different perspectives on the same factualities or questions. It is then obvious that ethnicity becomes only one of many factors generating diversity in human societies. Advocates of the universal diversity model support their arguments with empirical studies of organisations and companies. The basic idea of 'managing diversity' has its starting point in the assumption that the labour force consists of people who are diverse in many aspects. The diversity consists of visible as well as invisible differences which affect people's participation and performance in organisations and in working life. The idea of managing diversity also assumes that mobilising and using diversity generates a productive environment in which people feel valued, where their talents are being used and in which organisational goals are met. The universal diversity model stresses all types of differences, while the equal opportunities model basically focuses on ethnicity, gender and handicap.

The universal diversity model appreciates differences between individuals, and aims at using these differences optimally for the individual and the organisation in which the individual is working. An attempt to implement the universal diversity model in the field of social policy would, for example, mean that the social policy measures would be oriented towards stimulating the survival of diversity. Thus, social policy measures would support individuals as individuals rather than as members of a certain ethnic group. In social work, it would mean managing each client according to the client's personal needs, situation and preconditions without having any prejudice about the client's group affiliation.

APPLICATION OF THE MODEL

So far, it has been argued that migration has a dual role of problem-solving and problem-generating, and its effects should be studied at least at two levels, that is, the individual (and group) level and the societal level, which is a macro level. It has also been argued that within the framework of the modern state, more specifically the welfare state, three prominent, conceptually founded, approaches or models have been crystallised as responses to social problems generated by migration. These approaches are aimed to act at the individual and the societal levels, respectively. The individual level is covered by social work practice, while the societal level is approached by social policy measures. There is interdependency and complementarity between social work practice and social policy measures in this context.

What can more substantially be said about how these three models function through social work practice and social policy measures? Are there any concrete examples of models implemented in different immigration countries? The answer to these questions is an empirical issue. It could be argued that in certain instances it is possible to point out empirical examples of models which directly emanate from one of the three conceptual models of response to social problems generated by migration. In other instances, the models are still at a theoretical or normative stage and have not been directly implemented. Here, the purpose is not an attempt at a systematic empirical account, but rather to demonstrate possible, or whenever available, empirical consequences of each conceptual model of response. Figure 2.2 displays the state of the art in terms of what the three conceptual models mean in social policy and social work fields.

Let us follow the structure given in Figure 2.2. Categorical diversity appears in its modern shape in terms of 'equal opportunities', which basically is oriented towards legislating against discrimination, and in some cases towards a universalistic social policy. Swedish social policy is perhaps one of the best examples of the most active adaptation policies *vis-à-vis* immigrant populations (Gur 1996). Basic characteristics of the equal opportunities model are: It is driven legally and from top-down, that is, it is promoted by intellectual and enlightened segments of society. It aims at improving

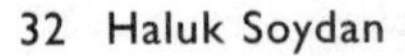

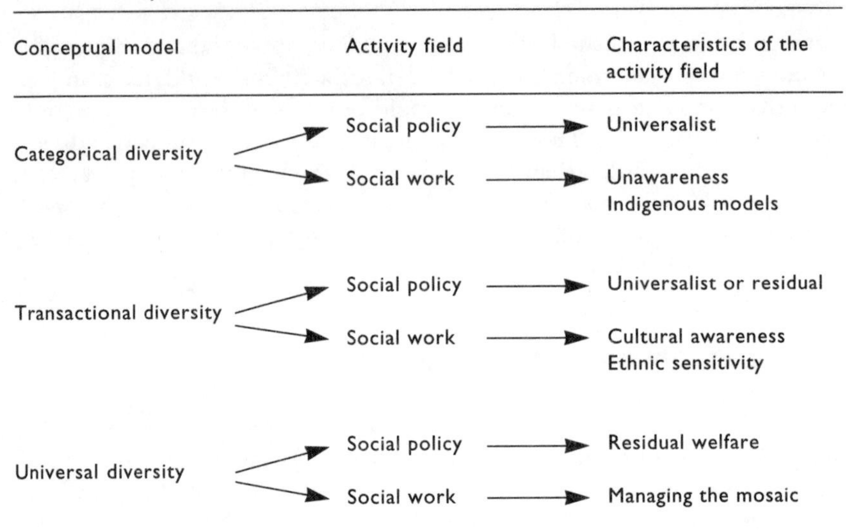

Figure 2.2 Social work and social policy in the shade of three conceptual models: a typology

the proportion of ethnic participation, for example through quota systems in schools and the labour market. It is reactive and tends to use positive discrimination. It is also important to stress that ultimately it functions within the premises of the dominant culture and basically assumes assimilation.

Categorical diversity seems more salient in the field of social policy. In social work practice, it is characterised by passiveness and *unawareness*. In social work practice, it is expected that indigenous models – middle and upper class, white-oriented – of social work are used for clients with immigrant and ethnic background. Social services are basically organised for the needs of the dominant population on a universalist or 'difference-blind' model. The situation may be aggravated when the perspectives of ethnic minority professionals are lacking and when the personnel lack multicultural training and understanding (see Green 1995; Juliá 1996).

Transactional diversity is expected to be either universalist or residual at the social policy level. In the field of social work, a number of models, recognising the transactional character of ethnic relationships, have developed, especially in the United States. However, this is not to say that they are widely used in human social services. These models appear under a number of names, but the label 'ethnic-sensitive' is perhaps the best characterisation of this genre of social work models for clients with immigrant and ethnic backgrounds. The best two examples of these models have been reported by Wynetta Devore and Elfriede Schlesinger (1996), *Ethnic-Sensitive Social Work Practice* and by James Green (1995), *Cultural Awareness in the Human Services. Multi-Ethnic Approach*.

Universal diversity has by definition an individual orientation. In the field of social policy, it is expected that this approach is harmonious with what Richard Titmuss called 'the residual welfare model of social policy', which is based on the premise that the private market and the family are the two natural arenas meeting an individual's needs. Only when these arenas break down should social welfare institutions become active. Thus, it might be said that the universal diversity approach would follow a passive, residual welfare model.

What about universal diversity in terms of social work? In the previous section, it was mentioned that this approach is designed for diversity management in institutions and companies. The results of implementation in institutions and companies are reported to be positive in many ways, such as recruiting from a wider range of talented candidates, retaining this talent, savings from lower turnover and absenteeism, efficient manpower utilisation, better resource utilisation (Kandola and Fullerton 1994). Managing diversity in institutions and companies is a relationship between managers and employees, while managing diversity in social work is a relationship between professionals and clients. Thus, in social work it has to do with professional–client encounters.

Implementation of universal diversity in social work would mean that the dimension of ethnicity becomes one of several factors assumed to have an impact on the results of social work intervention. In client encounters, not only ethnicity but also other aspects should be taken into consideration. Clients should be seen as individuals with specific personal characteristics rather than as members of a given ethnic group.

The choice of the dominant diversity model is a result of each country's historical characteristics, conditioned by social, economic and political factors. Migration being not only a problem-solving mechanism but to a large extent also a problem-generating mechanism, societies face the task of handling problems generated by migration. As one consequence of migration, social work is thus confronted with a challenge of great scope. The three models of conceptualising diversity have been the main approaches on which social work practice with minority clients is based. Theoretical and empirical considerations, as well as value preferences and power relations, will determine the set of social work models implemented for minority clients in any particular country.

CONCLUSION

This chapter has shown that migration is a complicated social phenomenon, especially within the framework of the intensified globalisation of social relations. In Europe, modern migration has implied huge and most probably irreversible demographic alterations. It is argued that migration has a dual character by being problem solving and problem generating for individuals as well as for communities. Social relations between ethnic minorities and majority populations are characterised as power relationships. The social consequences of migration are highly affected by the gender and age structure of the ethnic minorities. Formation of social policy and development of social work methods with relevance to ethnic minorities and minority clients are dependent on the kind of dominant conceptualisation of ethnic diversity in each society.

REFERENCES

Barth, F. (ed.) (1969) *Ethnic Groups and Boundaries. The Social Organisation of Culture Difference*, Boston: Little, Brown.

Buijs, G. (ed.) (1993) *Migrant Women. Crossing Boundaries and Changing Identities*, Oxford: Berg.

Castles, S. (1984) *Here for Good. Western Europe's New Ethnic Minorities*, London: Pluto Press.

Castles, S. and Kosack, G. (1993) *Immigrant Workers and Class Structure in Western Europe*, London: Oxford University Press. (1st edn 1973)

Comité des Sages (1996) *For a Europe of Civic and Social Rights*, Brussels: European Commission.

Devore, W. and Schlesinger, E. (1996) *Ethnic-Sensitive Social Work Practice*, Boston: Allyn and Bacon.

European Science Foundation (1980/1) *Human Migration* Contributions to the workshops organised by European Science Foundation, Strasburg: European Science Foundation, volumes I–IV.

Eurostat (1996a) *Statistics in Focus. Population and Social Conditions*, Luxemburg: Official Publications of the European Communities, no. 2.

—— (1996b) *Demographic Statistics 1996*. Luxemburg: Official Publications of the European Communities.

Giddens, A. (1990) *The Consequences of Modernity*, Cambridge: Polity Press.

Gitterman, A. and Germain, C. (1976) 'Social work practice: a life model', *Social Service Review*, 50 (4), pp. 601–10.

Green, J. W. (1995) *Cultural Awareness in the Human Services. Multi-Ethnic Approach*, Boston: Allyn and Bacon.

Gur, T. (1996) *Staten och nykomlingarna. En studie av den svenska invandrarpolitikens idéer*, Stockholm: City University Press. (English summary)

Juliá, M. C. (1996) *Multicultural Awareness in the Health Care Professions*, Boston: Allyn and Bacon.

Kandola, R. and Fullerton, J. (1994) *Managing the Mosaic. Diversity in Action*, London: Institute of Personnel and Development.

Kubat, D. (1997) *The Politics of Migration Policies*, New York: Center for Migration Studies.

Leyder, D. (1993) *New Strategies in Social Research*, Cambridge: Polity Press.

Lorenz, W. (1994) *Social Work in a Changing Europe*, London: Routledge.

Miles, R. (1993) *Racism after Race Relations*, London: Routledge.

Perotti, A. (1994) *The Case for Intercultural Education*, Strasburg: Council of Europe Press.

Rex, John (1992) 'Race and ethnicity in Europe', in J. Bailey (ed.), *Social Europe*, New York: Longman, pp. 106–20.

Soydan, H. (1998) *The History of Ideas in Social Work*, Birmingham: Venture Press.

Steinberg, S. (1989) *The Ethnic Myth. Race, Ethnicity, and Class in America*, Boston: Beacon Press.

Svanberg, I. and Tydén, M. (1992) *Tusen år av invandring – En Svensk Kulturhistoria*, Stockholm: Gidlunds.

Titmuss, R. (1974) *Social Policy*, London: Unwin Hyman.

Chapter 3

Multiculturalism, anti-racism and social work in Europe

Lena Dominelli

INTRODUCTION

The terms assimilation, integration, multiculturalism, ethnic pluralism, 'race'[1] and racism have had a contested history in European intellectual thought. However, these concepts have been used in racialised discourses to describe the dominant patterns of social interaction within 'race relations' across the European continent. Their importance in setting the parameters within which social policy and everyday practices, including in social work, are formulated is evident throughout European societies. The process of a racialised 'othering' or the casting of people as outsiders who are barely tolerated on the basis of skin colour and ethnicity is a significant dimension of this process.

In this chapter, I examine how social work practice has been implicated in the racist 'othering' of members of ethnic minority groups and the provision of inappropriate services to them as a result. I also consider how the struggles of groups who have been racially oppressed have contributed to broadening our understanding of the dynamics of racism in Europe and to the development of anti-racist social work services.

EUROPEANNESS: AN IDENTITY IN FORMATION

Even the terminology used to describe the phenomena of diverse ethnic groups living together in any given part of the European continent is subject to controversy and different usages. I will use the word 'European' only in the sense that it refers to a geographical location because I take the view that an all-encompassing vision of Europeanness as an identity has yet to be elaborated. What we have at the moment is a collection of national visions existing alongside each other with some attempts at developing a political and cultural unity driven by economic considerations.

The 'European', then, is in the process of being created. But the efforts to achieve such a vision will be realised only if they obtain the consent of the majority of the population in each constituent country. To achieve it, they will have to address the issues of diversity, heterogeneity and ethnicities which the peoples of Europe have struggled to maintain for centuries. Nonetheless, although their antecedents and current expression vary, there are themes which appear with depressing frequency across the continent. Sadly, racist discourses count amongst these.

There is no specifically *European* discourse around the issue of racism as it pertains to social work, if by European we mean a supra-national socio-economic formation. The European Union (EU), a legal entity which could in theory represent such a construct, is largely a regional grouping of economically diverse nation states which have harmonised certain of their economic activities to maximise their potential to compete in the global marketplace. However, the forces for political or social integration at the regional level have been strongly resisted by many of the nation states which form the EU. Ironically, the project of maintaining national identities unites many across the spread of the political spectrum from the social democratic Danes to the xenophobic members of far-right groupings such as Le Pen's National Front in France. At the same time, contradictory trends are evident in measures such as the issuance of ubiquitous 'European' passports. These indicate regional-level political affiliations addressing the topic of individual mobility albeit primarily for the purposes of seeking jobs, at least for the nationals of those states in the EU.

Despite claims to the contrary in some anti-racist writing which refer to a 'Eurocentric' (Blaut 1993) version of social work, the notion of a 'European' social work is illusory. Each European country has its own definition of what constitutes social work and its own set of cultural and legal traditions associated with it. The only claim which can currently be made about social work in Europe is that it is a vastly diverse profession (Lorenz 1994). This is not to say that there have not been certain tasks or functions which social work, however defined in different European nation states, has assumed and which may be found in all of them. However, this statement applies to activities at a fairly high level of abstraction, for example, enforcing social control, assisting deprived communities, and adhering to a liberal democratic value base. How social workers act in practice is a matter of specific description and analysis. Other commonalities are evident in the kind of social problems encountered by social workers in all European countries, for example child abuse, poverty.

At the level of macro-analysis, the issue of the forms of racism being transmitted through social work practice does become important. For it is at such points that the common thread of a value base which legitimates the idea of white European superiority, although it has been realised as a specifically constructed set of practices enshrined in the legislative norms, policy diktats and professional observances particular to each country, appears. Moreover, even in 'skin colour' terms, some intellectuals in Europe (see Adas 1989;

Barkin 1992) have differentiated the 'Caucasian race' by dividing it into three types – the Nordic, Alpine and Mediterranean, with the darkest being deemed inferior (D'Souza 1995). More recently, the British Home Office has introduced the category of 'Dark European' in its ethnic monitoring categories (Dominelli *et al.* 1995). Thus, the creation of a racialised social reality is one which is constantly changing and adapting to altered circumstances. In short, it is actively constructed and should not be viewed as either static or immutable. Furthermore, such constructions may have unintended consequences, despite being created by people exercising their sense of agency in particular circumstances. The positive side of this understanding is that racism can be deconstructed and eradicated. The negative side is that anti-racists have a point in referring to the notion of white European superiority as 'Eurocentrism'.

It would be erroneous to conceive of Eurocentrism as indicating a homogeneous European culture or even sense of 'white' identity. Indeed, one of the intellectual challenges to our understanding of racism in Europe, whether in past epochs or the present day, is the variety of ways in which it is expressed and the diverse ethnic groups that it targets and has targeted. Racism in Europe has not been, nor is it now, simply a question of black over white. For example, there is racism against people of Jewish descent, despite the fact that many of these are 'white' in skin colour. People of Irish descent in the UK, people of Finnish origins in Sweden, those of Italian ancestry in Germany, blond-haired and blue-eyed Muslims from the former Yugoslavia in Italy, to mention but a few, have all experienced some form of racism and racial hatred directed specifically against them, despite their membership of the 'Caucasian race'. Such categorisation, of course, begs the question of whether there is any factual basis to the notion of 'race'. Most scientists would argue that all human beings belong to the same 'race' – *Homo sapiens*.

Nevertheless, these insights call for a refined understanding of the ways in which racism is socially constructed so as to take account of its various forms and permutations, the way it has changed over time and the different personal attributes that it has focused upon. In this respect, some of the analytical tools which focus on the relevance of slavery in clarifying the forms of racism which have been directed against people of African descent may not assist us in making sense of the specific experiences of racism encountered by other ethnic groups. We may need to develop additional theoretical concepts to guide us in practice formulations affecting them. Additionally, we need to consider the interconnections between the different types of racism and how these are a reflection of the various positions that different ethnic groups occupy in the racialised hierarchies that currently exist in any particular country.

Paul Gilroy (1993), in *Black Atlantic*, demonstrates how the slave trade was implicated not only in forming 'black' identities,[2] but also 'white' identities, in all of the areas that were affected by it – Europe, America and Africa. bell hooks (1989) has clarified how black and white women's sexualities have been defined in relation to each other. This refrain is also taken up by Roediger (1991), who argues that the identity of the white American working class was constructed as part of a distancing of white workers from the conditions that slavery imposed on black workers, for in the early days of the institution in the USA there were both black and white slaves and black and white freemen. Ultimately, slavery became associated exclusively with people of African descent (D'Souza 1995), but the concept of racialised identities became a feature of modern life.

I define racism as a set of practices which assumes the inherent superiority of one 'race' over others and thereby the right to dominate (Lorde 1984: 115). Thus, racism is about relations of dominance and subordination which are rooted in the 'othering' of others as a social process of exclusion in which particular personal attributes are identified as the basis for a racialised 'othering' to occur. These characteristics are aspects of an individual's or group's identity which are castigated as 'inferior' by a dominant group which has the power to enforce its definitions of reality on others. They may be based on biological features such as skin colour and hair type, cultural practices, linguistic abilities, or religious observances which are adversely valued socially and weighted against the interests of the subordinated group.

The dynamics of power are central to the question of the value ascribed to those categorised as 'other', for it is the social power and resources wielded by the dominant group which enables it successfully to assert its views against competing claims about how society should be organised and the relationships between and amongst its constituent parts ascertained. The definition of inter-group relations involving 'racialised boundaries' is one of these areas (Anthias and Yuval-Davies 1993). 'Othering', therefore, lies at the heart of racial oppression.

THE 'OTHERING' PROCESS

However, the dominant group's racialised definition of their reality is constantly being challenged by individuals and groups that have been subjected to the 'othering' process. This reaction constitutes resistance to the subordinate place that has been assigned to oppressed people by the dominant group (Gilroy 1993). Resistance may take a variety of forms, which range from reluctant acquiescence to refusal to submit. Reluctance allows dissenting actors to undertake resistance within everyday activities, for example, working slowly when an oppressor is requiring the speedy completion of a job. Resistance behaviour, therefore, varies from reluctantly performing what is required of them as members of an 'inferior' group to widespread revolt. Moreover, the process of defining and redefining resistance and the struggles against oppression are ongoing because both the oppressor and the oppressed are constantly negotiating and renegotiating their realities in the light of events as they unfold. Thus, the two sides are in continual interaction. Both are essential to the process and each impacts upon and influences the behaviour of the other across all walks of life. In this way, the 'other' becomes integrated into the society, albeit on unfavourable terms. Thus, in the European context, as in the American one, albeit often in subordinate positions, people whose ancestors came from the former colonies of imperial powers are an integral part of the socio-economic and political formation of the country they reside in.

Despite the claims of Far Right ideologues and the notion of 'Fortress Europe' (or an equally fortified USA), visibly racialised minorities are as much part of Europe (or the USA) as the allegedly unracialised majority. Indeed, if we take Gilroy's (1993) analysis on board, there is no such thing as an unracialised group. We are all racialised now. The crucial thing is how racialised identities have come to be defined as limited to particular groups who occupy the margins of society and then taken as signifying inferiority. In this context, the efforts of Far Right ideologues to regain the upper hand in the process of defining and redefining others have to be seen as an attempt to reconstruct whiteness as a racialised category that is imbued with claims to being culturally and biologically superior (see Herrnstein and Murray 1994). This course of action has become necessary for them given their anxieties that those who have been othered are making successful claims for being considered their peers and equals as far as social, political and economic rights are concerned.

However, the attempt to redefine 'whiteness' as an exclusive category has not been limited to adherents of Far Right ideology. Indeed, one of the worrying aspects of racism in Europe in the present historical conjuncture is the legitimacy and normality granted to such attempts across the political spectrum. Much of this redefinition has occurred within the apparatus of the state, particularly through immigration policies and the construction of racialised discourses which have 'othered' ethnic groups on the basis of their place of origins, kinship connections and cultural attributes.

In Britain, for example, Margaret Thatcher lent political respectability to the notion of Britishness as a cultural attribute applicable only to white English people by claiming that they had a right not to be 'swamped by alien cultures'. In this way, she excluded black British people who had been maintaining that they too were part of Britain. The logic of this statement became enshrined in law a few years later under the 1981 Nationality Act, when being born in Britain no longer automatically qualified people as British citizens. The position that the Thatcher government subsequently adopted was not completely new. The 1971 Immigration Act had already set the scene by allowing unrestricted leave to enter the country to 'patrials' or those who had 'close' connections to the UK such as having a parent or grandparent born in the country. This legislation excluded primarily black

British people. Barker (1981) called the focus on cultural attributes the 'new racism'. But it signifies the struggle between those who sought to find inclusive ways of defining British so that black British people were included along with the vast variety of 'white' British people and those who were determined to keep alive the notion of British as referring solely to those with white Anglo-Saxon ancestry.

Consequently, members of Far Right groups in Britain began to talk about the *indigenous* population of the British Isles in such exclusive terms that they ignored even its recorded history of migration from the Roman conquests to the peaceful settlement of New Commonwealth populations of more recent times. This nostalgic search for a mythological identity is a reflection of the search for differences carried out in dichotomous terms to separate 'them' (the 'others' who do not belong) from 'us' (those who belong). It is a way of simultaneously claiming territory and identity. As such, it links in with the need to redefine the nation state, since it has lost its previously less penetrable boundaries. National boundaries, as a result of mass migration and globalisation, have become highly permeable. National policies are shaped as much by decisions taken by those outside its territorial limits as those within them, particularly if they are the holders of enormous quantities of financial capital or mobile labour. Seeking ways of clawing back this lost ground is an important part of the process of redefining ethnic identity. In a context of substantial racial intermarriages, dual nationalities, settled black populations and cross-cultural borrowings, cultural heritages cannot easily be defined in the exclusive terms possible when the nation state first held sway. Neither can citizenship.

A similar process is occurring in other European countries. For example, in Germany, German ethnicity is being redefined to exclude not only those called 'third' country nationals from outside the EU, but also those with Germanic ethnic origins from Eastern Europe. In Italy, the Lega del Nord has sought to exclude other Italians, particularly those from the South who it claims have polluted the ethnic purity of the Northerners. But more than this, its discourse is also conducted in terms of a corrupt body politic which has violated the social and cultural integrity of the North, or at least parts of it. The graffiti and public pronouncements which have been used to conduct this monologue, since the voice of the *meridionale*, as the Southern Italians are pejoratively called, is remarkably absent from public pronouncements on this subject, are similar in their abusive constructs of them as those utilised by white racists in the UK against people of African and Asian descent. Additionally, the Lega del Nord has sought to divide Italy into regional parts. Some of its adherents recently climbed the bell tower in Piazza San Marco in Venice to proclaim the Republic of Padania, a mythological creation of ethnic purity from non-existent times. Moreover, such attempts at redefining identity and citizenship have to be understood within the context of globalisation. This has made redundant the idea of a homogeneous nation state and of geographically restricted ethnic identities whilst at the same time increasing insecurities about who people are and what their role in the social and business affairs of the world is.

Indeed, the widespread migration of peoples across the globe, for a variety of reasons ranging from imperial conquests to refugees from areas devastated by war or natural disasters, has given rise to a broadened and deepened understanding of the spread of ethnic identities across geographic and temporal domains. This tends to be encompassed by the concept of ethnic diasporas (Brah 1996; Gilroy 1993). Enduring diasporas are manifestations of people's capacity to adapt to different circumstances whilst still retaining some sense of their original ethnic identity. In short, they have resisted racial annihilation.

SOCIAL WORK IN EUROPE

Social work in Europe has operated within the context of racialised identities and globalisation. However, social work as a profession has up to now defied a singular definition. Contested versions of terminology and meaning abound. Consequently, most allegedly comparative texts will settle for a catalogue listing the variety of forms which will fall under the social work remit, usually on a country by country basis (see Kramer 1989; Ely and Munday 1996). An attempt to transcend this limitation is currently being undertaken in a study by the International Association of Schools of Social Work (IASSW). Its prescription for getting out of this impasse, if it is to be worth following, should be inclusive by focusing on definitions of the tasks social workers undertake and noting the similarities and differences at this level, whatever local name or descriptor is given to their job.

If this proposition is followed through, social work becomes an activity which concerns itself with the details of people who live in society but have difficulty in dealing with the trials and tribulations of everyday life. Katherine Kendall, Honorary President of IASSW, formerly defined social work as a distinct professional activity

> which assess[es] the nature of the need and the problem, to estimate the capacity of the person to handle the problem, to foster every inner strength of the person towards the goal of finding his [*sic*] own solution, and to utilise all the outer resources of the environment and the community which might be of value in this problem-solving endeavour.
>
> (Kendall 1978:43)

Kendall's line of argument provides us with a definition of social work practice that occurs at a high enough level of theoretical abstraction to encompass the social pedagogue working in Germany, the youth worker in

Sweden, the community worker in Northern Ireland, the clinical social worker in Denmark, the health care social worker in France, the care manager in England or the probation officer in Wales. It is also independent of setting and encompasses the state sector, the private institution or voluntary sector activities. This is because the definition focuses on *what* practitioners do rather than *how* they do it and leaves out the context which is crucial to identifying the specificity of their interventions at the local level.

Whilst useful, this definition has the disadvantage of focusing on interventions at the level of the individual. It will, therefore, omit discrimination which is perpetrated on a group of individuals, or even individual members of a disadvantaged group through practitioner intervention. It also does not assist us in identifying the impact of racism in, on and through social work practice in the complex manner suggested by Dominelli (1988) and Ahmad (1990).

Another problem with Kendall's definition is that it assumes a benign intent on the part of the social worker and/or the service. The worker's integrity and professionalism are cast in neutral tones which suggest that their services are uncontroversial and will not give offence to people who are at the receiving end of their ministrations. In other words, social work's social control function and capacity to oppress those receiving its services are discounted. Moreover, in portraying the professional in this light, he or she is cast as *the expert* who has the skills and knowledge to determine what is the best path for the 'client' to follow. This understanding of the practitioner role runs the risk of making the 'client'[3] a passive receiver of professional ministrations which run counter to social work's avowed value of self-determination. Ignoring the right of the 'client' or recipient of these services to act on their own behalf and in their own interests denies agency to the individual concerned and increases his or her over-reliance on professional support.

Despite these reservations, Kendall's definition facilitates our engaging in a dialogue that enables us to examine those features which are common to the social work profession across national boundaries whilst at the same time allowing us to consider the different elements that make up the diversity which also needs to be addressed.

BELONGINGNESS AND OTHERING IN SOCIAL WORK

Social work occurs in the social, political, economic and cultural context of the nation state. It is subject to the same social forces as other elements of the body politic, whether these happen at the economic, political, social, cultural or ideological level. These include the forces of globalisation and social change. Moreover, social work replicates the same relations of power which prevail elsewhere in society within its own professional boundaries. This is because social workers share values, expectations and traditions with their compatriots. Their professional socialisation and ideology is predicated against the backdrop of these as either a confirmation of or challenge to those social relations which prevail more generally.

Racism in the broader society can be understood as a set of practices aimed at asserting the dominance of a particular racialised identity over others. Racism occurs at three levels – the personal, institutional and cultural. These are interconnected and interdependent upon each other (Dominelli 1997a). Social workers draw upon societal expressions of racism and perpetuate these through their own legislative prescriptions, policies and practices. In social work, the racialised 'othering' process is manifest through racist practices which can be quite subtle because they are not based on overt racial hatred. Racism expressed in social work provides a way of rationing scarce welfare resources by excluding racialised groups from services aimed at ensuring individuals' personal well-being whilst the pathologising of their attributes brings into play a social control function which results in their being disproportionately represented within society's punitive institutions (Dominelli 1991a).

Racism in Europe has gone through a number of manifestations linked to the extent to which ethnic minorities have been considered as belonging to or having a place in the body politic of the country in which they reside. Crucial to establishing a sense of belonging or being part of a nation state is being accepted for who one is, that is, having a self-defined identity considered legitimate and valid. European countries have responded to those people they have 'othered' by either accommodating them as outsiders or rejecting them. Racism is associated with rejection. Thus, it evokes powerful emotions in both those who perpetrate racism and those at its receiving end. For the perpetrators of racist actions in a democratic society, the idea that people can be rejected not for what they have done but who they are strikes at the core of their liberal democratic values and ideas about culpability. This, coupled with the 'wrongdoing' such behaviour entails, makes those who accept liberal ideologies of tolerance feel guilty when their behaviour has been demonstrated to contradict their views of themselves in these terms.

A study by Bagley and Young (1982) has indicated, with respect to Britain, that social workers are more tolerant and broad-minded than the general population. The study is limited in that it focuses only on overt forms of racism rather than the more subtle kinds which are manifest through social work (Dominelli 1997a). However, social workers' self-perception as generally tolerant opens up the possibility that they will seek to alter their behaviour so that it is more in keeping with their espoused values. Thus, they are amenable to take racism in their activities seriously, with the intention of doing something about it. This same strength becomes a weakness when they fail to transcend racism in their practice, for it will leave them feeling disempowered and paralysed by their attempts at securing change in both their behaviour and their employing agencies. Since progress on anti-racist social work has been limited, despite various initiatives to promote it, it would be useful to have detailed analytical research on why this has been the case. To date, we have had largely anecdotal explanations.

For overt racists, the realisation that people can be rejected for who they are serves to confirm them in their perceptions of themselves as superior. Feeling superior is an essential component in 'othering' individuals and groups in ways that deprive them of their humanity and turn them into objects that can be maltreated. That process of objectification allows them to commit acts of violence against the 'other'.

Responses to the arrival of different ethnic groups in Europe have been diverse, depending on the place of origins, manner of their entry and the reasons for it. In post-war Europe, Castles and Kosack (1972) argue that the need for additional labour to fuel economic recovery after the Second World War enabled different nation states to open their doors to in-migration from across the globe. Now that the need for labour power has been dramatically reduced and firms are exporting jobs overseas, these migrant workers have become redundant. There is no further need for importing labour power.

Moreover, the terms under which migrants have entered a particular European country have varied according to the relationship between the exporting countries and the importing ones, the history of colonialism, the degree of labour scarcity and many other factors. The words used to describe these entrants and the conditions under which they have been allowed to stay have also varied from country to country. Much of the discourse around the entry of non-European nationals into Europe treats them as 'migrants', that is, people who are expected to come to Europe for limited periods and then return to their countries of origin. National legislation tends to take this into account, but has nonetheless produced diverse responses. For example, in Britain, nationals from former Commonwealth countries had the opportunity of acquiring British citizenship through formal registration after five years of residence or through birth, until the early 1980s. They have also been able to vote in British elections at both national and local level after one year of residence. Meanwhile, in Germany, the *Gastarbeiter* (guestworkers), as migrant workers have been called, have not been able to obtain citizenship through these means. Indeed, until the mid-1980s, it was even difficult for other European nationals to do so. For example, the Italian migrant workers who sought employment in Germany in the 1960s and 1970s found that even their children who were born in Germany were excluded from citizenship and the rights of participation this implied.

These variations at policy level, particularly with regard to immigration, nationality and citizenship, and welfare entitlements have recently begun to diminish as European countries seek to harmonise their legislation on these subjects. Harmonisation in these areas has received a major boost through the Schengen Agreement which has sought to ensure that legislation and policies between the different nation states are harmonised to the extent that a decision about an application for entry by one country will be accepted by the others, whether it is in the applicant's favour or not.

The welfare state, of which social work forms a part, has been crucial in the debates about the rights of non-European or 'third' country nationals in Europe. Rightwingers in most European countries have insisted that 'foreigners' are attracted to Europe because of its welfare systems. Thus, migrants are alleged to seek entry to take advantage of benefits for which they have not paid and to which they are not entitled. Such portrayals of them seek to construct them as welfare abusers rather than as contributors and users. This constitutes another part of the othering process. Indeed, access to welfare benefits is specifically excluded in the conditions of entry of many types of entrants. In Britain, Michael Howard as Home Secretary recently denied even asylum seekers and refugees rights to social security benefits. Moves are afoot in other European countries to initiate similar legislation where it currently does not exist. Leftwingers, meanwhile, have protested against the failure of existing welfare states to meet the needs of people, regardless of their country of origins (Dominelli 1991b). Conservative debates have had an impact on social workers, many of whom are traditional in their outlook. Considerable anxieties have been raised for practitioners who wonder what to do when the legislation forbids their assisting people in need – a matter made more acute by their professional ethics, with their emphasis on responding to people's cries for help.

Social workers as a group do not have a strong reputation for placing the rights of an individual requiring assistance before the exigencies of the state. The most dramatic recent experience of this has been under Nazi rule. Large swathes of the German population, including social workers, were implicated in its genocidal preoccupations (Lorenz 1994). Such atrocities are by no means unique in the history of the profession, as the tales of First Nations peoples in Canada, along with the Aboriginals in Australia and the Maoris in New Zealand, to name a few, have testified (Haig-Brown 1988; Armitage 1996). This past has left another legacy: a reluctance to examine it and learn from it. For example, the experience of being occupied under the Nazi regime has engendered a great reluctance on the part of large numbers of individuals, including social workers in continental Europe, to discuss racism or 'race'.

In continental Europe, the idea of the 'stranger' coming to the 'host' country has dominated popular discussions about in-migration. In Britain, it has been about 'immigrants' (usually meaning 'black' people) coming to settle. These are 'code words' which mean that racism and 'race' do not have to be explicitly discussed. In this discourse, the realisation that the 'stranger' or 'immigrant' wants to be accepted as belonging to the body politic with full citizenship entitlements has been very difficult for the majority of white residents in any country in Europe to accept. This reluctance is evident even in the UK where 'black' people who have settled in the country for several generations are referred to as 'first, second or third generation immigrants'. Such terminology indicates the failure of the receiving country to accept that these people are full members of the country and there to stay. It is home, a place they would make their own by contributing to its social, cultural and political development, not a place of temporary abode.

ACCOMMODATIONIST, REJECTIONIST AND RESISTANCE STRATEGIES

The general strategies different European countries have used in responding to the entry of other nationals have been varied, but they have included the major ones of deportation, repatriation, assimilation, integration, multiculturalism, and anti-racism. Deportation and repatriation are rejectionist strategies. Assimilation, integration and multiculturalism are accommodationist strategies. Anti-racism is about seeking an egalitarian social order where 'race' is no longer a matter of social exclusion. As such, it is a resistance strategy. These strategies do not have to occur in linear order, and several of them can coexist at any particular point in time. Each of them has been problematic from the point of view of the incoming populations who have been 'othered' and therefore discredited (Gilroy 1987).

In some ways all these strategies, except for repatriation and deportation, have elements of an integrative approach if that is taken to mean the inclusion of different sections of the population into the body politic. What is different about each of them is their relationship to the ideology and practice of white supremacy. Adherents of repatriation refuse to accept that non-white nationals have any right to permanent residence in a given country. Nor do they have the right to retain their own cultural traditions and customs. This strategy is favoured by politicians of the Far Right. White supremacy is their ideology and practice. Openly endorsing the notion of white people's superiority, they maintain their right to keep their own white culture. Separation between the 'races' is desired. Under this schema, if repatriation is not possible, parallel separate provisions are preferred. The most extreme forms taken by this strategy have been evident in South Africa under apartheid.

If the Bagley and Young (1982) study reflects social workers' opinions on 'race', it is unlikely that they will endorse the overtly racist stances adopted by avowed white supremacists. However, as there has not been Europe-wide research on social workers' attitudes to 'race' and racism, it is difficult to comment on the actions they sustain in their practice in relation to repatriation and deportation as strategies for dealing with the presence of people with 'third' country origins. However, we do know that social workers and probation officers in Britain, for example, have had to deal with the deportation of individuals who have committed offences and been sentenced to it. But their behaviour has not been undertaken in the context of seeing it as a way of handling 'undesirable aliens'. Indeed, probation officers in the Inner London Probation Service have developed guidelines to ensure that issues of racism are addressed when they work with such prisoners (Towl 1993; Abernethy and Hammond 1992; Middlesex Probation 1991; Tarzi and Hedges 1990; Cheney 1993; Shaw 1993; Baker 1991).

Assimilation is the process of integrating people in ways that assume that the dominant culture is superior. Its proponents presuppose white supremacy, often without thinking about it, and insist that the subordinated group relinquishes its own specific cultural attributes and adopts the dominant group's ways. In short, the subordinated groups are required to 'melt' into the receiving society and become like the others. The power relations inherent in this approach are unequal and usually expressed in terms of what Parsons (1957) called 'zero-sum', that is, there is a winner and a loser.

The assimilationist ideology in social work is apparent in the treatment of people of different cultures as if they are the same as each other, that is, using the 'colour-blind' approach (Dominelli 1997a). In common parlance, it is articulated as 'I don't notice the colour of your skin'. The term 'colour-blind' is a misnomer. The issue is not that social workers from the dominant group do not notice the skin colour of their 'clients'. They do. But they discount its relevance to the work they are doing with them and the service that is being offered, thereby ignoring the impact of racism on their definition of where their 'clients' and they are starting from. What these social workers need to acknowledge is that racism has denied their 'clients' access to opportunities to avail themselves of social power and resources whilst it has privileged their own access to these. The problem, therefore, is racism, not skin colour. Skin colour has become a signifier of the object against which racist behaviours and attitudes may be perpetrated. The 'colour-blind' approach is usually verbalised as 'We are all the same. I treat them like us'. A level playing field is assumed when this is clearly not the case. Moreover, the subordinated groups are expected to follow in the footsteps of the dominant group. From the point of view of the subordinated minority, this approach means that their specificities, individually and collectively, become invisible. Subordinated ethnic minorities must lose their linguistic, religious and other cultural affiliations to be assimilated into the receiving country's social life.

In the assimilationist framework, the fact of migration itself is seen as a problem which the migrants also overcome by adopting the ways of the dominant society. Thus, any difficulties which individuals or families from other countries have are put down to the adjustment process. Triseliotis' (1972) book, *Social Work with Coloured Immigrants and their Families*, and Cheetham's (1972) book, *Social Work with Immigrants*, typify this approach.

The assumption is that there is something wrong with the 'immigrants', not the receiving society. The adjustment process is presented as a one-way street. Failure to carry it out in the terms set by the dominant group is defined as dysfunctional. The strengths held by the subordinate group are ignored whilst those of the dominant group are amplified and taken as the norm whereby the others are judged. This approach has been heavily criticised in the UK (see Dominelli 1988; Ahmad 1990), but it flourishes in continental countries such as Switzerland and Germany. Of course, the trauma of migration needs to be addressed by social workers who are dealing with newly arrived (im)migrants. However, the dynamics of racism and its impact on their lives should not be neglected.

The integrative approach is about the dominant majority being in geographical proximity to those from ethnic minority groups. It could, in theory, allow for cultural diversity. But tolerance under this strategy has its limits. It usually means that the subordinated group has to integrate on the terms set by the dominant majority. No real exchange of power has taken place. The (im)migrants are made to feel that they are visitors to the country and there on sufferance.

In social work terms, integrative approaches come across as a superficial acceptance of difference. Thus, social workers will eat 'ethnic' foods and attend 'ethnic' ceremonies to indicate their willingness to be friendly and understanding. There is also some emphasis on being aware of different cultures and being ethnically sensitive as a result. However, their comprehension of the issues involved is limited. Power relations remain unaltered. There is little acknowledgement of the right of the subordinated group to be full members of society, that is, to exist as people who belong on terms they have themselves negotiated. Such attitudes are evident in social work encounters between practitioners from the dominant group and members of subordinated groups. For example, this happens when a social worker asks a black British person, 'Which part of Jamaica are you from?' The young person replies, 'Brixton'. This interaction reveals that the white social worker assumes that any person with a dark skin is not really British, that is, a person who is an integral part of the country and has equal rights to belong, but a transient in the country because the majority group is tolerant.

Similar convictions are held on the continent. In Holland, I have heard a white Dutch social worker say to a young person of non-white Dutch origins, 'What part of Surinam are you from?' The young person answered, 'Amsterdam'. The message that is being conveyed in these two interactions, despite the social workers' assurances to the contrary, is that, although the individuals concerned have been born in the particular country mentioned, they have not been accepted as belonging to it. They have been given the message that they are too different and rejected as inferior. All that the white social worker has seen at the point of contact is the person's physical appearance. A racialisation of visible biological features has taken place.

The multicultural approach is more explicitly predicated on the idea that all cultures are worthy objects of study and knowledge. As such, they are equally valid. A number of activities deliberately attempt to reach out to other people and get to know them through their culture. The observance of religious festivals, dietary habits and names symbolise a willingness to take note of the cultural attributes of others. Multicultural activities have been particularly important in schools in Britain. Many continental European countries are also showing interest in this approach to race relations. In countries like Canada, multiculturalism is the official government policy for safeguarding the place of different ethnic minorities in Canadian society. People's right to their cultural identity is acknowledged. And, politicians pride themselves on producing a 'mosaic' in which each culture has its own place. Attempts to preserve the cultures of ethnic minority groups, increase the representation of different ethnic minority groups in the employment stakes, and develop more ethnically relevant services in social work are examples of multicultural initiatives at work. However, there has been no real transfer of power between the ruling group and the excluded ones. That is, the basic framework within which ethnic minorities are accepted has not changed. It is still the dominant groups who make the crucial decisions about the country's social, political and economic life.

A further problem with this approach is that of cultural relativism. This refers to the assumption that no culture can be judged except on its own terms (D'Souza 1995). That is, only those from a given culture can criticise either it or the behaviour of its adherents. Being unable to criticise others is problematic for social workers since it conflicts with the exercise of their professional judgement and their views about forms of behaviour which should be universally observed. These conflicts are most evident in such situations in which social workers from the dominant group pass value judgements on inappropriate forms of behaviour involving a member of a subordinated ethnic minority group. As a result, they tend to avoid making any decision, wrongly believing that this is the best way to deal with the dilemma of which value should be given priority over the other. Anything is excused if it is a 'matter of *their* culture'.

Such an attitude can be arrogant if the social worker assumes '*our* culture does not have these problems, therefore, *our* way of behaving is superior'. However, the matter does not have to be solved in these terms if social workers remember two crucial facts in their work across cultures. One is the issue of human rights. These, at least as defined in the relevant United Nations Conventions, have been agreed by most countries. Their observance can be used as common ground for initiating discussion about what is going on in any specific situation and would allow the social worker to make a full assessment of what is taking place within it. The other is that no culture is homogeneous. There are differences of opinions and views about what it consists of and what the culturally accepted forms of behaviour are. It may be that what is happening in a particular case is that there are disagreements about appropriate forms of conduct between people or generations who share a culture. Again, the social worker should be familiar with the diversity of views and not stereotype a given culture. Sensitivity of this nature can be very important in interventions around spouse abuse, for example. One does not have to be a Western feminist to know that Latin American, African, Indian, Chinese, Arabic and Pakistani women have also taken up this issue. But social workers do have to keep abreast of the relevant research and literature to know what is going on in communities other than their own. Finally, social workers have the responsibility of exercising critical judgement, not as a means of putting other people down, but as a way of engaging in discussions aimed at resolving disputes about appropriate behaviour and being clear about where the line is drawn, by whom and why. Ultimately, social workers are professionally bound to protect lives and people's right to a decent life.

However, there are additional problems with the multicultural approach than simply the question of power relations at the cultural level. One of these is the analysis problem that Shama Ahmed (1982) called the 'everything is racism' approach to black families in Britain. In this, white social workers feel very insecure in their knowledge base about other cultures. But the problem is social workers' fear that they might be labelled 'racist' for exercising their critical faculties and questioning any aspects of their work with an individual or family from a subordinate ethnic minority group which might undermine and devalue the cultural attributes of the person they are assisting. But instead of checking this out and informing themselves of what the actual problem is – their fears or the 'client's' behaviour – they do neither. They do not even ask the 'client' for further clarification about aspects of their relationship or interventions that do not 'add up'. Adopting this stance may mean that crucial aspects of social workers' responsibilities are neglected. And it could jeopardise the life chances of the person(s) they are supposed to help. One of the best publicised cases in which this has happened in Britain is in the murder of Jasmine Beckford. Jasmine Beckford was a young black child in care who was killed by her step-father because, not wanting to be seen to be acting in a racist way, the white social worker working with the family did not feel able to challenge the family's refusal to allow the examination of the child even when abuse was suspected (see Blom-Cooper 1986). Had the white social worker in question acknowledged that there are some truths which extend beyond cultural boundaries (D'Souza 1995), professional self-empowerment could have occurred. The unacceptability of child abuse, wherever it happens, is one of these truths. Instead of being paralysed into inaction, a white social worker armed with such understandings and insights could have more effectively discharged the responsibility to protect the black child.

Another problem of multiculturalism is its failure to tackle the issue of institutional and organisational power disparities. Consequently, people from subordinated ethnic minority groups who have been appointed to social work positions have either been sidelined in specialist jobs dealing with other members of their group and thus work outside the mainstream career grades, or they have been employed at basic grades with limited prospects of promotion and expected to act as experts on all subjects affecting ethnic minority groups on top of their normal workload (Rooney 1987). In short, they have had the task of tackling racism 'dumped' on their shoulders, whilst their white colleagues get on with their work as normal (Dominelli 1997a). 'Dumping' is one of the ways in which white people avoid confronting their role in eradicating racist practices. Dominelli (1997a) describes the various subtle but complex strategies white people use to deny the existence of racism and their responsibility for dealing with its impact as omission, denial, decontextualisation, avoidance, dumping, colour-blindness, patronising attitudes and exaggeration. Each of these acts as a rationalisation for white people doing relatively little to challenge overtly the enduring capacities of racist power dynamics.

Anti-racism is concerned with the structural position of subordinated ethnic minority groups and its psychological impact on both the oppressor and the oppressed. This places questions of power, equity and transformative social change at both the structural and personal levels at the heart of anti-racist activities. Unlike accommodationist approaches which focus on the 'other' as the problem, anti-racist social work concentrates on racism and the role that the perpetrators of racist behaviour play in maintaining a racist system. Anti-racist social work seeks to alter existing social relations by securing change at the personal, institutional and cultural levels (Dominelli 1997a) to bring about equality amongst cultures and diverse peoples within an egalitarian framework. Equality is a goal to be obtained, not presumed. Moreover, anti-racist social work is also committed to enabling those from subordinate ethnic minority groups themselves to shape the social work agenda, develop appropriate services for their use and mainstream their concerns. Power is acknowledged as multifaceted and to be shared through processes of negotiation.

This commitment to a fundamental change in the current social order has contributed to the strength and widespread nature of the backlash against anti-racist social work. In Britain, the backlash has become the focus of an intense power struggle in which the state, through its government ministers and legislative programmes, has played a key role in seeking to dismantle anti-racist social work. Both anti-racist education and practice were subjected to antagonistic scrutiny by the Major government and labelled 'politically correct'. This is unfortunate because an opportunity for open dialogue about the crucial issues that societies must face in addressing complex matters of racial justice has been missed. An important dimension of this would have been a discussion about the limitations of multiculturalism as it is currently practised, for anti-racist social work arose as a considered critique of its failures.

The backlash against anti-racist social work has also to be considered in terms of globalisation and the role of the state in the process of managing the domestic economy for the purposes of enhancing its international competitiveness on the one hand and providing safe places for the accumulation of capital on the other. From this point of view, social work is deeply implicated in maintaining the social control edifice within the welfare state. Indeed, theorists such as McKnight (1995) have argued that social workers are not in the business of liberating their 'clients' because they have built their career structures around other people's misery. This claim would be strongly disputed by anti-racist theorists, who argue that the aim of anti-oppressive forms of practice like anti-racist social work is explicitly to empower oppressed people whether as members of society, workers or 'clients'.

Anti-racism has been critiqued by black Britons for not giving credit to the role that 'black' people have played in challenging racism and in developing constructive alternatives to the appalling services that have been made available to them by mainstream society (see Gilroy 1987). This has been because some anti-racists, particularly those in local government, have presented black people as passive victims in the face of racist onslaughts (Gilroy 1987). Black Britons have also developed black perspectives on social work through which they have sought to present their views of their experiences of racism and the strategies that they have used to cope with its ravages and transcend its limitations (see Ahmad 1990). They have also sought to teach their white colleagues how to work more appropriately across racialised divides. Black perspectives have many features including the adoption of a resistance strategy in common with anti-racists. That is, they too have structural analyses at their core. But they go beyond this in focusing on black people's sense of identity; how racism has structured their experiences; and their attempts to change societies which have sought to oppress them (see Robinson 1995; Dominelli *et al.* 1995).

The concern that white people are responding to the term 'black' as a homogeneous category has recently begun to fragment the more collective approach previously adopted by Britain's black population in their struggle against racism in social work. As a result, Asian probation officers, for example, have separated from the Association of Black Probation Officers to create the National Association of Asian Probation Officers. And, as a conference held at Sheffield University in October 1995 demonstrated, Britons of African origins have also begun to consider Africentric approaches to social work and drawn on the writings of Molefi Asante (1987), an African American to assist them in this task (Thomas Bernard 1995).

The situation is somewhat different in continental Europe, where anti-racism has yet to be adopted in any substantive way. Indeed, there is great reluctance to use terms like 'race' and racism in several nations, for example, Switzerland, Germany, Austria. Multicultural/transcultural/cross-cultural approaches are much more in tune with the discourses being pursued there. This has led to a flourishing of voluntary sector welfare organisations catering for the specific needs of ethnic minority groups. These groups have proliferated greatly because many cater for their own specific ethnic enclave. At the same time, it seems that these societies are in massive denial about racism, particularly its structural elements, which derive from cultural and institutional racism.

Social workers are responsible for enforcing social discipline and forms of acceptable behaviour. Thus, in their role as 'agents' of society, social workers practise social control and reinforce its dominant values and norms. Anti-racists have reason to reprimand social workers for working uncritically in this regard. For their approach perpetuates forms of social work practice which endorse the status quo and reinforces assimilationist norms and other types of behaviour which are racist in outcome if not intention. In short, the only yardstick whereby both individual and family patterns of behaviour are measured and judged as adequate or inadequate is that of the dominant group. The family patterns of those in subordinated ethnic groups are found wanting and pathologised in consequence. This sets up a vicious circle in which they have been declared incapable of caring for themselves and their children. This can be the outcome regardless of whether the 'othered' group's behaviour is modified to suit the prediction, or whether they reject the label and get into trouble for being 'troublemakers' or 'difficult to work with'. Methods of assessment can also endorse the priorities of the dominant group when they are carried out in 'client'–worker relationships where the imbalance in power relations between the professional and the 'client' favours the worker. For the worker has a panopoly of legal mechanisms, resources and customs which can be drawn upon for either legitimating his/her position or ensuring the execution of the task in hand on his/her terms.

CONCLUSIONS

Social work in Europe is a varied and disparate profession. Its record on working with people across cultural divides but, more importantly, in anti-racist ways is mixed. Although there are exceptions, much of the work done by social workers from the dominant group with those from subordinated ethnic minority groups is of poor quality. It often reflects the relations of inequality and subordination which prevail in the society at large and those at the receiving end of their ministrations find that they have not received the services they need. As a result of this, people from subordinated ethnic groups have had to develop their own services and to ensure that these services are capable of meeting their needs and can be used to challenge inadequate mainstream provisions. Meanwhile, globalisation has exacerbated this situation. Its emphasis on making nation states increasingly more competitive has meant that attempts to divert resources to training social workers to work in anti-racist ways are less likely to receive a sympathetic hearing in today's cost-cutting environments. The simultaneous collapsing of their boundaries has given the nation states less control over their internal affairs.

The redefining of Europe's racialised boundaries as a result of the Single European Treaty makes it imperative that the debate about the acceptance of subordinated ethnic minority groups as equal participants in the European project is conducted openly. Only by identifying the social relations through which racism is perpetrated and seeking to change them in egalitarian directions can non-European nationals feel that they belong on this continent just as much as those who have 'othered' them. Social workers, such as those who are working with the day-to-day realities experienced by excluded people, have a significant role to play in creating a truly non-racist society.

NOTES

1 I use the word 'race' in quotes to denote that the terminology is problematic and that I am referring to the ways in which issues of 'race' and ethnicity are socially rather than biologically constructed.
2 'Black' is used in the UK to refer to people of Asiatic or African descent to indicate that they have been at the receiving end of racism. For me, it does not imply that they constitute a homogeneous group. Their diversity occurs on a range of dimensions – historical, cultural, political, linguistic, religious, ethnic, which makes the specificity of their experience of racism important when this is being discussed in detail. However, this chapter is concerned with the dynamics of racism at the macro level where the commonalities of their experiences are more significant than their differences. It is not seeking to make points about any aspect of their particular ethnic identities.
3 The word 'client' is also problematic. I use it in quotes to denote the difficulties with it. However, I still find it the most 'universal' word in the social work lexicon and preferable to consumer or service user.

REFERENCES

Abernethy, R. and Hammond, N. (1992) *Drug Courier: A Role for the Probation Service*. London: Middlesex Area Probation Service (MAPS).
Adas, M. (1989) *Machines as the Measure of Men: Science, Technology and the Ideologies of Western Dominance*. Ithaca: Cornell University Press.
Ahmad, B. (1990) *Black Perspectives in Social Work*. Birmingham: Venture Press.
Ahmed, S. (1982) 'Social Work with Minority Children and their Families' in *Ethnic Minority and Community Relations*. Buckingham: Open University Course no. 354, Unit 16.
Anthias, F. and Yuval-Davies, N. (1993) *Racialised Boundaries*. London: Routledge.

Armitage, A. (1996) *Aboriginal People in Australia, Canada and New Zealand*. Toronto: McClelland and Stewart.
Asante, M. (1987) *The Afrocentric Idea*. Philadelphia: Temple University Press.
Bagley, C. and Young, L. (1982) 'Policy Dilemmas and the Adoption of Black Culture' in J. Cheetham (ed.) *Social Work and Ethnicity*. London: Allen and Unwin.
Baker, P. (1991) *Interpreters in Public Services*. Birmingham: Venture Press.
Barker, M. (1981) *The New Racism: Conservatives and the Ideology of the Tribe*. London: Junction Books.
Barkin, E. (1992) *The Retreat of Scientific Racism*. Cambridge: Cambridge University Press.
Blaut, J. M. (1993) *The Colonizer's Model of the World: Geographical Diffusionism and Eurocentric History*. New York: Guildford Press.
Blom-Cooper, L. (1986) *Child in Trust: The Report of the Panel of Inquiry into the Circumstances Surrounding the Death of Jasmine Beckford*. London Borough of Brent: Kingswood Press.
Brah, A. (1996) *Cartography of Diasporas*. London: Sage.
Brooks, D. (1996) *Backward and Upward: The New Conservative Writing*. New York: Vintage Books.
Castles, S. and Kosack, G. (1972) 'The Function of Labour Immigration in Western European Capitalism', *New Left Review*, 73, May/June, pp. 8–21.
Cheetham, J. (1972) *Social Work with Immigrants*. London: Routledge and Kegan Paul.
Cheney, D. (1993) 'Prison Race Equality', *Prison Report*, 23, Spring.
D'Souza, D. (1995) *The End of Racism: Principles for a Multiracial Society*. New York: Free Press.
Dominelli, L. (1988) *Anti-Racist Social Work*. 1st edition. London: BASW/Macmillan.
—— (1991a) '"Race" and Gender in Social Work' in M. Davies (ed.) *The Sociology of Social Work*. London: Routledge.
—— (1991b) *Women across Continents: Feminist Comparative Social Policy*. Brighton: Harvester/Wheatsheaf.
—— (1997a) *Anti-Racist Social Work*. 2nd edition. Originally published in 1988. London: BASW/Macmillan.
—— (1997b) *Sociology for Social Work*. London: Macmillan.
Dominelli, L., Jeffers, L., Jones, G., Sibanda, S. and Williams, B. (1995) *Anti-Racist Probation Practice*. Aldershot: Arena.
Ely, P. and Munday, B. (1996) *Social Care in Europe*. London: Prentice-Hall.
Gilroy, P. (1987) *There Ain't No Black in the Union Jack*. London: Hutchinson.
—— (1993) *Black Atlantic*. London: Verso.
Haig-Brown, C. (1988) *Resistance and Renewal: Surviving the Indian Residential School*. Vancouver: Tillacum Library, Arsenal Pulp Press.
Herrnstein, R. and Murray, C. (1994) *The Bell Curve: Intelligence and Class Structure in American Life*. New York: Free Press.
hooks, b. (1989) *Talking Back: Thinking Feminist, Thinking Black*. Boston, Mass.: Southend Press.
Kendall, K. (1978) *Reflections on Social Work Education: 1950–1978*. New York: International Association of Social Work.

Kramer, D. (1989) *Social Work in Europe*. Vienna: IASSW.
Lorde, A. (1984) *Sister Outsider*. New York: Crossing Press.
Lorenz, W. (1994) *Social Work in a Changing Europe*. London: Routledge.
McKnight, J. (1995) *The Careless Society: Community and its Counterfeits*. New York: Basic Books.
Middlesex Area Probation Service (Middlesex Probation) (1991) *Corporate Strategy, 1991–94: Race Issues*. London: MAPS.
Parsons, T. (1957) 'The Professions and Social Structures' in *Essays in Sociological Theory*. New York: Free Press.
Robinson, L. (1995) *Psychology for Social Workers: Black Perspectives*. London: Routledge.
Roediger, D. R. (1991) *The Wages of Whiteness: Race and the Making of the American Working Class*. London: Verso.
Rooney, B. (1987) *Resistance and Change*. Liverpool: Department of Sociology, Liverpool University.
Shaw, S. (1993) 'Race Issues: Brickbats or Bouquets?', *Prison Report*, 23, Spring.
Tarzi, A. and Hedges, J. (1990) *A Prison within a Prison: A Study of Foreign Prisoners*. London: Inner London Probation Service.
Thomas Bernard, W. (1995) 'Black Masculinity: Success or Failure?' Ph.D. thesis, Sheffield University.
Towl, G. (1993) 'Groupwork in Prisons', *Probation Journal*, 40(4):208–9.
Triseliotis, J. P. (1972) *Social Work with Colored Immigrants and their Families*. London: BASW/Batsford.

Chapter 4

Controls, rights and migration

Mark R.D. Johnson, Martin Baldwin-Edwards and Claude Moraes

INTRODUCTION

Migration controls and legislation relating to nationality and the rights of refugees can have a disproportionate effect upon minorities, both those who are 'of' Europe, and those who are 'in' Europe. The development of European-wide structures has, while creating a notionally 'common travel area' for free trade, generated barriers and difficulties for minorities and set limits upon the enjoyment of hard-won privileges or rights for those who are seen to be different. As Lorenz (Chapter 14) shows, population diversity is the more typical state of being for most of the great cities of Europe, but the after-effects of the wars in the first half of this century have created a false sense of homogeneity and unity, which has led to political pressures to reduce the mobility which creates and sustains that richness. In this chapter, without seeking to provide a complete description of the law and nature of migration control, we attempt to indicate some of the key features which may be relevant to the social professions. In this we are conscious that there is no single source of guidance or experience relating to its impact on social welfare – all we can do here is to raise the issue as an area which requires development!

Key considerations for ethnic minorities in Europe are the issues of migration, immigration and free movement, and their relationship to social welfare matters. Migration, immigration and free movement go to the heart of matters such as national identity and sovereignty as well as affecting economic, social and demographic objectives. Immigration policy in Europe is simultaneously too sensitive for most governments to include in democratic dialogue, yet too important for them to neglect. Throughout the 1990s European governments have been constructing a partial international regime of immigration controls, albeit one located in different fora and with fundamental problems of consistency and enforcement. In tandem, southern European states have been obliged to respond to increased immigration by developing their own immigration policies. With little experience of immigration control and regulation of resident aliens, southern policy initiatives inevitably have been influenced by northern European norms. At the same time, northern states have found new moral panics, or 'folk devils', and challenges to their sense of solidarity, through the arrival of refugees, some from close to home and travelling by land, others apparently (and in immensely pejorative phrasing) 'penetrating the soft underbelly of Europe' through those southern states.

THE CONSTRUCTION OF EU CITIZENSHIP

From a relatively early stage of the European Community, there has been discussion of an incipient form of European citizenship. This has focused on the free movement provisions of the Rome Treaty, although it was not until the Tindemans Report of 1975 that political rights for nationals of member states were advocated. Plender in 1976 argued that there were three features upon which Community citizenship could be built: a class of persons defined by some common European criterion; the enjoyment of privileges by such persons (including free movement throughout EC territory); and the abolition of discrimination based on nationality (cited in Closa 1992:1141). By 1985, the second Addonino Report on 'A People's Europe' was addressing a whole range of issues from education to the image and identity of the Community, whilst the actual meaning of the term 'Community citizen' was unclear and hardly discussed (O'Keefe and Twomey, 1994:87). It was really only in the buildup to negotiations on the Treaty on European Union that the debate on citizenship became significant, with the 1990 Dublin summit including citizenship in the framework of the overall objective of political union (Closa 1992:1154). The Rome summit of 1990 accepted the principle of European citizenship, and saw the idea as based around three groups of rights. These were civic or political rights, social and economic rights (similar to the EEC Treaty), and protection of Community citizens outside Community borders. More general human rights were not considered to be appropriate for the citizenship section, but are separately referred to in the Treaty. The Maastricht Treaty, in Title II Part Two – Citizenship of the Union – announces that 'Citizenship of the Union is hereby established'. Despite a certain amount of mainly legal analysis, there has been no debate or consideration given to the issues of inclusion in and exclusion from this status. No doubt, this was in part due to a problematic debate about the 'competence' of the Union to discuss such matters, and the political sensitivity within individual states of questions of national citizenship and immigration. With the adoption of the Maastricht and now the Amsterdam treaties, and the movement of migration issues into the 'First Pillar', we may see some movement on this and on the attached questions of 'human rights'.

The actual Citizenship provisions of the Treaty on European Union are fairly meagre, despite being accorded their own section. A Citizenship of the

Union is established, to be conferred on every person holding the nationality of a member state. Seven rights are listed:

- the right to free movement;
- the right of residence;
- the right to vote and stand in local and European Parliament elections;
- diplomatic or consular assistance where one's own member state is not represented;
- the right to petition the European Parliament and to apply to the Ombudsman.

Several problems are immediately apparent. First of all, Citizenship of the Union appears to require nationality of a member state. Even this is unclear, since the attached Declaration on nationality of a member state continues the practice adopted by Germany and the UK. Both submitted Declarations defining nationals for EC purposes differently from domestic purposes, more widely in the case of Germany and more narrowly with the UK. Thus the provisions do not create any new juridical or political subject (Martiniello 1993), nor do they break the previous citizenship–nationality link but renew it in a slightly different way. Furthermore, the Treaty would appear to rule out the possibility of the EU granting citizenship to third-country nationals, at the same time as allowing member states to grant their nationality – and thereby EU citizenship – to aliens according to the many and varied national practices (see Baldwin-Edwards 1991b; Closa 1994). Third, whilst proclaiming a right of free movement and residence for all, the Treaty makes implicit provision to continue the requirements of three 1990 Directives (affecting students, pensioners, and the economically inactive), which allow free movement only where it can be shown that such persons will not make welfare or other claims. Thus free movement is not a universal right for EU citizens. Manifestly, non-citizens – 'guest workers', 'third-country nationals', or by whatever term they may be called – are even further marginalised and at risk – and those who appear to be 'in' but not 'of' Europe, according to the stereotypes and suspicions of state functionaries, may be exposed to the dangers of internal policing designed to reinforce the privileges of membership.

THE EUROPEAN LEGAL FRAMEWORK

European co-operation in immigration matters has emerged in many different fora in the post-war period: initially the two most important were the OECD and the Council of Europe (for its international conventions safeguarding immigrants' rights). The process of European integration inevitably has led to pressure for the development of European Community policy in the areas of immigration, immigrant policy and citizenship. These pressures were resisted by national governments, even as recently as 1985 when five member states challenged in the Court of Justice a Commission Decision requiring co-ordination of immigration policies in the EC. The Single European Act (1987) had appended to it a General Declaration (allegedly at the insistence of the UK) which purported to deny any implicit transfer of sovereignty in this area and, in the Amsterdam Treaty signed in 1997, Britain negotiated an 'opt out'.

Immigration as an explicit policy area in the EU treaties emerged only in the Maastricht revision – the Treaty on European Union (TEU). However, its precursor lies clearly in the intergovernmental Ad Hoc Group on Immigration, formed in 1986. This forum operated outside the scrutiny of the Parliament, Commission and Court of Justice; its activities were predicated on the 'threat' posed by asylum seekers, illegal immigrants and international crime; its secrecy was modelled on the TREVI group formed a decade earlier to deal with terrorism and other cross-border criminal activities. The first initiatives at a European level are correspondingly one-sided: they emphasise control of immigrants and asylum seekers whilst offering little in the way of immigrants' rights or measures to combat racism or xenophobia.

Upon joining the Community every member state has (in various ways) recognised Community law as a supreme body of law creating a 'new legal order' with rules covering a diverse range of economic objectives aimed at establishing a common market. The best known cover imports and exports, customs tariffs, and common policies on commerce and agriculture. A major theme is free movement. This concept covers not only goods, capital and services but persons – both workers (Article 48) and the self-employed, and in most cases also their dependants. However, there are clear limits to the privileges that go with free movement – not the least of which are restrictions on access to welfare support. 'Immediately necessary' help, such as medical care following an accident, may be universally provided under some notion of human solidarity, but the majority of welfare services are, if not designed to be 'control' measures or there to protect the general public, based upon insurance and subject to complex reciprocal agreements such as those attached to the form E111: 'Certificate of entitlement to benefits in kind during a stay in a member state'. It is clear that there are careful safeguards designed to prevent 'welfare tourism' – a parasitic existence of dependency without contribution facilitated by the differences between national bureaucracies! Thus, unemployed people do have the right to residence in another (non-'home') state for six months (established by case law), but to unemployment benefits (*revenue minimum d'insertion*) paid by their home country for only three months (Regulation 1408/71). Nowhere does there appear to be provision for the definition of their entitlement to a social worker's assistance in making such a claim!

Community immigration law

Under a complete system of 'European citizenship', Community nationals might gain the same freedom to move across the borders of other member states as they presently enjoy within the territory of their own EC countries. The present Community regime does not establish any *general* rights of freedom of movement, but it does establish specific rights, including:

- A right of entry.
- A right of residence. EC law also requires that member states must recognise the right of residence even without issuing a residence permit in respect of:
  - a worker pursuing an activity as an employed person, where the activity is not expected to last for more than three months;
  - frontier workers; and
  - seasonal workers.
- Recent directives have extended a right of residence to:
  - nationals of member states (and members of their families) who do not enjoy this right under other provisions of Community law; and
  - certain retired persons; and
  - certain students.
- In all three cases the right of residence is subject to these people being able to support themselves without becoming an unreasonable burden on the resources of the host member state. These reflect a trend away from treating the right of residence as simply a prolongation of the original right to stay for work.
- A right to remain in the host state on termination of employment within that state.
- Various procedural rights including rights of appeal.

Community recognition of such rights constitutes a system of protection which is quite different from that traditionally adopted at the national level. Whereas the latter generally denies rights of entry and abode to aliens, the Community system confers such rights on Community nationals and requires any restrictions on them to be justified in accordance with carefully specified criteria. Further, the European Court of Justice (ECJ) has made it clear that within the sphere of free movement of persons the existing Community rules have direct effect. This means that:

- they can be treated as binding in law whether or not they are restated in national laws or rules; and
- in the case of conflict between them and national immigration rules, they must be given precedence over the latter.

Free movement can also come into play in special circumstances for employees of some providers and nationals covered by EC treaty agreements.

The status and rights of migrant workers

With the cessation of unskilled labour recruitment in the 1970s, new forms of immigration have emerged: family reunification, asylum seekers and clandestine migrants. Whereas there has always been some degree of illegal immigration tolerated, this has now reached very high levels – especially in southern Europe. For 1991, the ILO estimated 2 million illegals across Europe (Baldwin-Edwards and Schain 1994); subsequently, despite massive regularisation programmes and deportations, these numbers have escalated. Thus in addition to denizens there are two new major issues relating to permanent residents – how to incorporate illegal aliens and refugees. Layton-Henry suggests the following typology of rights:

Very few rights	Illegal entrants/ illegal workers
Few rights	Seasonal/ temporary workers
Some security	Workers recruited under bilateral treaty
Considerable rights and security residence	Foreign workers with permanent [denizens]
Full rights including political rights	Post-colonial workers with citizenship; naturalised citizens; native-born second generation with citizenship

(Layton-Henry 1990:14)

The welfare service most readily given is school education for migrants' children, although access to higher education is much more restricted. Healthcare also is generally available – even to illegal migrants. Unemployment benefits are available if the migrant satisfies the conditions of the scheme; social assistance (means-tested) is rarely available and can threaten the residence status of the applicant. Public housing is sometimes available in principle, but in practice immigrants are given low priority. Looking at benefits by category of migrant, the best-protected are Convention status refugees and those with permanant residence rights (denizens). The least protected are illegal immigrants and workers, followed by 'tolerated' refugees.

Generally, recognised refugees are given substantial rights approximating those of denizens. Thus the major new challenge is that of illegal migrants and illegal workers: there is no European consensus on how to approach this matter. Most countries, with the major exceptions of Germany and Greece, grant regularisation to illegals satisfying certain conditions; equally, attempts are made to prohibit illegal employment, and to prosecute employers and deport illegal workers (Miller 1994). Nevertheless, illegal immigrants and workers now form a substantial part of nearly all European economies, particularly in certain sectors. This is partly through the attraction of reduced labour costs for employers, partly through the reluctance of the indigenous workforce to accept dirty, low-paid and dangerous work, and partly through the cessation of legal imported unskilled labour.

Clearly, the great bulk of activity has been in the areas of asylum seekers and illegal immigration. The effect of the measures for dealing with asylum seekers, when taken in combination with the visa requirements, has been either to prevent applicants from ever reaching Europe, or disqualifying them on the grounds of abuse if they should do so by means of false documents. The implication is that non-EU countries bordering the EU will bear the brunt of the burden; indeed, the readmission agreements both bilateral and Schengen-based reinforce that effect.

In terms of illegal immigrants, there is a presumption that this phenomenon is necessarily harmful and that the actors are not deserving of rights. This goes against the long-debated UN Convention of 1990 on the Protection of the Rights of all Migrant Workers and Members of their Families. This, along with the Council of Europe 1977 Convention on the Legal Status of Migrant Workers, has the provision of attributing substantial rights to long-term illegal workers. The UN Convention has not yet entered into force, owing to insufficient signatories; the Council of Europe Convention was effective from 1983, and has six EU signatories. The European Commission recommends that member states should sign the UN Convention as a means of guaranteeing protection of third-country nationals – both legal and illegal (CEC 1994:29).

As mentioned in several chapters, the main agreement within the Union affecting migration and travel has been the so-called 'Schengen Arrangement', which has the following as its main components relating to migration (Brochmann 1996:80):

- common rules for control at external borders of the Schengen area;
- adjustment of conditions for border crossing and visa policy;
- sanctions against air companies which carry people without proper documents;
- criteria for which country should handle asylum applications;
- exchange of information on asylum seekers.

It had been claimed that this agreement would in fact facilitate the right to travel within Europe for third-country nationals, but this does not appear to have been realised in practice, and because of disagreements between individual states, it has also not led to significant gains in mobility for many of the 'majority' population either.

The Amsterdam Treaty

More recently, and following intensive lobbying by NGOs concerned with the rights of migrants and minorities, as well as bureaucratic developments within the Commission, the third major revision to the Treaty of Rome, the Amsterdam Treaty, has brought about some very significant changes. In particular, the 'European Coordination', supported by such groups as the UK-based Joint Council for Welfare of Immigrants (JCWI), and the 'Starting Line' group, won support for declarations on race equality and the enactment of Article K9 of the Treaty which allowed immigration and asylum matters to pass from the competence of the 'Third Pillar' (justice and home affairs) to the 'First (Single Market) Pillar'. Consequently, subsequent immigration rules will have to follow the anti-discrimination rules which were also incorporated in the Amsterdam Treaty. Other proposals from the Commission, including a convention on the rights of third-country nationals including a right to travel and work, remain in the pipeline and will have to be reformulated in the light of these changes.

The Treaty embodies a new article, 6A, which is a general anti-discrimination provision. It is sufficient to serve as a treaty base for secondary legislation to outlaw discrimination on the grounds of sex (*sic*), racial and ethnic origin, religion and religious belief, age, and sexual orientation. However, it is unclear that this provision can be applied to non-citizens of the Union.

A new title – Free movement of persons, asylum and immigration – is to be inserted into the Treaty. Within five years after entry into force of the Treaty, measures must be adopted which achieve free movement of persons (Article A), measures on the crossing of external borders including rules on visas, a common visa list, procedures for a uniform visa, and free movement for up to three months of third-country nationals (Article B). Also within five years measures must be taken on various aspects of asylum, temporary protection, illegal immigration and residence, including repatriation of illegal residents (Article C); excluded from this five-year requirement are the relative burdens of refugees admitted across member states, conditions of entry and residence to member states, and the residence rights in other member states of third-country long-term residents (Article C 2(b), 3(a) and 4). Similarly, there is no change in the granting of Citizenship of the Union – this is still predicated on nationality of a member state.

BRITAIN: A CASE STUDY

The application of such law, and the debates about its extension and development, can only be understood properly within the context of an understanding of national history: and for each state, as other chapters in this book have made clear, this will be different. We may summarise, briefly, certain key elements of the British approach – which demonstrates clearly the role of law and its interaction with national politics! To this should be added an understanding of conceptions of national and ethnic identity – self-image, which underlies, and may indeed also be in conflict with, the formal statements which appear in either national or Community legislation.

Immigration and nationality are often talked about as though they were synonymous: this causes great confusion, as people often talk about 'citizenship' when they mean 'right of residence'. In fact, immigration and nationality are two separate areas of law, each with its own major primary legislation. In Britain, for example, these include the Immigration Act 1971 (as amended by the Immigration Act 1988, the Asylum and Immigration Appeals Act 1993 and the Asylum and Immigration Act 1996) and the British Nationality Act 1981. The history, and the confusion, date well before these, to at least the beginning of this century with the passing of an 'Aliens Act' which perhaps began the process of codification and exclusion, not unrelated to the beginnings of the possibility of mass travel, a phenomenon we now take for granted.

In UK law, *nationality* simply defines the country of which people are citizens, and which usually issues them with passports. Nationality law sets out the ways in which people can become citizens (usually by being born in a country, being born abroad to parents who are citizens of the country, or taking out citizenship by naturalisation after a period of residence in a country). On the other hand, *immigration* is the system of laws and rules by which the state decides who shall be able to live in its territory and under what conditions. Immigration law sets out the categories of people who are allowed in automatically (usually citizens of the country) and the mechanisms and officials who decide whether and on what conditions others may enter and enforce the departure of people who are not supposed to be in the country.

The Aliens Act 1905 was passed, after two decades of intermittent agitation, in order to prevent refugees, mainly Jewish, poor and fleeing from Eastern Europe, from seeking refuge in Britain. The Act only applied to boats with more than twenty passengers and to those travelling steerage class who could be excluded if 'undesirable' – defined mainly as being unable to support themselves and their dependants. The Act only applied to 'aliens' – people not from any part of the British empire – but it set up the first rudimentary machinery for checking entry which was expanded and developed through the rest of the century.

In Britain the simple distinction between nationality and immigration is complicated by the fact that not all those who have British nationality are automatically able to enter Britain. There are six categories of British nationality of which only one, the British citizen, has an absolute right to enter Britain. The other five are people originating from British dependencies or ex-colonies who had their right of entry to Britain taken away in 1962 or 1968, even though they travel on British passports. The British Nationality Act 1981 (which needs to be read with the Immigration Act 1971) sets out the conditions for acquiring five of those nationalities (British citizenship, British Dependent Territories citizenship, British Overseas citizenship, British subject status and British Protected Person status). It was slightly amended, for Falklanders, by the British Nationality (Falkland Islands) Act 1983. The sixth kind of British nationality, British National (Overseas) status, was created for people from Hong Kong in the Hong Kong Act 1985 and the Hong Kong (British Nationality) Order 1986, in anticipation of pressures that might (but do not seem to) have arisen following the reversion of the territory to Chinese rule in summer 1997.

At the same time, a small number of people who do not have British nationality, but are citizens of independent Commonwealth countries, do have an automatic right of entry and are therefore free from immigration control. They are people who have the *right of abode* in the UK. Right of abode does not mean the same as the right to live in the UK, which many foreign nationals have. It is a special status, available only to Commonwealth citizens born before 1 January 1983 to a person who was a British citizen or had the right of abode in the UK, as defined in the Immigration Act 1988.

Before 1993, the UK had no specific asylum law and asylum was mentioned almost as an afterthought in the immigration rules, after all other ways in which people might qualify to come to the UK had been listed. There are now two laws, the Asylum and Immigration Appeals Act 1993 and the Asylum and Immigration Act 1996, voluminous immigration rules explaining the separate procedure and listing the factors which the specialist Asylum Directorate at the Home Office must take into account in considering asylum applications, and a separate system of appeals against refusal of asylum. The 1993 Act states that 'nothing in the immigration rules, shall lay down any practice which would be contrary to the Convention' but the Home Office can still make far-reaching administrative changes in how it deals with applications, often giving people no notice about them.

EUROPE, NATIONS AND THE STATUS OF REFUGEES

The UN Convention defines a refugee as

> a person who has a well-founded fear of persecution for reasons of race, religion, nationality, membership of a particular social group or political opinion and who is outside the country of his nationality and is unable or, owing to such fear, is unwilling to avail himself of the protection of that country; or who, not having a nationality and being outside the

> country of his former habitual residence . . . is unable or, owing to such fear, is unwilling to return to it.

The Convention was signed in 1951 and was prepared in the aftermath of the Second World War, mainly in the context of the thousands of displaced people in Europe. In 1967 a Protocol was added to it, extending the definition of refugees to non-Europeans and to people forced to seek refuge because of events that took place after 1945. Surprisingly perhaps, there are no internationally agreed procedures or standards in deciding who falls within the UN definition. Governments which have signed the Convention and Protocol choose the criteria they will use to decide whether people qualify and what standard of proof is necessary. This varies between countries of refuge and according to the countries from which people are fleeing.

European definitions

The Justice and Home Affairs Council of the EU agreed a joint position of the interpretation of the definition of a refugee in November 1995, to inform the decisions made by individual countries. This stressed that

> persecution is generally the act of a state organ . . . in addition to cases in which persecution takes the form of the use of brute force, it may also take the form of administrative and/or judicial measures which either have the appearance of legality and are misused for the purposes of persecution, or are carried out in breach of the law.

These may be 'general measures to maintain public order' which are implemented in a discriminatory way or to camouflage measures against particular groups, measures directed against specific categories which have been 'condemned by the international community, or where they are manifestly disproportionate to the end sought', or measures taken against an individual for a Convention reason, in particular where the action is 'intentional, systematic and lasting'. Persecution not by the state will only be considered if it is 'encouraged or permitted by the authorities'. This clearly creates problems for those in danger from non-state authorities, for example the Liberation Tigers of Tamil Eelam, or in a situation where the state itself has broken down, such as happened in Somalia or Zaire. The Convention has been interpreted to mean that there must be a danger to the person individually, though the reason for this may be membership of a particular group.

In most cases, except where the seeker of asylum is able to obtain prior clearance through taking shelter in a diplomatic compound or embassy, the majority of decisions relating to refugee status depend upon an application as the asylum seeker arrives at the borders of the state of refuge – otherwise known as on-entry control. This function is carried out by immigration officers, who have enormous power to grant or refuse entry, to detain, to search people and their luggage, to read papers and letters and to require people to submit to medical examination. Because of the sensitivity of their role, in many (but not all) EU states, they undergo specific training in 'human rights' awareness – although this may not be apparent to the traveller! The problem, in social work terms, is that similar powers may be available to social workers, and the migrant may perceive the workers as being members of the same bureaucracy, with similar objectives. Indeed, in many cases it is also true that social workers and other welfare staff are expected to act in this 'policing' role, and to report cases of suspected illegality or dependency. Evidently, this can cause a conflict with the duty (or professional sense of it) to care, and to support those in need. Where stereotypes, and complexities of entitlement, enter into the equation, we may be sure that it will be the rights and dignity of people of minority background which are the most at risk.

Acquisition of – and enjoyment of – citizenship

We have discussed the rights of citizens, and the case of refugees – but these categories suggest that there is an absolute and static situation, while the truth is naturally more complex. There are, under certain circumstances, ways in which people may obtain membership or citizenship. Increasingly, too, this situation is being challenged by migrants and their descendants, who feel that they have given something to their state of residence, and that they should be entitled to appropriate recognition of their commitment to the land of their residence. Recently, indeed, there have been (unsuccessful) attempts to change the rules in several countries. Citizenship, notwithstanding Citizenship of the Union as adumbrated in the Treaty on European Union, is still solely a matter of national prerogative. Naturalisation of foreigners is an important, if marginal, matter since it provides the only secure means of full incorporation into the society and polity. Three southern European countries are heavily dependent upon *ius sanguinis*; Portugal, on the other hand, has a tradition more nearly resembling the former British *ius soli* (Rule 1996:12). This reliance on nationality by descent (*ius sanguinis*) has serious implications for the descendants of immigrant families, effectively denying them straightforward access to citizenship.

The citizenship laws of the two largest two states, France and Germany, are directly traceable to the end of the last century. In the case of France, the 1889 law was a consolidation of the assimilationist approach dating from the Revolution, but in fact extended nationality automatically to second-generation immigrants, partly to enable their participation in military service. The German 1870 law, on the other hand, was a product of the distinctive political and cultural geography of Central Europe. Citizenship by descent was viewed as a specifically national principle, unlike the feudal ties of *ius soli*, and had the desired effect of excluding Poles and Jews.

The rates of naturalisation/acquisition for most European countries range from 0.9 to 5.6, although Germany has a rate of 0.6 (Bauböck and Çinar 1994) and Portugal (0.1), Italy and Greece (0.5) provide examples of even greater difficulty in obtaining national citizenship. Further, examination of the facts suggests that most of those who do manage this feat are in fact 'family members' and/or nationals of other (existing) EU citizenships. On the other hand, many aliens have been resident illegally in Southern states, almost unnoticed for decades across the region.

What is perhaps more surprising than the actual naturalisation rates is that three southern European countries have made access to citizenship more difficult in the 1990s. In 1993 Greece increased its residence requirement for spouses of Greek nationals from effectively zero to five years; for other aliens the residence period was increased from eight to ten years, with the application examined five years after declaration of intent. Italy also reformulated its nationality provision in 1992, raising the residence period from five to ten years for non-EU nationals, and reducing it to three for those of Italian descent (Zincone 1994:136). Portugal's 1994 revision increased the period of residence from six to ten years for children born in Portugal of foreign parents, at the same time as stipulating that their parents must have been lawfully resident for that period (Rule 1996). This trend, particularly in the south, goes against moral and pragmatic arguments being proposed in certain circles for easier access to citizenship, increasing acceptance of dual nationality and gradual relaxation of naturalisation requirements. Further, the hardening of rules has been enacted in the complete absence of public debate. Third, this trend appears to deny the reality of permanent immigration into these countries by refusing to facilitate incorporation of immigrants into society.

TOWARDS THE FUTURE

Throughout Europe, countries are strengthening their common external border (by increased visa controls, common visa procedures, fines on airlines and the automatic refusal of entry by one country to anyone previously refused entry, or deported, by another member state). They are also anxious to improve internal controls (by checks on people within a country to find out whether they have the right to be there, and by linking immigration status to access to work, benefits and services). Governments of all countries are debating their response to refugees and asylum seekers coming to their borders, to try to ensure uniformity in dealing with applications and that asylum seekers should not be drawn to particular countries, where they think it might be easier to remain.

On the other hand, European harmonisation provides opportunities for co-operation between non-governmental organisations in different countries. This may include attempts to use European freedom of movement legislation for European nationals and for nationals of countries which have formal association or co-operation agreements with the EC, or trying to use the European Convention on Human Rights more creatively to support family unity rights. Examples of this can be found, and seen to have been effective. Recently, the 'European Coordination for Foreigners' Right to Family Life' has been actively campaigning for amendments to the European Treaty, and produced its own draft, 'Convention on the Right to Live as a Family'. Regrettably, the overall trend seems to be one of increasing harshness, so that even in the southern states which had traditionally been more liberal, at least towards illegal migrant settlers, there has been a tendency to absorb the control elements of immigration control from European collaborative fora (Baldwin-Edwards and Schain 1994:14). Unfortunately, the policies of the EU and Schengen have been completely one-sided, concentrating on crisis management of migrant flows. These new policies have been in the context of long-standing protection of migrants' rights under both domestic and international law: thus northern European national practices have, to some extent, been tempered by judicial control. The effect of asymmetrical policy creation – that is, control of immigrants without a corresponding development of immigrants' rights – has been to modernise immigration policy at the cost of dehumanising it.

Increasingly, immigration is blamed for the financial crisis in sustaining generous welfare arrangements, particularly with the highly visible assistance given to asylum seekers and refugees (Bauböck 1994). Almost all available evidence suggests that immigrants contribute far more than they receive from welfare arrangements (e.g. Barabas *et al.* 1991; Ruland 1994). Another related claim is that immigration causes unemployment; yet both legal and undocumented migrants work in highly segmented labour markets with little or no competition from the indigenous labour force. Significantly, as immigrants have a high concentration in vulnerable industries such as textiles, there has been rising unemployment amongst the immigrant populations (Bauböck 1994). This is sometimes taken as clear evidence that immigration itself causes unemployment.

As almost all European countries approach their predicted demographic crisis, with its problem of many pensioners to be supported by few of working age, it may seem that immigration would be an ideal solution. There are three major problems with this, however. First, the level of immigration would have to be phenomenally high – and this would be unacceptable politically. Second, inevitably these 'guestworkers' too would remain – thus changing the ethnic composition substantially after some time. Third, the pension schemes of at least Germany have been sustained for some time by migrant workers' contributions: Ruland (1994:85) comments that for 1989 immigrants' contributions exceeded payments by a factor of 3 or 4, thus bringing short-term relief to the system.

Finally, it is worth noting that, whereas expanding European economies thirty years ago were able to absorb immigrants and also develop extensive welfare systems, today unskilled labour is mostly unwelcome whilst those welfare systems are undergoing major reform. The underlying forces are, of course, economic; yet the question of policy options remains open and largely ignored with respect to migrants. What of the future? The mobilisation of migrants, particularly through migrant associations at both national and European level, must be a major possible mechanism for reform. Non-governmental organizations (NGOs) can be not only a socio-political force, but also have the unique capacity to incorporate and represent illegal migrants. Furthermore, the migrant groups may well constitute an unattached electoral force in a future 'federalised' Europe: such political power – along with NGO self-help, albeit with state and EU financial support – constitutes the most likely route for the emancipation of Europe's migrant communities.

SUMMARY

- Migration, nationality and asylum laws have significant effects on the lives of people of minority origin.
- Recent changes to the EU 'constitution' introduce opportunities to protect citizenship rights of minorities, which are at the same time threatened by restrictions on migration.
- Because 'free movement' provisions are based on expectations that migrants will not claim welfare, social workers may find themselves acting as immigration police.
- The 'crisis of solidarity' is linked to a domestic politics of immigration and nationality.
- There is, in effect, a hierarchy of citizenship existing within Europe, with minorities and migrants having significantly worse access to welfare entitlements.

REFERENCES

Baldwin-Edwards, M. (1991a): 'The socio-political rights of migrants in the EC', in G. Room (ed.): *Towards a European Welfare State?* Bristol: SAUS pp. 189–234.

—— (1991b): 'Immigration after 1992', *Policy and Politics* 19(3), pp. 199–211.

—— (1995): 'Citizenship of the Union: rhetoric or reality, inclusion or exclusion?' in Pekka Kosonen and Per Madsen (eds): *Convergence or Divergence? Welfare states Facing the European Integration*. Brussels: Commission of the EC, Cost A2 Series.

Baldwin-Edwards, M. and Schain, M. (1994): *The Politics of Immigration in Western Europe*. London: Frank Cass.
Barabas, *et al.* (1991): 'Gesamwirtschafteliche Effekte der Zuwanderung 1988–91', *RWI-Mettelungen* 4 (2), pp. 133–54, Rheinisch-Westfälisches Institut für Wirtschaftsforschung.
Bauböck, R. and Çinar, D. (1994): 'Naturalisation policies in western Europe', in M. Baldwin-Edwards and M. Schain (eds) *The Politics of Immigration in Western Europe.*
Bauböck, R. (1994): 'The integration of immigrants', mimeo report prepared for the Council of Europe.
Brochmann, G. (1996): *European Integration and Immigration from Third Countries*. Oslo: Scandinavian University Press.
CEC (1994): *Communication from the Commission to the Council and the European Parliament: On Immigration and Asylum Policies, COM (94) 23 final*. Brussels.
—— (1995a): *Proposal for a Directive on the Right of Third-Country Nationals to Travel in the Community, COM (95) 0346 final*. Brussels.
—— (1995b): *Communication from the Commission to the European Parliament and the Council on the Possible Application of Article K9 of the Treaty on European Union, COM (95) 0566 final*. Brussels.
Closa, C. (1992): 'The concept of citizenship in the Treaty on European Union', *Common Market Law Review* 29, pp. 1137–69.
—— (1994) 'Citizenship and nationality', in D. O'Keefe and P. Twomey (eds) *Legal Issues of the Maastricht Treaty*. London: Chancery Law Publishing.
ISSA (1994): *Migration: A Worldwide Challenge for Social Security*. Geneva: International Social Security Association, Studies and Research No. 35.
Layton-Henry, Z. (ed.) (1990): *The Political Rights of Migrant Workers in Western Europe*. London: Sage.
Martiniello, M. (1993): 'European citizenship, European identity and migrants: towards the postnational?' ECPR Workshop 'Inclusion and Exclusion: Migration and the Uniting of Europe', 1991, printed and circulated, Leiden, April 1993.
Miller, M. (1994): 'Towards understanding state capacity to prevent unwanted migrations', in M. Baldwin-Edwards and M. Schain (eds): *The Politics of Immigration in Western Europe.*
O'Keefe, D. (1995): 'Recasting the Third Pillar', *Common Market Law Review*. 32, pp. 893–920.
O'Keefe, D. and Twomey, P. (eds) (1994): *Legal Issues of the Maastricht Treaty*. London: Chancery Law Publishing.
Ruland, F. (1994): 'Impact of international migration on social security: the example of old age insurance in Germany', in ISSA, *Migration*, pp. 77–96.
Rule, E. (1996): 'Portuguese nationality law in outline', *Immigration and Nationality Law and Practice* 10 (1).
Soysal, Y. (1994): *Limits of Citizenship: Migrants and Postnational Membership in Europe*. Chicago: University of Chicago Press.
Zincone, G. (1994): 'Immigration to Italy: data and policies', in F. Heckmann and W. Bosswick (eds): *Migration Policies: A Comparative Perspective*. Bamberg: European Forum for Migration Studies.

Chapter 5

Ethnic monitoring

Bureaucratic construction of a 'minority' entity or identity

Mark R. D. Johnson

INTRODUCTION

This chapter discusses an issue which has proved problematic in many settings: the recording of information about individuals which includes reference to their minority status. It is argued that services, particularly those of a personal, social service, type cannot be satisfactorily delivered in the absence of such information. A number of different types of information can be considered as essential. Since some data may not be available or allowable, other types of information can sometimes be used as proxies. At the same time, the sensitive nature of such data is acknowledged, and the debates which have been held around this issue, particularly in Britain, are reviewed. 'Good practice' in collecting and using this information is described and discussed.

It is not necessary here to retrace the arguments about what a minority is, or why minority status is relevant to the planning and delivery of social services: these have been explored elsewhere in this book. We do, however, start from the assumption that these distinctions are salient, and that action is required to ensure that individuals receive suitable services to meet their needs. It is also assumed that the reader will be generally in agreement with the hypothesis (also laid out by Lena Dominelli in Chapter 3) that European traditions of social work have historically focused on the treatment of the individual, around a personalised assessment of that individual's needs. However, we would contend that this fails to acknowledge that in most cases such individuals are members of collective entities within society (which is itself a collective entity). Membership of a group provides benefits and access to certain resources, notably collective support and some form of identity. It also generates needs – whether concrete or abstract, and affects the ways in which the individual accesses 'goods'. Location within a group can also be, from certain perspectives, a problem or at least a risk. It is the case that power relationships mean that in most societies the needs of the majority are those around which the edifice of welfare support is constructed – in terms of training, planning, and even physical provision. Vegetarians fare badly in a carnivorous environment, and wheelchair users prefer ramps to stairs!

A complex circle develops, whereby that which is not demanded is not provided, that which is not recorded is not planned for, and that which is not planned for has no resources allocated to its provision. Then, when it is not available, no one thinks of asking for it.

More simply, the hegemony of uniformity or of uniform provision – the so-called 'republican' model of society – imposes its own tyranny on members of minorities: 'General policy is not however necessarily neutral. If policy favours one language, one religion or (more generally) one view, or even imposes them on all the people, that policy is general but not neutral' (Vermeulen 1997:10).

A complex situation then arises, since it is necessary to take account of difference, without necessarily being seen to approve of, or support, the issues around which groups form. A state like France, which is explicitly forbidden in its constitution to take account of religion, or one like Sweden, where 'race' is such a sensitive issue that it cannot be asked about in official forms, may find it difficult to make such differences 'visible' in the collection of information about members of its society – and yet:

> To develop, implement and evaluate general or target group policy when they are aimed partly or wholly at ethnically defined categories in society, it is essential to gather reliable information about the composition of that multi-ethnic society. This is no simple task, because if dissimilar criteria are used, the available data cannot be compared . . . the only truly comparable data available are those based on the criterion of nationality . . . [but] people who have taken on the citizenship of their new country do not appear in the statistics.
>
> (Vermeulen 1997:10–12)

It is clear that, as Soydan and Williams have indicated above, there are many ways of defining a 'minority'. Frequently one characteristic or another is used as a proxy (or a signifier) of the difference: this may provide a solution to the would-be monitor of the needs and experiences of service clients, but that is not certain. We have already in this book discussed the confusion between the notion of migrant and minority: the crucial issue is that any categorisation used is relevant to the delivery of a service and recognition of a 'client's' need. One of the least threatening and most commonly used identifiers, is that of 'mother tongue' or 'language most commonly used in the home'.

> The trouble with using nationality, birthplace, ethnic origin or language spoken at home as indicators of ethnic categories is that this implicitly assumes that such criteria all refer to the same clear-cut entities. . . . It is more effective to use different criteria to pursue different policy objectives.
>
> (Vermeulen 1997:12)

It is apparent from this dictum that social workers or others seeking to deliver a service must first consider what factors are relevant to their work and the ways in which 'ethnic' differences affect the ways in which people need or use their service.

WHAT IS ETHNIC MONITORING?

It will be clear from the discussion so far that 'ethnic monitoring' requires the identification of individuals as belonging to one or more groups, defined in terms of culture and origin. However, were it nothing more than this, it would be no more than the sort of casual categorisation that can lead to discrimination and harm based on stereotype. To be effective and useful, ethnic monitoring must rely upon the individuals concerned being given the opportunity to define their identity in terms that are meaningful to them – and hence which reveal something about them which is of value to the care-giver. Further, this information should be recorded somewhere within the data management systems of the agency, otherwise there will be a continual need to seek this information, and no way of using it for planning specific services or allocating relevant resources.

The terms 'ethnic monitoring' and 'ethnic record keeping' are often used interchangeably. This is a serious mistake. The keeping of records is necessary, and a part of the process, but it is not, and should never be allowed to become, the totality of the action. Bureaucracies thrive on collection of information, but too often we have found in researching the commitment of agencies to equality of opportunity that the statement of a policy, and the recording of some data, are thought of as sufficient evidence of a change in the way the organisation operates. Ethnic monitoring is not some form of magic panacea that guarantees instant equality of opportunity. Rather, it is one of a number of strategies (including surveys) that can be used to examine service uptake and outcomes. The information thus gained must then be related to some objectives and standards which have been set as part of a policy for the allocation of resources and expected outcomes. Record keeping without monitoring is a pointless exercise. The collection of information without its use is not merely wasteful of resources but can be actively harmful to the operation of an agency. In particular, it can lead to:

staff disillusionment: Why should they bother to collect data (and perhaps face questions and irritation from clients) if the data are never used?

community disillusionment: Why should co-operation be given when there is no 'pay-off' or end result in terms of an improvement of service?

If information is collected and nothing done to analyse it, or consider the implications of the patterns of use that it shows, it becomes a redundant exercise. This cannot be done without some cost – even if that is only slight. Further, the staff involved will query the value of their effort in collecting the information, and minority communities will question why the data are being collected and whether they have any relationship to a programme or commitment to equal opportunities. This can lead to future mistrust of other well-meant initiatives, and render the job of the care-supplier more difficult.

Thus, while ethnic record keeping is *necessary* if monitoring is to take place, it is not *sufficient*. Ethnic monitoring is a *process* whereby information about the relevant aspects of people's ethnic origins is collected, recorded, and used to establish patterns, which can be compared with other information about their relationship with society and 'need'. In the best cases, this information is used to set targets and establish policies which will overcome disadvantage and lead to improvements in service delivery and the material circumstances of the members of minorities. At the very least, it can be used to establish the facts and make a case for such changes to be attempted.

> 'There are three kinds of lies,' said Mark Twain in his autobiography, 'lies, damned lies, and statistics.' Local authorities which keep no kind of statistics cannot evaluate how big a lie they are telling when claiming to be equal opportunity authorities. And few authorities collect, process and evaluate statistics effectively enough to enable them to make such a claim with confidence or conviction.
>
> (Roper 1990:25)

In some services, furthermore, a direct functional value can be adduced for the maintenance of ethnic monitoring and related information systems. There is clearly a direct link between the proportion of Muslims in a community and the likely demand for halal meat, or a Muslim burial ground. Planning for efficient as well as equitable operation requires the agency to know these sorts of thing! Similarly, in health services certain diseases (while not *exclusively* confined to certain minorities) are much more commonly encountered in certain groups. The association between sickle-cell anaemia and African or Afro-Caribbean populations is one such; certain South Asian and Mediterranean communities have similar needs in relation to thalassaemia (another genetically determined blood disorder). On the other hand, European people from Sweden are five times more likely than the Dutch to carry the 'Factor V Leiden' gene which can raise their risk of (potentially fatal) deep-vein thrombosis (Vandenbroucke *et al.* 1996). While some data on birthplace may be available from the census, this does not help with religious orientation, nor can census data give information about changing population profiles or the arrival in an area of refugees from a particular group after the census has taken place. As Europe becomes increasingly a society of settled migrants, with third and fourth generations born in countries to which their grandparents may have moved, inheriting the risk of diseases less common among the autochthones, this sort of question will become more rather than less urgent.

Further, inefficiencies can be exposed through ethnic monitoring, as well as new opportunities to deliver service or to recruit 'customers' and thereby justify expenditure. 'Minority' clients, it should be remembered, have 'majority' needs as well.

WHAT SHOULD BE MONITORED?

We may start to consider certain specific issues around which groups may be differentiated, and the implications this has for monitoring service users. Clearly there are various ways of defining minorities, which are discussed elsewhere in this book. The implementation of ethnic monitoring requires careful consideration of the characteristics which are of most relevance to the delivery of service. It may be that the 'ethnic group' labels such as those used in the UK Census – 'Black-Caribbean', 'Asian-Pakistani' and so on – are sufficient to identify the existence of discrimination on broad, racialised grounds. For many purposes, this will be enough, at least to alert policy makers to the need to investigate matters more closely. On the other hand, for planning services and allocating resources, as suggested above, more detailed information is likely to be needed. While some categories such as 'Pakistani' may be associated fairly closely with particular cultural characteristics such as language (Urdu), religion (Muslim) and perhaps certain aspects of life-style, it is dangerous to assume that this will always be the case – the language and social preferences of Pathan (Pushto-speaking) people from the north-west of Pakistan are quite distinct from those who sometimes describe themselves as Kashmiris or Pakistani Punjabis from the north-east of the same state. Their children too may describe themselves by different labels. On the other hand, when numbers are small, the 'ideal' solution of allowing everyone to self-identify their preferred label may lead to inaction on the basis that there are too many differences to plan for. In such cases, it is best to offer broad categories ('Asian', 'African-Caribbean') to establish overall patterns, supplemented by additional questions about issues such as language, religion and diet, which may require the provision of specific services in order to meet genuine personal needs.

Language

In some European countries, linguistic diversity is tolerated, and in others it is at best ignored (Drakeford and Morris, Chapter 6, has a more detailed discussion). The motto of the French Revolution, 'One State, One Nation, One Language', had the laudable objective of national unity but led to the devaluation of the status of regional languages – even the major Occitan

('Langue d'Oc') of the southern half of the country. Minority languages such as Breton are rarely taught in school and the concept has little official recognition in France save for the existence of German speakers in Alsace. German Sorb (Saxon) and Danish (Schleswig-Holstein) speakers are recognised as official minorities in Germany. We may therefore suggest that in many European countries there may be some scope for the use of language as an accessible means of estimating the numbers and needs of at least certain minority groups. This is perhaps best exemplified in Sweden, where over 130 'home-languages' have been identified. Indeed,

> boards of primary schools are legally obliged to carry out the following activities every year: make an inventory of home languages other than Swedish spoken by any of the pupils of the school; provide information for parents of non-Swedish-speaking pupils . . . and provide IMLI (mother-tongue instruction).
>
> (Broeder and Extra 1997:88)

The result of this activity is that the Swedish Board of Statistics can publish quite detailed and presumably accurate figures of minority pupils in the country, thereby enabling some estimate of the relative importance of (say) Albanian, Arabic and Vietnamese. (For 1994, the relative sizes were 2,838 Albanian-, 11,688 Arabic- and 918 Vietnamese-speaking pupils in primary schools: Swedish Bureau of Statistics 1995.) On the other hand, although Belgium, with three national official languages, might be expected to be rather more sensitive to the recording of linguistic identity, it has found, as in other states, that this can become an issue which reopens divisions within the 'majority' community: the Belgian Census had to abandon the inclusion of a language question as it was 'too politically sensitive' (Extra and Verhoeven 1992:12).

Religion

Western European society draws for much of its cultural heritage upon a history which has been dominated by Christianity – indeed, the first unification of Europe was under the banner of the 'Holy Roman Empire'. Even in those states such as France which explicitly term themselves 'laïc', it is hard to escape notions which are founded in Christian ideology, such as the 'family', or the relation between 'charity' and the 'state'; in all the discussions about the right of young Muslim women in France to wear the 'veil' to school there were few objections to the right of others to wear crucifixes or other religious symbols. Religion can play an important part in the care of people in distress – the role of hospital chaplains is well established, for example, and it is very important to observe the correct procedures in respect of the care of the dying and the treatment of bodies after death. The situation in

Germany, where a voluntary 'church tax' can be levied on those who self-identify as adherents of an 'official' religion, is perhaps the most clearly defined, but similar arrangements for the formal recognition of 'churches' (including Islam and Judaism) exist in a number of European states: rights of Muslims in Greek Thrace are explicitly protected by the Treaty of Lausanne (1923). In others, it appears to be more problematic to ask this question.

Birthplace

The most common indicator of difference, or the size of 'minority' populations, in census data and other official records, is birthplace. This information is recorded in nearly every state, and is used to analyse data such as those collected on death certificates. Unfortunately, it provides a poor indicator of cultural or 'ethnic' origin: many well-known British figures were born in parts of the former empire, and have little in common with the autochthonous populations of those places. Equally, it is now true that more than half of the 'minority' ethnic population of Britain which can trace their parents' or grandparents' origins to India, Africa and the Caribbean were actually themselves born in Britain. A similar situation now obtains in Germany, where significant numbers of German-born young people of Turkish origin are not yet regarded as German citizens. Some states, notably the Netherlands and Sweden, are able to produce information about those whose parents were born abroad – but eventually this too will become as redundant as the (1981) proxy used in analysing the UK census – of the 'head of household's birthplace'. In terms of ethnic monitoring, birthplace data are probably of no value whatsoever.

Nationality

This is probably one of the most problematic categories. Too often the notion of nationality is confused with that of citizenship, i.e. passport. Indeed, in some of the 'newer' states of Europe such as Lithuania, it is possible to have one's ethnic origin recorded on the national passport, and many other states recognise 'national minorities' such as the Sami of Finland and Norway. In such cases, as with Czechs in Austria and Germans in the Czech Republic, there are protections and privileges (notably in respect of schooling in a minority language) which are guaranteed by the constitution. To others, the notion of nationality implies a homogeneous category, and 'foreigners' may have lesser protection under the law. In ethnic monitoring, it is essential not to confuse the idea of identity with the question of the rights of the citizen to state-funded services.

WHY MONITOR?

A number of reasons for the introduction of monitoring have already been put forward in the discussion, including those of organisational efficiency, allocation of resources, and the making explicit of the patterns of use of a service. In some states, there are also legal reasons – it may, for example, be necessary to demonstrate explicitly that one is not discriminating, and this can only be done by the production of data from monitoring exercises. Formal investigations in the UK conducted by the Commission for Racial Equality frequently end by serving a legal 'enforcement notice' requiring agencies to set up systems of ethnic monitoring and to produce periodic reports relating to their progress. At a national level, the British 1991 Criminal Justice Act laid a duty on the Home Office (equivalent to other countries' ministry of the interior) to produce a regular report on both gender and ethnic equality in the activities of the criminal justice system. An earlier statute (the 1966 Local Government Act) had set aside certain funds to pay for provision of 'special services' required for the cultural or linguistic needs of minority populations (in this case, explicitly 'immigrants' from the 'new' Commonwealth countries of Africa, Asia and the Caribbean): these could only be claimed if the authority could demonstrate the size of such populations using its services – again requiring monitoring. Examples of similar provisions, notably in respect of the provision of schooling and other language needs or religious observance, have already been given from other European states.

On the other hand, it has to be admitted that there have been voices raised in opposition to the introduction of monitoring. Most frequently, it has been suggested that by monitoring and thus drawing attention to difference, one is somehow discriminating. Ethnic monitoring has come late to the European scene despite a long history of its usage in the United States of America, where it was a key recommendation of the Kerner Commission after the disturbances of 1967 (NACCD 1968). In America, ethnic monitoring was linked to contract compliance and the provisions of the 1964 Civil Rights Act and hence clearly linked to the supply of resources by the state, which was a much more radical approach than has ever been attempted in Europe. It is also true that American society had long been divided by race, socially, legally and in common discourse. These factors have been critical in the acceptance of 'ethnic' or 'racial' monitoring.

The position of accepting the value of monitoring has not been universally accepted. Resistance characteristically makes reference to the misuse of ethnic or racially categorised records and to issues of civil liberty. Most evidently perhaps, and quite understandably, such anecdotes refer to the Holocaust and the use made of records by the Nazis to identify Jewish individuals and families. It is not surprising that this particular issue is still sensitive, although it may be argued that the identification of most ethnic minorities does not require such bureaucratic assistance – even where 'visibility' is in the 'eye of the beholder', members of most minorities are aware just how easily they can be identified and discriminated against, without recourse to documentation. Much opposition is founded upon a belief in the value of a 'colour-blind' approach – an attitude characterised by the British MP Anthony Steen in a parliamentary debate: 'To continue to identify second and subsequent generations by an ethnic label, where this is avoidable, is to negate the policy of integration' (Official Report 1979: col. 72).

To this, other speakers replied that avoidance of such labelling would not necessarily prevent the perpetuation of discrimination. An equally pertinent observation was made by the veteran Labour MP Sid Bidwell, criticising those white people who opposed ethnic monitoring 'on behalf of' black sensitivities:

> This is a nerve spot affecting people who are not very closely related. . . . My experience is that black or brown people do not object to such a record, and that this is objected to by people who think that they are their closest friends.
>
> (Official Report 1979: col. 155)

The chief objection to the use of ethnic monitoring, however, came from those who saw it as a covert means of giving preferential treatment to a particular group:

> The basic principle remains that a certain section of the community is being identified by its ethnic origin or colour. The word 'colour' has been avoided and the definition 'ethnic' has been so widely extended that it embraces practically everyone. The words 'a group of persons distinguished by colour, race, nationality or ethnic or national origins' include practically every inhabitant of any large city, but we all know what is meant. . . . 'Ethnic' is written but we know in the House that what is meant is 'coloured'. The Bill provides that certain categories of people are to receive preferential treatment.
>
> (Official Report 1979: col. 100)

Most objections have been justified on administrative or practical grounds or made by 'gatekeepers' arguing that they were protecting the interests of minorities or the community as suggested by Bidwell (see above). It is also argued, as it has been for many years, that there is no intentional discrimination in the system: 'we operate a fair access system, colour-blind: none of our staff would discriminate in a racist fashion' is a fair summary of the typical response. The argument that only through the introduction of ethnic monitoring can *accidental* (a term many seem to prefer to *institutional*) discrimination be identified and dealt with is therefore an appealing and generally convincing one.

There remains one more recent issue, not unconnected with the debate over civil rights and the fear of excessive power becoming concentrated in the hands of the state and others who collect data, particularly using the modern technological power of the computer. That is a general objection to the collection of personal data without the explicit consent of the individual. Indeed, in 1995 the European Council agreed a Directive which comes into force in 1998, that relates to this issue and explicitly mentions 'ethnic origin': this places significant restriction on the processing of data:

> . . . any processing of personal data must be lawful and fair to the individuals concerned . . . and not excessive in relation to the purposes for which they are processed, whereas such purposes must be explicit and legitimate and must be determined at the time of the collection.
>
> (Directive 95/46/EC: para. 28)

> . . . data which are capable by their nature of infringing fundamental freedoms or privacy should not be processed unless the data subject gives his explicit consent.
>
> (para. 33)

It is, however, also important to recognise that the ministers and officials involved in drawing up this ruling were aware that such data would be required, and should be used for the public interest. Thus the Directive continues:

> . . . member states must also be authorised when justified by grounds of important public interest to derogate from the prohibition of processing sensitive categories of data where important reasons of public interest so justify in areas such as public health and social protection . . . especially in order to ensure the quality and cost-effectiveness of the procedures used.
>
> (para. 34)

In 'Section III – Special Categories of Processing', particular attention is paid to questions of 'sensitive data', which includes the sorts of information here considered as relevant to ethnic monitoring:

> Paragraph 1: Member states shall prohibit the processing of personal data revealing racial or ethnic origin, political opinions, religious or philosophical beliefs, trade union membership and the processing of data concerning health or sex life.

Again, there are explicit exclusions from this prohibition, which include such situations as those where the 'data subject' has given his (*sic*) explicit consent, or where it is necessary to be able to demonstrate that other national laws, such as those relating to discrimination, are not being broken. It may be expected that future attempts to introduce ethnic monitoring may be resisted, perhaps by reference to this Directive: it is equally certain that a good case can be made for appealing to the derogations included in the Directive specifically because there are occasions where it is necessary or desirable to do the monitoring in the interests of members of minority groups.

A CASE STUDY

Before concluding, we may take as a case study the use of ethnic monitoring in social work departments in Britain. Many of them would argue that they have a well-developed level of 'good practice' in respect of ethnic sensitivity and 'anti-racist practice' but this is not always true in respect of the implementation of ethnic monitoring in social work. A Commission for Racial Equality study published in 1989, to which only 70 of 116 targeted departments responded, found little improvement over the situation described ten years previously by a joint working party with the Association of Directors of Social Services (ADSS/CRE 1978; CRE 1989). Even the 70 responding departments were not all following formal equal opportunity policies, and a mere 10 (14 per cent) reported having introduced 'comprehensive ethnic monitoring', with a further eight running pilot schemes in selected areas. None apparently had at that point 'been doing so long enough' to have produced comprehensive analysis reports. A major obstacle was the reluctance of staff to collect the data, or other elements relating to a lack of commitment among staff and management. Many reported that the introduction of computerised record keeping was expected to improve the situation.

It should be noted, as Connelly has observed, that the provision of personal social services tends to come at critical and stressful points in people's lives. The nature of this provision must affect the way in which information is collected. As she says, 'the combination of vulnerable people and need for information raises a number of questions about power and relationships' (Connelly 1988:30). There has also been a history of interventions related to 'race' in this profession, some of which have left bad feelings on both sides, including many *ad hoc* surveys and exercises and a wider range of efforts to meet black community needs and demands. Any innovations must take this history into account. That is not to say that ethnic monitoring is such an innovation in some areas of social work. The collection of ethnic background has, in fact, been a regular feature of the standard at-risk register since 1983:

> Prior to 1983 the register forms had asked for information on the country of birth of the child's parents and details of any cultural factors which were thought to be relevant. This latter section was very rarely filled in. . . . When the form was redesigned in 1983 it was decided that ethnic background would be a more useful indicator. . . . There was a certain amount of initial opposition [which] . . . has been replaced by a desire to establish some baseline of information in order to ensure that any under or over reporting of abuse . . . is not due to the lack of services provided.
>
> (Creighton and Noyes 1989:17–18)

Another significant factor has been the introduction of a new law relating to the protection of children. The Children Act 1989, Schedule 2(11) states that:

> Every local authority shall, in making any arrangements –
> a) for the provision of day care within their area; or
> b) designed to encourage persons to act as local authority foster parents,
> have regard to the different racial groups to which children within their area who are in need belong.

This duty is (as defined in law) 'absolute' and requires each local government body to identify the extent of children in need in the area. In order to take this further and establish their racial origin, an authority must either introduce blanket policies of 'in need' criteria based on ethnicity, or be able to identify each individual child and her or his ethnic origin. Clearly, this duty cannot be carried out without the extensive application of ethnic monitoring and accurate knowledge about the ethnic composition of the whole area.

CONCLUSION

The principal reason for undertaking any form of monitoring must be a desire to improve performance by gaining understanding about current outcomes. Implicit in this is the expectation of action. Equally, because the introduction of ethnic monitoring is unlikely to occur without either controversy or consultation, the very fact of its being undertaken will raise expectations in certain quarters (not least amongst ethnic minorities) that action will be taken to improve access, allocation and the overall quality of service experienced by those minority groups. While it may, of course, provide a stimulus for action subsequently, it would be wrong to enter into the collection of data (with the consequent implications for resource allocation) without the expectation and planning of change.

It must be emphasised that ethnic record keeping and monitoring do not of themselves lead to greater equality or increased take-up (or less over-use) of services. They are tools which can be used in devising and implementing plans of action. Information may be power, but it is unfocused and ineffective without a policy context: nor is it of any value unless it is obtained carefully, professionally, and in a context.

Ethnic monitoring *is not an end in itself* nor is it a magic wand whose implementation will solve all problems; nor, indeed, should it be seen as operating in isolation. Rather, it should *form part of an integrated service delivery system* designed both to ensure that agencies are not acting in a discriminatory way in the delivery of their services, and to ensure that those services are reaching, and relevant to, the communities that those agencies exist to serve. Ethnic monitoring will not provide all the answers, but it will highlight areas of possible concern, and enable the right questions to be asked.

The prerequisites for effective monitoring

- Monitoring should be introduced only after an extensive process of consultation and consideration, so that it has the full support of those who are to conduct the collection and analysis of the data – and, indeed, to act on its findings; and also the agreement of the minority groups and general population who are to be monitored. Otherwise, refusal to supply information will render the exercise useless.
- Monitoring should only be introduced in the context of an explicit policy for the development of equality of opportunity, to justify its existence and provide a basis for the implementation of change arising from any observed inequalities.
- What exactly is to be monitored and why it must be established.
- Who is to collect the information, when, how and from whom, and how the data are to be stored and protected from illicit processing must be clarified.
- Benchmarks or targets for the comparison of the data, and procedures to report on the findings and make appropriate adjustments to future data collection and targets, are also needed.

REFERENCES

Association of Directors of Social Services / Commission for Racial Equality (1978) *Multi-racial Britain: The Social Services Response*. London: CRE/ADSS.

Broeder, P. and Extra, G. (1997) 'Language' in H. Vermeulen (ed.) *Immigration Policy for a Multi-cultural Society*. Brussels: Migration Policy Group.

Connelly, N. (1988) *Ethnic Record Keeping and Monitoring in Service Delivery*. London: Policy Studies Institute.

Connelly, N. and Young, K. (1981) *Policy and Practice in the Multi Racial City*. London: Policy Studies Institute.

CRE (1989) *Racial Equality in Social Services Departments: A Survey of Equal Opportunity Policies*. London: CRE.

Creighton, S. and Noyes, P. (1989) *Child Abuse Trends in England and Wales 1983–87*. London: National Society for the Prevention of Cruelty to Children.

Cross, M., Cox, B. and Johnson, M.R.D. (1988) *Black Welfare and Local Government: Section 11 and Social Services Departments*, Policy Paper 12. Coventry: CRER, University of Warwick.

Edwards, J. and Batley, R. (1978) *The Politics of Positive Discrimination*. London: Tavistock.

European Parliament and Council, Directive 95/46/EC (24 October 1995): On the protection of individuals with regard to the processing of personal data and the free movement of such data. *Official Journal of the European Communities* (OJ) L 281/31 Volume 38 – 23 November 1995.

Extra, G. and Verhoeven, L. (eds) (1992) *Ethnic Community Languages in the Netherlands*. Amsterdam: Swets and Zeitlinger.

Home Office (1992) *Race and the Criminal Justice System: CJA Section 95*. Report published under Section 95 of the Criminal Justice Act 1991.

MacDonald, S. (1991) *All Equal Under the Act? – A Practical Guide to the Children Act 1989 for Social Workers*. London: Race Equality Unit, National Institute for Social Work.

NACCD (1968) *Report of the National Advisory Commission on Civil Disorders* (Kerner Commission); Summary Report. New York.

Official Report (1979) 'Local Government Grants (Ethnic Groups) Bill' Debate, *Official Report* (Hansard) 12 March cols 55–170.

Roper, S. (1990) 'Bringing the facts to light', *Local Government Chronicle*, 25 May: 25–6.

Swedish Bureau of Statistics (1995) *Hemspråk och hemspråksundervisning*. Orebro: SCB.

Vandenbroucke, J.P. *et al.* (1996) 'Leiden University Study', *British Medical Journal* 313:1127–30.

Vermeulen, H. (ed.) (1997) *Immigration Policy for a Multi-cultural Society*. Brussels: Migration Policy Group.

Part II

Case studies of some common themes

Right across Europe nation states are experiencing the profound contraction of welfare at the same time as being required to respond creatively to the new and growing demands of culturally diverse populations and the increased presence of refugees and asylum seekers. An offshoot of this combination of factors is the growth of hostilities towards migrants, minorities and refugees as individuals and communities fear that outsiders will take privileges away from those who are more entitled to them. This compounds the often perilous and disadvantaged position of minorities which is too often characterised by unemployment, economic hardship, educational disadvantage and ghettoised and deprived living conditions. Some of these problems faced by 'immigrants' and refugees are part of the structural and political context in particular European countries. High unemployment rates, poverty and housing shortages, for example, may be general features of specific countries but these are features which hit migrant and ethnic minority communities disproportionately hard. The welfare needs of illegal immigrants and of refugees and asylum seekers are also a key concern for public authorities. State services are largely impotent in relation to illegal immigrants, whose living and working conditions are notoriously dangerous and insecure, and different countries vary in respect of provision for the immediate needs of refugees let alone their responses to the particular traumas and stresses that many of these peoples carry with them. Romany life-style poses its own particular challenges to social service delivery in that there is often a mismatch between mainstream expectations and ideas about what is a 'good life' for these communities' own perceptions of welfare.

If social service provision is to be appropriately attuned to these circumstances European states will have to move beyond the picture of liberal paternalism, ethnocentrism, indifference and fear that currently characterises their responses. An appropriate response to the realities of cultural diversity requires a holistic and inclusive approach on many different levels and sectors of society. Equal opportunities cannot be left to the operations of the free market. They require design and intervention to right inequalities and imbalances. Central to this activity is the 'need to know', the need to quantify and monitor the extent of these imbalances. But knowing and acting are not axiomatic and, as Johnson argued in Chapter 5, assessing the extent of the 'problem' must imply remedies.

What is clear from the chapters that are to come is that members of ethnic minority communities are resourceful and capable people who have survived often extreme economic constraint, oppression and marginalisation with a resilience that has equipped them to order and shape their own lives in ways meaningful to them given the appropriate framework. Arntsberg, Segerström and the Hessles all illustrate powerfully the wish and the ability of these communities to 'do it their own way' and question Western models of intervention. The social professions have lessons to learn from the design and delivery of these community responses. It is these 'ways of doing' that must be legitimised within social work theory and practice; these emergent methodologies should provide the basis of the knowledge we construct for social work with ethnic minorities.

These chapters and others such as the work of Powell and Hirsch illustrate some of the tensions evident in building partnerships between state agencies and autonomous community organisations which so readily appear in all countries in response to the need for sensitive and appropriate service delivery. Authorities in various European countries have seen the activities of these organisations as marginal and transient and failed to offer appropriate resourcing to them in ways that allow them to retain their autonomy and specialisms.

The notion of sensitive service delivery is taken up by Drakeford and Morris and later by Patel, Naik and Humphries in respect of linguistic and religious minorities. The issues here are legion, not simply in terms of appropriate pragmatic interventions but in terms of contributing to the retention and formation of individual and collective identities within a society. To many workers language barriers, cultural differences and the traditions and practices of certain communities become sources of uncertainty and fear and appear insurmountable and overwhelming. The reaction is to retreat into the certainty of ethnocentrism or trite formulas for action or to labelling, categorising and pathologising the minority individuals or groups as 'difficult' or 'evil' or 'the problem'. The search is constantly to make certain the uncertain, to quantify and ossify culture and therefore to control it. This must be resisted. This collection of chapters forcefully illustrates that we cannot reduce complex phenomena to ready prescriptions for action, that these communities are dynamic entities, characterised by change and transformation that is both regenerating and unsettling to these communities themselves. Rather than 'managed' diversity, the aim must be 'negotiated' diversity.

In most European countries some type of response is emerging, most usually in the form of special projects. Such special provision is no excuse for the failure of mainstream providers to recognise and address the needs of minority communities. What underlies this approach of 'special provision' is an attitude that these minority communities are not an integral or permanent part of society in these countries. The problems facing minority communities often have structural, political or organisational causes which require not individualised and pathologising responses but collective and strategic solutions. Social work alone cannot address these ills and social development models must be deployed that engage many partners in relationships that are empowering to all participants. What is clear, however, is that social work does have an important role to play in the development of anti-oppressive, anti-discriminatory practice and that the challenge posed by work with ethnic minorities means that in many very fundamental respects social work is forced to re-examine its methodolgical base and the way in which it constructs knowledge in conditions of multiculturality.

Chapter 6

Social work with linguistic minorities

Mark Drakeford and Steve Morris

INTRODUCTION

This is a chapter concerned with social work in European communities where more than one language is in daily use, but where these languages are spoken by greater or lesser numbers of people and have a different status in a series of important spheres including the legal, cultural and social. It deals with mainstream European experience. Almost every state in Europe is at least bilingual, in the sense of having more than one indigenous language, as well as languages spoken by migrants from other places. The issues which arise in the design and delivery of social welfare services in such contexts, therefore, are part of the daily fabric of civic life across the whole continent. As such, these concerns have received attention at a European Union level. The Council of Ministers, on 5 November 1992, adopted the European Charter for Regional or Minority Languages, which set out steps to be taken by member states through which the use of regional or minority languages in public life might be promoted. These principles were further endorsed in the 1993 Vienna Declaration of the Heads of States and Government of the member states of the Council of Europe (see Council of Europe Report, 1996, for further details, and application of such developments in social work services, in particular).

In this chapter we concentrate upon the experience of delivering social work services in Wales, a country which is characterised by many of the traits outlined. The chapter will, however, attempt to draw into its discussion two other main features. First, whereas the Welsh language is essentially territorially confined to Wales itself, there are many other localities where a lesser used language may be spoken which is very widely, and indeed dominantly, used in other places. This chapter will attempt to consider both territorial and non-territorial examples of minoritised languages. Second, we will aim to place the Welsh example specifically within a European context, considering ways in which experience here exhibits points of similarity to and difference from those to be found elsewhere. The case of the Catalan language provides a comparison.

WALES: SOME BACKGROUND INFORMATION

In Wales, a country with its own history and culture, two languages are spoken by half a million people, on a daily basis. One is English, the first language of possibly some 85 per cent of the population; the second is Welsh. The Welsh language is the oldest living language in Britain and one which, until this century, was the language most often spoken by a majority of its inhabitants. Yet for almost a century Welsh speaking has been in decline, its often-heralded demise (see, for example, Durkacz 1983) attributed variously to the impact of industrialisation, mass communication and a pervasive feeling that the language stood in the way of both personal and national 'progress'. Against this background, perhaps the most remarkable feature of its history may justifiably be held to be not its decline but its survival, sharing as it does 'a relatively small island with one of the world's most influential, powerful and predatory of languages – English' (Casson *et al.* 1994).

The enduring salience of received wisdoms concerning the language remain powerful. Untutored perceptions continue to regard it as a dying and rustic anachronism to which elderly and crafty peasants are able rudely to resort in order to get the better of the visitor from outside. In fact, the current state of the Welsh language ruptures every stereotype which is commonly held to be true about it. It is a language spoken by at least 20 per cent of the population of Wales – or about half a million people, although the 1992 Welsh Social Survey would suggest that as many as 40 per cent – are either fluent speakers or able to understand the language. It is also a growing language. The 1991 Census showed a growth in the absolute number of Welsh speakers in some of the more anglicised areas of Wales and the number of adults learning the language has increased substantially during the late 1980s and early '90s (see Morris 1996). The growth was most dramatic in the percentage of young people able to speak the language, which has surpassed that of the over-65 age group: indeed, between 1981 and 1991 the numbers of young Welsh speakers increased by over 22 per cent (Aitchison and Carter 1994:104). Although concern has been expressed regarding actual language use by young people (Gruffudd 1996), Welsh will nevertheless enter the twenty-first century as a language of the young, rather than the old. There are parts of the country where it is in daily use by more than 90 per cent of young people. It is also an industrial and urban language. More people are able to speak Welsh in the city of Swansea, for example, than in towns such as Caernarfon. It is, finally, a language spoken by thousands of people who have no other. The 1981 Census returns – the last occasion upon which such a question was asked – showed over 20,000 people for whom it is the only language of communication. Most significantly, for this chapter, monolingual Welsh speakers are most often very young children, the elderly and individuals with learning disabilities – or, in other words, amongst groups most likely to be in need of social welfare services. The worn-out and discredited cry of 'They All Speak English Anyway' (see Davies 1994) is not only offensive in itself, but for social welfare workers it is untrue. Moreover, for many individuals who are able to use English, the language of *choice* may be Welsh, and their right to use it is as unqualified as that of any monolingual speaker.

What explanations may be offered for the enduring vitality of the language and the turn-around in its most recent fortunes? A leading academic commentator (Williams 1996) suggests a five-fold process in which, over a period of more than a century, idealism and protest produced a statutory recognition of Welsh linguistic rights and a broader public acceptance of bilingualism. The present phase is one described by Williams as 'institutionalisation', a period when new domains, especially in the para-public sector of government and the local authorities, has created new employment and social opportunities, thus ensuring the representation of the language within the main strategic agencies of the state. The future, according to this analysis, has to be one of 'parallelism', in which use of the language is extended to the widest range of social situations, producing 'an all-encompassing reflection of bilingualism in most areas of everyday life'. The effort towards 'normalisation',[1] in which language choice will be freely and unproblematically available, demands a series of investments, for example from government, professions and individuals, if it is to be realised. It also demands, as Williams suggests, a shift in which minority languages free themselves of a self-image of protest and deal directly with a new status 'as a service language, a language of influence, a language of power, a language of governance'.

The achievement of natural bilingualism in the Welsh context remains, then, an aspiration, albeit one which shows greater signs of achievability than would have seemed possible even twenty years ago. Even in a relaxed and confident bilingualism, however, language choice would remain significant, for in societies where more than one language is in daily use, choice of language is not a neutral selection, like the choice between tea and coffee. It is, rather, a basic shaper of power relations within communities, carrying with it a whole resonant set of cultural and political phenomena (Caroll 1956). Thus, as Thomas (1994:157) suggests:

> it is not size that defines a language-group as a minority, but power and status. Catalan . . . has more speakers than Danish, which is a nation state language and therefore an official language of the EU. More than twice as many people speak Welsh as speak Icelandic, but it is Welsh that is the minority language. *It may therefore seem as if the nation-state is the guarantor of a language and that nothing less will secure a language against discrimination* [emphasis added].

Social workers are, by and large, employees of the state and, even if to a disputed extent, its agents. The choice of language in which a social work encounter takes places is therefore resonant with wider implications of citizenship and social worth.

NON-TERRITORIAL CONTRASTS

Later in this chapter we deal with Wales in the context of other European communities where two or more languages are spoken. Before doing so, however, it is important to draw attention to a related but distinct set of questions which arise in relation to languages which are spoken by a minority within a local population, but which may be spoken by many millions of other people in dominant cultures elsewhere. In the Welsh context such languages would include Bengali, Urdu, Hindi and others. A recent survey of languages used on the playground of one inner-city Cardiff school, for example, revealed that more than a dozen different languages may be in use at any one time – including Turkish, Portuguese, Chinese, Arabic, English, Welsh and six Indo-Pakistani languages (Drakeford 1997). In a European context there are minority communities where the language spoken is the official language of another state. Hungarian speakers in Austria or German speakers in Denmark, France and Italy are examples of such communities. As the European Union Mercator project suggests, 'while these languages are not themselves likely to decline, on account of their official status elsewhere, the language and associated cultural heritage of these regions and territories are subject to similar pressures as those of the minority languages'.

Do such non-territorial languages have the same claim on state protection and promotion as languages such as Welsh? In this chapter, we advance an admittedly problematic distinction between principle and practice. In principle, as Thomas (1994) and others have argued, there are important differences which are defined by territoriality. In day-to-day social work, as we suggest below, the demands of good practice exhibit fewer differences. The principled distinction, however, may be set out in this way. Territorial minority languages are threatened by what Thomas, quoting the philosopher J.R. Jones, describes as a kind of reverse exile – 'not leaving your country, but your country leaving you'. In-migration by speakers of a dominant language, and the penetration of that language into institutional life, means that the local language is forced into retreat. The consequences of this retreat for the language and its culture are catastrophic: were it to disappear from its own territory, it would disappear altogether. Non-territorial minority languages, by contrast, face fewer threats at this macro level. Individuals and communities which bring their own language with them have, albeit to varying extents, made a choice to enter a locality where another language will be in daily and dominant usage. Sources of support – in terms of cultural material, literature, newspapers and so on – will continue to be available from other places where the language is unproblematically in use. A Hungarian speaker in Austria, for example, would be able to draw upon all these resources. It is even possible that more specialised needs could be met. By contrast, should a social work user in Wales wish to receive services through the Welsh language, then such services are only likely to be available from within the territory where the language is spoken. Where languages are not territorially confined, then speakers of minority languages may obtain services from other places where the language continues to be spoken by a majority. Most fundamentally, the fate of the language itself does not depend upon its continuation in the non-territorial context.

These arguments are most relevant at a state level. At the level of individuals and families, where social workers ply their trade, a rather different set of considerations apply. We return to these arguments below.

MINORITY LANGUAGES OR MINORITISED LANGUAGES?

Languages spoken by a 'minority' within a specific nation state or languages spoken within a territory which are not the official state language are frequently referred to as either 'minority languages' or 'lesser-used languages'. These categorisations can, however, be perceived by many of the speakers of the languages in question to be factually and politically incorrect. One example which has been previously cited is the Catalan language, which is spoken by 7 million people. In Spain as a whole it is a 'minority' language, but in the territory of Catalonia it is the language of the majority of the inhabitants and clearly not a minority language in the sense of the number of speakers able to use it. In addition, it has already been stated (Thomas 1994) that there are more speakers of Catalan than speakers of many other 'majority/state' languages in Europe such as Danish or Finnish. Concepts of 'majority'/'minority' can therefore be misleading and can serve to reinforce the very sense of being treated as a 'minority' group amongst speakers of that particular language. In a country like Wales, the Welsh language is spoken by a numerical minority but in many parts of the country it is nevertheless spoken by a majority of the inhabitants. In that respect, English could be classified as a 'minority language' in those particular communities. The term favoured by the European Community is 'Lesser Used Language', which again could be argued to be something of a misnomer in many circumstances. The term we have employed in this chapter is 'Minoritised Language' as this possibly describes more accurately the political situation of the language and the fact that, albeit in some communities the mother tongue of the majority of the inhabitants there, it is still not the majority language for most of the linguistic domains encountered by those speakers.

The experience of the Welsh language, and those who speak it, is not unique. Rather, its history shares important traits with that of other indigenous communities which have found themselves dominated by a more powerful and incoming culture. A recent series of studies (Dixon and Scheurell 1995:ix) draws common trends across the whole of the globe, tracing what the editors cite as a common process: 'political subjugation; negligence; shifting focus of social policy; social and legal discrimination; provision of social services; and ethnic, cultural and political rejuvenation'. In the Welsh context, these common patterns ring strikingly true. To use their five-fold division, the Act of Union of 1536 had as its purpose the *subjugation* of Wales to England in all significant spheres – political, administrative and cultural. A long period of *isolation* followed, before the Victorians embarked upon an active campaign of *assimilation*, based upon the belief most notoriously expressed in the 1847 Report into the condition of education in Wales that 'The Welsh language is a vast drawback to Wales and a manifold barrier to the moral progress and commercial prosperity of the people. It is not easy to over-estimate its evil effects' (Report known as *Brad y Llyfrau Gleision: The Treason of the Blue Books*). The twentieth century has witnessed a shift towards *protection* of the indigenous language, culture and welfare of Wales, as evident in the Welsh Courts Act of 1942 and the Welsh Language Act of 1967, which attempted to provide for the equal validity of Welsh and English in legal and public administration in Wales. In the final two decades of the century there has been clear evidence of *ethnic/cultural and political rejuvenation*, to be found, for example, in the tremendous growth in Welsh-medium nursery and school education, the successful foundation of the partly Welsh language television channel S4C and the widened sphere of rights to use the language and receive services through it as embodied in the 1993 Welsh Language Act.

Within Europe, where welfare provision has formed a more explicit part of the industrial settlement, these issues have some particular features. Catalonia forms an autonomous region of Spain and – like Wales – the indigenous language, Catalan, is spoken within that territory in tandem with a very powerful world language, Spanish (or Castilian). During the Franco years, the Catalan language and culture were severely oppressed and banned from almost all public spheres at a time when huge numbers of Castilian speakers were also moving into the area for employment. In addition, public social services in Catalonia and Spain barely existed before the establishment of a democratic constitution following the end of the Franco dictatorship in 1978 (Casas 1997). What is, to a certain extent, unique about the Catalan experience is that the development of a social welfare system and the resurgence of the language have occurred during the same period of time. Catalan is spoken by nearly 4 million people in Catalonia proper (64 per cent of the population), with a further 2 million speakers in the autonomous regions of Valencia and the Balearic Islands (Leprêtre 1992) as well as substantial linguistic communities in the *département* of Pyrénées-Orientales (Perpignan) France and the city of Alghero in Sardinia.

In Catalonia itself, the status of the Catalan language has been transformed during the ensuing years of democracy and is afforded complete official and legal status with Castilian. Catalonia passed a law of language normalisation in 1983 and ever since has actively legislated and planned for the spread of the social and public use of the language in all domains. The move from *subjugation* to *ethnic/cultural and political rejuvenation* (Dixon and Scheurell 1995) has occurred at an astonishing rate in Catalonia and at the same time a social welfare system has been developed throughout the region which has endeavoured to use as its medium the Catalan language. The situation in Spain is of particular interest as each autonomous community has responsibility for the creation and improvement of social services and this process had begun earlier in Catalonia than in other Spanish communities. This development has consequently facilitated the use of Catalan within the social welfare system and problems similar to those experienced in Wales – for example, the establishment and standardisation of terminology (Williams 1988; Prys 1993; Sitjà 1988) – have had to be faced. The Catalan experience is interesting from both a linguistic and a social work perspective as the term 'normalisation' is readily employed in the context of discussion of both areas: the concept of normalisation of a once minoritised language and of the provision of social welfare services has much to offer those engaged in the study of the interface between the two. Catalan can also be considered a non-territorial minoritised language, for example in the Perpignan region of France and Alghero in Sardinia, whose speakers nevertheless are able to avail themselves of the positive strides towards normalisation of the language within Catalonia proper and – to a lesser extent – the Valencia and Balearic communities.

Many other minoritised languages in Europe are still suffering from a lack of status and consequent social and legal discrimination. A sister language to Welsh is the Breton language spoken in the *département* of Finistère and the western parts of Côtes-d'Armor and Morbihan in France. It is currently estimated that about 450,000 people understand Breton, 300,000 of whom also speak the language (the French government does not undertake census enquiries into the numbers of speakers of its minoritised languages). Breton has no official legal status in Brittany and its speakers have no automatic right to use the language in their dealings with public administration there. It is virtually unknown for official documents – including those relating to the field of social welfare – to be available in Breton; there is no legal requirement for civil servants to speak the language and only limited use of Breton is allowed in the courts. Those speakers most likely to have difficulty in communicating through the medium of their second language (French) are also most likely to be either elderly people or – to a lesser extent – young children, with obvious implications and disadvantages for those citizens when they need to use the social welfare system. The situation of the Breton language reflects more accurately that of the many other indigenous minoritised languages of Europe than the more open and embracing developments witnessed in Catalonia, for example.

SOCIAL WORK RESPONSES IN WALES

Against this general background, a number of specific questions arise concerning the interface between social welfare and language which we now intend to explore within the Welsh context: (i) how have social work services in Wales come to meet the challenge posed by operating in a bilingual context? (ii) what are the issues which are specifically of importance to social work as a discipline? (iii) which concerns are relevant to social work as part of wider public services? (iv) what is the current state of response to these challenges?

The case for providing services in the Welsh language is not simply one of the numbers established earlier in this chapter: it is also emphatically one of good, effective and sensitive practice. Communication is the core of what social workers are about – and communication, very often, carried out in crisis. Even in more routine encounters welfare workers are engaged with people who need help with personal and private concerns. These are hard to talk about at any time, let alone while translating feelings and events into a language through which such personal material is never otherwise expressed. Such everyday encounters as helping someone who has been bereaved, or a teenager struggling to come to terms with changes in family life, are all damaged and devalued if sensitivity to language is not ensured. Within the day-to-day exchanges of social work there are, moreover, very important powers at play which allow workers and services to intervene in the lives of other people. A probation officer writing a report upon someone who may go to prison or a community nurse deciding whether or not someone is mentally ill, and thus contributing to his/her compulsory admission to hospital, are both involved in major decisions. The discussions which surround them are often difficult and stressful. How much more so – and how much more likely to be mistaken – if these discussions have to take place in a language which is one in which the person on the receiving end would not normally conduct her or his life. The outcomes for service users in these circumstances are potentially dangerous, as well as disadvantageous, if decisions are made on the basis of linguistic errors or misunderstandings. Finally, we need to remind ourselves that, at an individual level, users of social welfare services feel a stigma from the fact of being a user (Holman 1988). When these services are provided in a way which denies or devalues the basic experiences of such individuals, this adds to their feeling of being stigmatised (Allen 1983) and adds to the problem of achieving a positive outcome from these inherently difficult exchanges.

Attempts to have these principles recognised within the professional training and culture of social work have not always been easy and, although broadly successful, have only been so as the result of the united and determined efforts of individuals and groups within the profession with those of wider campaigners outside. The British experience is unusual, in this way, as it lacks the formal, written constitutional guarantees through which continental European countries have most often provided for language choice in formal circumstances – such as legal proceedings. In Wales, a series of Acts of Parliament now embody obligations placed upon agencies to provide services in a linguistically sensitive manner. The 1989 Children Act, for example, contains a requirement that due consideration be paid to 'race, religion, language and culture' when decisions about services for young people are being made (for a recent and useful account of the operationalisation of these concepts in Wales, see Colton *et al.* 1994). The Mental Health Act of 1983 and Section 95 of the 1991 Criminal Justice Act contain analogous obligations in their own spheres. More broadly, the 1993 Welsh Language Act, widely regarded as the single most significant piece of legislation this century in its implications, places new and significant duties upon public bodies to develop and deliver services which are fully and equally available in both Welsh and English.

The resulting principle, that service users, wherever they may be in Wales, have a right to receive that service in the language of their choice embodies, as a consequence, not only essential civil and political rights but, in the social welfare arena, is a fundamental of worthwhile practice.

NON-TERRITORIAL CONTRASTS

In an earlier section we suggested that lesser-used languages which are non-territorial – that is to say that are widely and dominantly spoken elsewhere – have certain differences in the call they are able to make upon public policy and promotion. In direct social work practice, however, these distinctions are possibly less significant. Evidence from the United States, perhaps the supreme example of non-territorial language diversity, suggests that use of a minority language has important cultural and identity connotations at the individual level. Stevens (1992:183), for example, suggests that

> the strong association between non-English languages and ethnicity . . . means that whether non-English language Americans use their minority language or use English in their daily social interactions sends messages about the ethnic cultures embodied in the language used and in the one not used.

Alba (1990) goes further in suggesting that knowing and using only a very small and grammatically unconnected amount of a non-English language is sufficient to affirm and give content to an ethnic ancestry. In Britain, recent research across three generations of Punjabi families has also emphasised the importance which use of the mother tongue plays in the transmission of core cultural values (Dosanjh and Ghuman 1997).

Against this background, it is our suggestion that many of the practice issues which occur in providing services for first-language Welsh speakers are of equal importance, at an individual level, in work with people who speak other minoritised languages. These are summarised by Pugh (1992) as including difficulties of basic access – what is available, from whom and where – problematic use of interpreters, difficulties in transposing the conceptual framework of one language into another and the obstruction of clarity of expression in one language of patterns of speech learnt in another. In Britain, the practical consequences of these difficulties have been highlighted more in the field of health care than social work. Hayes (1995), for example, in considering maternity services for women from an ethnic minority in the English Midlands, described them as 'inappropriate, inaccessible and inadequate'. Literature was most readily available in English, and where efforts had been made by organisations to provide material in a range of other languages the supply of that material in hospitals was often inconsistent. Audio-visual material was mostly written and spoken in English. Interpreting services were limited by lack of understanding and by the complexity of linguistic needs. Respondents to the survey were asked, 'What languages are spoken by the women who use the maternity services?' As Hayes says, 'The reply of "Indian" from one respondent suggests a remarkable lack of knowledge of the spoken Asian languages. More disturbingly, it may be indicative of covert racism.' It is not surprising, perhaps, in this context, to find that children were used to interpret for mothers attending for maternity care and that bilingual staff were expected to set aside their own duties in order to act as interpreters. In some health district hospitals records were not even taken of the language spoken by the service user. Nor can such deficits be explained entirely by lack of suitable information concerning good practice in such circumstances. Within the Health Service itself information has been commissioned and published which deals with the issues which arise in translation of written material from one language to another (Dada 1992). Good practice in working with interpreters has also been actively explored in a number of social work contexts, such as Abdulla and Payne's (1997) account of a Probation Service and County Council initiative in Nottinghamshire which aims to improve translation and interpretation services in the courts. The conclusion which Hayes draws, however, could still be replicated in many social work situations in Wales and other places where a territorial minoritised language is in use:

> Good maternity care requires intimate and sensitive communication between women and those who care for them. A woman whose medical advisers cannot speak her language is not only likely to be lonely and confused; there is also a danger that she will not be properly treated. Thus it should be the responsibility of the health services to ensure that proper communication is possible.

These findings have been borne out in other health-related research. In a specifically Welsh context, Roberts (1994) explored the communication between nurses and patients in a hospital setting, finding, for example, that many adults think in their native language, even while speaking their second language. Johnson *et al.* (1996) concluded that there were significant variations in minority ethnic community use of occupational therapy services. Carr-Hill and Rudat (1995), in an analysis of a national survey of health issues and ethnic communities, confirmed serious inequalities in the system and in its ability to respond to different language and cultural needs. Dickinson and Bhatt (1994), looking in more detail at the nature of these needs, concluded that absence of basic information and understanding concerning ethnic communities contributed significantly to health services' inability to combat inequality in uptake and outcome. Many of these findings are apparent in social welfare generally. Sandra Rennie (1993), working in Bradford and specifically in the field of social welfare services, concluded that, while the difficulties of providing mother tongue services were real, the disadvantages to service users of alternative methods were more formidable. In the end the choice returns to the basic question of where the balance of disadvantage should rest – with the powerful, in the shape of relatively large and rich service organisations, or with the powerless, in the shape of relatively small and impoverished users? The answers suggested by Rennie, and in this chapter, are unequivocally in favour of the responsibility falling to the former.

WELSH EXPERIENCE IN THE EUROPEAN CONTEXT

Being the speaker of a minoritised language – especially where that language is confined to a single geographical area – can lead to feelings of isolation and, conversely, accusations of insularity from majority language speakers. One refreshing consequence of the move towards a more integrated Europe has been the realisation that the Welsh speaker or the Catalan speaker is not alone. In fact, being bilingual is more of a global norm than being monolingual and it is estimated that 50 million citizens of the European Union use a language in their everyday lives which is different from the language of the state in which they live. The European Bureau for Lesser Used Languages set up by the European Commission has been active in promoting mutual understanding and fostering information exchange between linguistic minorities within the Union and there is a growing feeling of shared experience between the different language communities which has resulted in increased cross-fertilisation of ideas and developments, including some within the field of social work.

One example of this is the realisation that the level of literacy within minoritised language communities is often much lower than that amongst speakers of the official state language. Older Welsh and Catalan speakers, as a result of the previously monolingual education policies of the governments of Britain and Spain, are often literate only in English or Castilian whilst being far more articulate in Welsh or Catalan. There are, once again, obvious implications for social welfare services here, especially when these service users are required to complete forms. Similarly, as has already been mentioned, practitioners in the field who are speakers of the minoritised language may lack the appropriate professional vocabulary to be able to communicate through the written medium (for example, preparation of reports) and may therefore have additional training needs in order to become fully conversant with this aspect of their work. This has been addressed in Wales through the training and publication programme of the Central Council for Education and Training in Social Work Cymru/Wales, which has increased the material available to social workers through the medium of Welsh in addition to producing materials to raise awareness of practitioners in general of the importance of language sensitivity. Similar developments have been observed in Catalonia although, as indicated previously, the development of a social work framework in Spain has been much more recent than in Britain.

In recent years, there has been a growing consensus that language use and provision has to be planned for in the same way that other services are planned. The general language normalisation plan approved by the Generalitat of Catalonia in 1995, for example, sets general targets and sectoral targets for the normalisation of the Catalan language within Catalonia. Under Health and Care, for example, there is the specific target (55) to *stimulate language normalisation in health and care institutions, guaranteeing the use of Catalan in all public coverage services and in dealings with the users*. Further targets include normalising the use of Catalan in public and local administration and strengthening the rights of service users to receive those services through the medium of Catalan. As we state below, developments in Wales have been more makeshift but the passing of the 1993 Welsh Language Act has brought about a legal requirement for all public bodies (including Local Authorities) to produce language plans which have to be approved by the statutory Welsh Language Board. Many of these have yet to reach the more specific target-led approach witnessed in Catalonia but they will undoubtedly strengthen the provision in Welsh and the status of the language within Wales.

Language planning – although much more developed in Catalonia and the Basque Country in Spain – is still in its infancy in Wales and the lack of a devolved decision-making body until now has hampered developments in this direction. There is a specific language directorate within the autonomous communities of Catalonia and the Basque Country able to inform and influence not only language planning policies throughout their respective territories but also – and possibly more significantly – able to impact on the work of other governmental departments such as education, local administration and health/social care. Other minoritised language communities in Europe are often not so fortunate – as has been observed in the case of the Breton language – and the languages spoken by them have little or no official status. The situation of the Irish language (an official language in Ireland with some million and a half able to speak it but far fewer actually using it as the medium of their everyday dealings) should also be heeded in as much as successful language planning in any community must be carried out with the *active* support of the overwhelming majority of the speakers of that particular language as well as the good will of that section of the community which does not speak the minoritised language. Certainly in Wales, positive public attitudes towards the language from amongst non-Welsh speakers has contributed to a consensus which is willing to reverse previous trends of antipathy towards the language from some quarters and encourage a revival in its use and an improvement in its status.

What lessons might therefore be drawn from the Welsh experience to date and what features of this experience might be relevant to other bilingual European communities possibly aspiring to assert their language more successfully and gain greater status for it? The experience of Welsh in the public domain points to a very particular way of planning – both language and service provision planning – for the future and one which stands in direct contradiction to traditional understandings of public administration where the planning of public services is demand-led. New schools, for example, are built in areas of housing development where it is already known that a demand will arise. Use of Welsh language services operates in precisely the opposite way to these market models. Demand for public services in Welsh follows supply. Where there is no availability of Welsh language services, or where access to such services can be obtained only on special request, the level of demand remains very low. Once services are provided in a convenient and non-stigmatising manner, however, demand emerges where none had been suspected and at a level which exceeds the provision which has stimulated its appearance in the first place.

Social welfare services are no different. Where language choice is genuinely and freely left to the consumer, rather than determined by the service provider, not only does demand for Welsh increase amongst existing users but new approaches are made by those who previously had considered such services too remote from their own experience to benefit. This has been implicitly recognised in Catalonia, for example, where the setting of specific targets for provision of services through the medium of Catalan, as we have commented previously, has enhanced and increased language choice as well as normalising the use of the language within these domains which had previously been dominated by only the official state language. Recent experience in the Basque Country, where a policy is in place to enable every service user to have the choice of whether to use Castilian or Basque, has thrown up an interesting dichotomy, with Basque speakers still often opting for Castilian (Siencyn 1995). Research there has shown that Basque speakers wish to receive services with a minimum of 'fuss' and without being considered to be a 'nuisance'. This highlights the need for changes to be introduced in a gradual and sensitive manner without the service user necessarily being expected to have to keep to one language choice throughout – i.e. offering the possibility of being able to conduct a meeting through the mother tongue (Basque or Welsh) but of completing written forms in the state language (Castilian or English).

The second set of general lessons to be drawn from this account of social work in Wales centres around the question of responsibility for ensuring the sort of policies, services and practices outlined here. It is worth beginning with a restatement of the most obvious corollary that responsibility should not be left with the service user. The idea that 'they can have it if they ask for it', or even 'available on request' will not do. Service users come to social welfare agencies already vulnerable and ill at ease. They are most unlikely to add to their burdens, as they perceive them, by holding out for services which mark them out as demanding or difficult. Even within the general progress outlined in this chapter, there is much ground still to be made up. Sian Howys, a social worker describing the experience of service users in North Wales, suggests that on the ground this is still often characterised by 'negative or indifferent attitudes towards cultural circumstances of service users' which quickly escalates into an 'attitude towards those who insist on having their needs and experiences recognised of hostility, even when these are enshrined as a right. Such users come to be regarded as arrogant, awkward people, creating a deliberate difficulty' (Howys 1993).

The climate for linguistically sensitive services has to be created by the powerful, not the powerless, in social welfare encounters. This means that agencies and employers have to be in the forefront of the action. It also means that workers have to assume their responsibility, both in their own work and in resisting the harmful legacy of the 1980s which has seen a retreat from organised pressure and campaigning.

CONCLUSION

In this chapter we have tried to illustrate, from the Welsh example, some of the most significant contemporary issues which arise when we attempt to apply the principles of linguistic sensitivity to the particular context of social welfare practice. Social welfare encounters bring into sharp focus those qualities which characterise the relationship between an individual and the state in which she or he resides. Consideration given to language issues in the design and delivery of such services tells us much about the state of settlement between the powerful and the relatively powerless, between the governing and the governed in particular societies. Our conclusion has to be that, against a gradually improving background, developments in different parts of Europe remain very mixed. Wales emerges as a locality where, in comparison with other European nations, much has recently been achieved and yet where important lessons remain to be learned. In that sense, the experience explored here stands as a metaphor for the future needs of all minoritised languages in Europe, if the fundamental linguistic rights of its citizens are to command the priority they deserve.

Key summary points

- Concept of minoritised languages and the role of power in the creation of minority status.
- The right of the user to the language of choice as good practice.
- Bilingualism the 'norm' in Europe, with examples of minoritised languages.
- The distinction between territorial and non-territorial minorities.
- Language as fundamental to the individual's identity and culture.

NOTE

1 We use the term 'normalisation' throughout as employed in Catalonia, i.e. that the language in question – invariably a less used language – may once again be used normally in every situation or domain where use of the majority or state language is currently dominant. The Catalan Language Normalisation Act 1983 states that it 'proposes to overcome the current situation of linguistic inequality by stimulating the normalisation of the use of the Catalan language throughout Catalan territory. In this sense, the current law guarantees the official use of both languages in order to ensure that all citizens may participate in public life; establishes knowledge of both languages as an educational objective; balances them in the communication media; eradicates discrimination for reasons of language; and specifies the means of channelling linguistic normalisation in Catalonia.'

REFERENCES

Abdulla, M. and Payne, D. (1997) 'Good practice in working with interpreters', *Probation Journal*, 44:2, 86–8.

Aitchison, J. and Carter, H. (1994) *A Geography of the Welsh Language 1961–1991*, Cardiff, University of Wales.

Alba, R.D. (1990) *Ethnic Identity: The Transformation of White America*. New Haven. Yale University Press.

Allen, R. (1983) *Can We De-Stigmatise Social Work?* Social Work Monographs 13, University of East Anglia, Norwich.

Carr-Hill, R. and Rudat, K. (1995) 'Unsound barrier', *Health Services Journal*, 105, 28–9.

Caroll, J.B. (1956) *Language, Thought and Reality: Selected Writings of Benjamin Lee Whorf*, Cambridge, Mass., MIT Press.

Casas, F. (1997) 'Child welfare in Catalonia', in *Stigma and Child Welfare*, Aldershot, Avebury.

Casson, M., Cooke, P., Jones, M. and Willliams, C. (1994) *Quiet Revolution? Language, Culture and Economy in the Nineties*, Aberystwyth, Menter a Busnes.

Colton, M., Drury, C. and Williams, M. (1994) 'Policies on ethnic, linguistic and religious needs in Wales under the Children Act 1989', *Social Work and Social Sciences Review*, 5:1, 45–63.

Council of Europe (1996) *Report of the Study Group on the Initial and Further Training of Social Workers, Taking into Account their Changing Roles*, Strasburg, Council of Europe Steering Committee on Social Policy.

Dada, M. (1992) *Multilingual AIDS: HIV Information for the Black and Minority Ethnic Communities*, London, Health Education Council.

Davies, E. (1994) *They All Speak English Anyway*, Cardiff, CCETSW/Open University Press.

Dickinson, R. and Bhatt, A. (1994) 'Ethnicity, health and control: results from an exploratory study of ethnic minority communities' attitudes to health', *Health Education Journal*, 53:4, 421–9.

Dixon, J. and Scheurell, R.P. (eds) (1995) *Social Welfare with Indigenous Peoples* London, Routledge.

Dosanjh, J.S. and Ghuman, P.A.S. (1997) 'Punjabi childrearing in Britain: development of identity, religion and bilingualism', *Childhood*, 4:3, 285–304.

Drakeford, M. (1997) 'What's in a name?', Cardiff, unpublished paper.

Durkacz, V.E. (1983) *The Decline of the Celtic Languages*, Edinburgh, Donald.

Gruffudd, H. (1996) *Y Gymraeg a Phobl Ifanc*, Research Papers in Continuing Education, Department of Adult Continuing Education, University of Wales, Swansea.

Hayes, L. (1995) 'Unequal access to midwifery care: a continuing problem?' *Journal of Advanced Nursing*, 21, 702–7.

Holman, B. (1988) *Putting Families First*, London, Macmillan.

Howys, S. (1993) 'Welsh speakers and social work: a case of discrimination in action'. Paper given to CCETSW seminar, 'Race, Culture, Language and Social Work', Cardiff.

Johnson, M.R.D., Petherick, R., Jeffcoat, M. and Wright, A. (1996) 'Local authority occupational therapy services and ethnic minority clients', *British Journal of Occupational Therapy*, 59:3, 109–14.

Leprêtre, M. (1992) *The Catalan Language Today*, Barcelona, Generalitat de Catalunya.

Morris, S. (1996) 'The Welsh language and its restoration: new perspectives on motivation, lifelong learning and the university', in *Communities and their Universities – The Challenge of Lifelong Learning*, ed. J. Elliott, H. Francis, R. Humphreys and D. Istance, 148–63, London, Lawrence and Wishart.

Prys, D. (ed.) (1993) *Geirfa Gwaith Plant / Child Care Terms*, Cardiff, University of Wales.

Pugh, R. (1992) 'Lost in translation', *Social Work Today*, 13.8.92.

Rennie, S. (1993) 'Language differences and social work – muddling through the confusion'. Paper given to CCETSW seminar, 'Race, Culture, Language and Social Work', Cardiff.

Roberts, G.W. (1994) 'Nurse/patient communication within a bilingual health care setting', *British Journal of Nursing*, 3:2, 60–7.

Siencyn, S.W. (1995) *Sain Deall: Cyflwyniad i Ymwybyddiaeth Iaith*, Caerdydd, CCETSW Cymru.

Sitjà, M. (1988) *Terminologia dels assistents socials*, Barcelona, Collegi oficial de diplomats en treball social i assistents socials de Catalunya.

Stevens, G. (1992) 'The social and demographic context of language use in the United States', *American Sociological Review*, 57, 171–85.

Thomas, N. (1994) 'Welsh-speakers as a territorial linguistic minority in the European Union', in *Social Work and the Welsh Language*, ed. R.H. Williams, H. Williams and E. Davies, 155–72, Cardiff, CCETSW/University of Wales Press.

Welsh Office (1995) *1992 Welsh Social Survey: Report on the Welsh Language*, Cardiff, Government Statistical Service.

Williams, C. (1996) 'Welsh, social work and the future of the language', Cardiff, CCETSW.

Williams, H. (1988), *Geirfa Gwaith Cymdeithasol/A Social Work Vocabulary*, Cardiff, University of Wales.

Chapter 7

Non-governmental organisations and the welfare of minority ethnic communities in Britain and Germany

Maureen Hirsch and Diana Powell

INTRODUCTION

Our discussion in this chapter is based on our joint professional experiences of community social work with and for minority ethnic group interests and our many years as tutors in social work education. We draw on our own research studies in the British West Midlands region and in and around Berlin, Germany, as well as on the recently published work of others.

Despite the fact that the post-war history and processes of immigration are very different in the two countries, we have been intrigued to discover that minority ethnic organisations in Britain and Germany have many similar functions and experiences. In both cases they are extremely important sources of support, advice and social care for their members. They are also expected to explain their cultural norms and values to the wider society in order to counteract racism and to act as helpful community representatives and advisers to many ethnic majority organisations. The work of these groups is rarely evaluated and publicised by social scientists and their contribution to the development of European Community work theory and practice is widely ignored. We hope that this discussion will encourage others to acknowledge the integrity of minority ethnic welfare groups, accept the need for them to be self-determining and explore with them ways of developing and supporting their valuable work.

BRITAIN

In this section we have used the term Black when we specifically refer to people of African Caribbean descent and Asian when we refer specifically to people whose families originated in the subcontinent of India. The generic term 'black' is adopted when we refer to non-white sectors of the population collectively.

Immigration and citizenship

Ethnic diversity through migration has been a factor in British society over many centuries, including a long history of black people settling in Britain. The dynamic contributions to British cultural, economic, political and social life made by migrant communities has been well documented (Fryer 1984). However, many migrant groups have also been subjected to hostile, phobic and oppressive reactions by the 'receiving' societies of the time and some groups, such as Irish people, Jews and black people, have experienced persistently negative social relations with white Britons, at least in part due to the incorporation of ideologies about supposed racial categories and hierarchies into all aspects of the British social system (Husband 1982).

However, the importance of these historical migrations is generally conveniently disregarded by those who espouse simplistic notions of 'national' character and identity. Contemporary ethnic diversity in British society is popularly ascribed to the post-Second World War period, when what is often characterised as a largely homogeneous society received substantial numbers of people of visibly different appearance and geographical origin. From 1948 to the 1960s immigration from the so-called 'New Commonwealth' countries, most notably the subcontinent of India and the British West Indies, was, at least in part, encouraged by certain government departments, whose efforts to rebuild the British economy were hampered by grave labour shortages. Commonwealth citizens had a right to enter Britain to work and to settle, a right which was to be steadily eroded as white racism in various shapes and forms transformed immigration and 'race relations' into major national issues that would affect the British political agenda for the rest of the century. However, the majority of these groups of Commonwealth immigrants and their descendants were and are full British citizens.

Throughout this post-war period, migrants and refugees from countries all over the world have continued to widen the ethnic diversity of the British population. There have been two significant responses to this trend, both underpinned by legislation and characterised by successive governments as interdependent social policy goals: severely to restrict further immigration in order to legitimise efforts to promote racial integration and equality. Drastically curbing rights of entry to Britain, especially of those people deemed to be 'racially' different from the white majority, has been the major aim of the increasingly restrictive nationality and immigration legislation enacted since 1961. Outlawing racial discrimination was facilitated through the enacting of specific Race Relations legislation in 1965 and 1976 and through incorporating equal rights clauses into the regulations governing a range of social institutions, including employment, health and welfare.

Immigration, social deprivation and social policy

The majority of Black and Asian post-war migrants settled in the inner-city areas of large conurbations, where many of the manufacturing industries needing cheap labour were located and where, due to demographic changes, low-cost housing was increasingly available to rent or buy (Rex and Tomlinson 1979). These neighbourhoods were run down and neglected, the very environmental conditions which led to cheap housing coming onto the market in the first place, as indigenous families sought to improve their standards of living. However, in the 1950s and '60s, the presence of immigrant communities became popularly associated with and were frequently scapegoated for the downward spiral of inner-city poverty and deprivation. At the same time, overt racial discrimination in its crudest forms made it extremely difficult for black families to move away from these 'receiving' areas. Low wages, due to gross discrimination in the labour market, public and private housing agencies and associated financial institutions such as building societies, all contributed to a process of inner-city 'ghettoisation'.

From the mid-1950s a number of black and multiracial non-governmental organisations were active, lobbying government for legislation to curb the increasing violence of racist groups and to tackle widespread racial discrimination. Labour MP Fenner Brockway's Bill to tackle such discrimination was defeated in 1958 and it was not until the election of a Labour government that Home Secretary Roy Jenkins successfully introduced the first Race Relations Act (1965), which outlawed overt forms of racial discrimination and incitement to racial hatred. The shortfalls in this legislation became increasingly evident and Labour brought forward further legislation (the 1976 Race Relations Act) which introduced the important concept of 'indirect discrimination', allowing British researchers and institutions to trace patterns of discrimination and to enable the development of focused policies to tackle racial disadvantage.

Subsequently, equal opportunities and fair treatment requirements have also been incorporated into other legislation, for example laws regulating local government services, mental health and child welfare. During the 1990s, formal equal opportunities policies and codes of practices have become increasingly adopted by a growing number of public and commercial institutions in the UK. Many equal opportunities specialists perceive legal sanctions to have made a particularly significant impact on discrimination, resulting in many positive improvements to the life chances of British people of minority ethnic descent (Taylor, Powell and Wrench 1997). However, recent research data continue to demonstrate that minority ethnic identity can still be a highly significant factor in the aetiology of social and economic disadvantage (Jones 1996).

In 1966 the Labour government's Local Government Act provided for grant aid to those local authorities able to demonstrate the presence of 'New

Commonwealth' populations. This funding, widely known as 'Section 11 funding', provided very modest sums of money to 'top up' funding for additional services to meet their needs. It was initially taken up almost exclusively by local education authorities, for 'English as a second language' teaching and some 'mother tongue' work in the classroom, but eventually became the means of funding specialist initiatives in many local authority services, such as housing departments, planning, public health and, as will be discussed later, social services.

Section 11 funding and the other packages of 'urban aid' and 'urban renewal' funding introduced by successive governments since the 1960s largely perpetuated this mixture of developing limited access to mainstream welfare services through special 'ethnic minority' projects and sponsorship of community groups by the local state to deliver mainly small-scale, ethnically discreet 'meeting and eating' social provision. Minority ethnic communities, families and individuals continue to be regarded as an additional burden to service providers rather than part and parcel of normal society.

Currently, central and local government funding are 'farmed out', sometimes to new partnership schemes, sometimes as grant aid to independent projects, sustaining the claim that equal opportunities goals are being met through grant-aiding minority ethnic services. There are usually strict constraints governing such funding, including time-limitations on its availability. Like most white voluntary organisations (Marshall 1996), black and minority ethnic organisations are struggling to resolve the serious confusion arising from the dramatic changes to their role, income and management systems resulting from the privatisation of health and welfare in Britain.

The role of non-governmental organisations in British welfare provision

Voluntary welfare bodies have a long and remarkable history of campaigning and pioneering work on behalf of many minority groups in British society. These roles were legitimised in the Beveridge Report in 1948, which underpinned the ideology of the British welfare state, while underlining the continued importance of the voluntary sector for its professionalism and 'independence from public control'. From the 1950s to the 1970s, voluntary organisations argued that their greatest strength lay in their independence from government, their ability to respond very quickly to new or changing needs and the intrinsic moral and psychological value of unpaid, reciprocal relationships based on care and compassion (Titmuss 1973). Charities and voluntary groups flourished as political watchdogs and campaigners, specialist service providers for specific minority groups, and as pioneers identifying and seeking to alleviate previously unmet needs. Thus, while the state met the welfare needs most commonly found in society, non-governmental organisations concentrated on raising the money to provide additional specialised services for people with particular needs, research, advice and advocacy services, and developing public awareness of and responses to 'new needs'.

During the 1960s, Enoch Powell MP fanned the flames of racial tension about the possibility of an escalation of violence in British cities, his famous 'rivers of blood' speech (1968) reinforcing the alarm caused by the American experience of inner-city disturbances associated with the struggle for civil rights. As early as 1967, the Home Office signalled its concerns about the growing evidence of the ill-treatment of black people by the police, issuing a circular to all Chief Constables (The Police and Coloured Communities) which advised them to appoint liaison officers in areas of black settlement. The local Community Relations Councils (now Racial Equality Councils) which were established from 1965, under the auspices of the new quango, the Community Relations Commission, have been condemned as '"buffer institutions" heading off a direct assault on the Establishment by the black community' which diverted the most able black community leaders from leading radical organisations such as the Campaign Against Racial Discrimination (CARD) (Ben-Tovim and Gabriel 1982). Nevertheless, in the late 1960s and the 1970s, Brixton CRC and others were included in a growing number of independent anti-racist bodies and individuals producing studies and reports about racial discrimination and the failure of front-line public services to meet the needs of minority ethnic groups, fuelling demands for remedial action (e.g. Smith 1977). However, these groups were, by and large, not sponsored by or connected to any of the main national voluntary organisations or their umbrella organisations, such as the National Council of Social Service (now the National Council for Voluntary Organisatons – NCVO).

The ethnocentricity and insidious racism of British voluntary organisations has received relatively little attention. Even the current literature on non-governmental welfare agencies only exceptionally includes information about the specific experiences of minority ethnic welfare organisations, their workers or their users (e.g. Davis Smith, Rochester and Hedley 1995). However, the continued marginalisation of the needs of minority ethnic groups by British welfare organisations has made it even more necessary for minority groups to put their best efforts into building their own community organisations to meet the needs of community, family and individual. In 1988, the Black People in Volunteering Group claimed: 'The Black voluntary sector is booming – but this is because black people have had to create their own organisations,' and continued with the magnanimous view that 'White voluntary agencies have not responded to black needs because for the best of reasons black people are seen as marginal because of their small numbers, or for the worst of reasons because there is real prejudice and racism'.

Today, British ethnic minorities sustain a sophisticated network of local and national voluntary organisations and networks covering, *inter alia*, information and advice services, day-care centres, educational initiatives, women's support groups, youth clubs and residential elder-care (e.g. Phaure 1991). They are also still the main protagonists to campaign on behalf of the black and Asian victims of a range of social and legal injustices.

Community work and inner-city deprivation

The limitations of interpersonal forms of social work intervention were widely debated in the 1960s and '70s, especially in relation to the social problems thrown up by poverty and social deprivation. The Labour governments of the period were committed to tackling poverty and the American 'War on Poverty' programme provided a model for alternative approaches to what was, at the time, characterised as a 'cycle of poverty' passed on from one generation to the next. Government funding to mobilise local action to tackle local social and economic problems has been a major plank of social policy for several decades, although each new government redefined its urban renewal ideology and goals. With hindsight it seems self-evident that the scale of this support could make only a marginal difference to the position of disadvantaged communities, but for a while, from the late 1960s to the late 1970s, community work flourished as a new, distinctive and exciting approach to social problem-solving.

Community work projects were based on the belief that promoting community participation and mobilisation could 'unlock' a hidden reservoir of resources in deprived areas, generating social and economic improvements through helping people to identify local social needs, develop self-help skills and negotiate for additional resources. This in turn would lead to a new sense of neighbourhood pride, strength and commitment, and paid community workers could then leave voluntary community activists to get on with their new agendas. The best known of the government-funded initiatives, the Community Development Projects, set up in a number of inner-city and other communities, had a short and controversial life. The research studies which ran alongside the projects identified the main weaknesses of the programme as arising from the government's (erroneous) belief that poverty and deprivation were the result of dysfunctional individual and group characteristics. The CDP workers and researchers developed an alternative analysis which suggested that people in deprived areas were the victims of unfair local and national government systems, keeping them in ignorance of their legal and income rights. The government became disillusioned with the initiative and did not extend their funding beyond the initial experiment (Edwards and Batley 1978).

Poor families, then and now, struggle to meet the costs and demands of even the most basic life-style The well-worn political belief (echoed in more recent Conservative government policies) that solving complex social problems can readily be achieved through somehow releasing significant 'untapped community resources' in deprived neighbourhoods really is a modern myth. Setting up local advice and support services requires a huge effort by disadvantaged communities and running projects thereafter requires an exceptional commitment from what invariably turn out to be very few key individuals. Additionally, such initiatives almost always need external financial support, not only to get them off the ground, but also to keep them going. From 1978 to 1981, this flourish of British community work activity formed the basis of an influential series of paperback books sponsored by the Association of Community Workers, including one on community work by and with black people (The Community Work Series).

However, many community work projects espoused a colour-blind approach, defining and subsuming the needs of Black and Asian communities under those of the wider white society, and many white community workers regarded racial discrimination and disadvantage as a product solely of class division. They invited immigrant residents to join white-dominated community groups to tackle what were seen as common problems for the working classes, such as poor housing conditions and unresponsive public institutions; the widespread failure of minority communities to become involved with these initiatives was ascribed to their inability or unwillingness to participate because of language barriers, cultural differences, or a desire to 'keep themselves to themselves' (Harlesdon Community Project 1980). There was also a real inability on the part of many white community workers to get to grips with white racism in the disadvantaged communities in which they operated.

These perspectives dominated the content of community work literature of the time, marginalising the contribution of minority ethnic community groups to British community work theory and practice for many years. They underpinned an increasingly racially divided voluntary and community work environment, where white groups mainly allied themselves to the local Councils of Social Service (now Councils of Voluntary Service) while black organisations became members of the local Community Relations Councils (now Racial Equality Councils). This divide is still very marked in some of the urban areas in which we have worked in recent years. However, the NCVO has gradually developed its work with black groups and in 1991 it launched the national Organisational Development Unit to support and represent more than 2,000 black voluntary groups across the country.

Until the 1980s, social workers and services virtually ignored the presence of minority ethnic groups in Britain as a policy or practice issue, failing to recognise the racism and ethnocentricity which pervaded their attitudes, decisions and intervention techniques.

During and since the Thatcher years, professional community work was drastically curtailed and today most state-funded community development work, at least in the provinces, seems to be located in the youth and community education services of Local Education Authorities, concerned mainly with home–school liaison and various forms of adult education. The inner-city disturbances of the 1980s also engendered a range of palliative youth-oriented community-work responses, offering social and educational development opportunities to disaffected black people who were failed by the school system (Cross and Smith 1990).

Social welfare and community care in the multi-ethnic society

For some twenty-five years, the social welfare needs of minority ethnic families continued to be subsumed under the rubric of 'universal provision' to the population at large and it was not until 1976, when the Association of Directors of Social Service drew attention to the availability of Section 11 monies to help develop minority ethnic social work projects that many Social Services Departments made bids for funding (ADSS/CRE 1978). This funding was seen as a way of gaining additional resources both to cover Social Services projects, such as employing minority ethnic social workers, and to support voluntary initiatives such as luncheon clubs for minority ethnic elders, based at community and religious centres (Johnson, Cox and Cross 1989). Section 11 funding allowed most local authorities to continue to reserve mainstream budgets for the white majority. By the mid-1980s, notably, but probably not only, in Bristol and Birmingham, evidence was emerging about the way that even Section 11 funding was being subverted to provide services to largely white neighbourhoods.

This failure of the mainstream state welfare system to meet the needs of minority ethnic communities effectively during those decades and the need for change has been well documented since the early 1980s (e.g. Cheetham *et al.* 1981). In 1981, the Scarman Report on the origins of the so-called 'Brixton Riots' by young Black people in London unexpectedly provided a powerful insight into some of the effects of racial discrimination on the experiences and life-chances of Black and Asian people (Scarman 1981). Since the further serious inner-city disturbances of 1981 and 1985, official concern about the position of minority ethnic groups in British society has waxed and waned, but health and welfare agencies have largely avoided any spotlight on their slow pace of change in relation to racial equality, probably because public attention has been distracted by the other fundamental changes imposed on these services by recent Conservative governments.

Today, despite the emphasis that current Child Care, Mental Health and Community Care legislation places on the need to meet appropriately everybody's ethnic and cultural needs, mainstream state and non-governmental welfare agencies still provide relatively few genuinely multicultural, ethnically sensitive universal services able to reach and help all the communities they serve. Services specifically geared to meet the needs of ethnic minorities are largely located in the non-governmental sector and run by minority community groups themselves. Indeed, during our recent studies, this has been presented to us by Health Authorities and Social Services Departments as a deliberate policy, justified both by the pressure to privatise services and by the difficulty of providing mainstream, ethnically sensitive services for the range of ethnic groups in their area. In our study areas, some funding for this diversification is commonly allocated from mainstream budgets, but at least matching and often majority funding has to be raised through applications for central government grants under schemes such as the Single Regeneration Budget and/or to charitable sources.

In fact, constantly thrown back on their own resources (and despite the racial discrimination and poverty which circumscribed those resources), black and other minority ethnic community organisations flourish in many cities, fanning the vital sparks of creativity, self-determination and political sophistication which characterise their individual members and organisations today. It is in such groups and associations that many Black and Asian welfare professionals gain the early experience which leads them into their chosen careers. However, only a minority of community activists get the chance of professional training; most community-based welfare service projects are staffed by ordinary people, who have restricted opportunities to access training courses, even those designed for voluntary workers. Courses aimed at minority ethnic volunteers are an even rarer commodity (Billis and Harris 1996).

During the stringent welfare cutbacks and reappraisals of the 1980s and '90s, social work also redefined its professional goals, establishing a new qualification with a strong managerial bias and excluded community work entirely from its repertoire of strategies and skills. The emphasis on an anti-discrimination code of practice was hailed as a great breakthrough and Social Services Departments have certainly been key players in the promotion of equal opportunities policies and codes of practice in many local authorities. It is also true that the transformation of social work theory and practice into a new multiracial and anti-discriminatory activity is, perhaps inevitably, proving to be a slow process.

Section 11 funding had been used by many SSDs to fund the employment and secondment for training of Black and Asian workers. These recruits are now experienced social workers, many of whom are now rising up the management ladders of social work agencies. It is to be hoped that, with their advancement, the commitment to racial justice and ethnic sensitivity in social welfare will enjoy a renewed impetus.

Purchasers, providers and partnerships

A new system of community care has been introduced, predicated on dividing welfare bodies into 'purchasers' and 'providers'. Central and local government departments now concentrate on policy development and public resource allocation, acting as the service purchasers. Internal statutory services, private companies and voluntary organisations compete to win contracts as service providers.

The emergence of competitive contracting as the main mechanism for determining who is going to implement government policies, and the greatly enhanced role of non-governmental organisations as direct service-providers, have placed a huge burden on the voluntary sector, especially on smaller, community-based bodies. Success in this arena requires a sophisticated grasp of formal tendering and accounting procedures, experience of professional styles of management and service delivery and the ability to sustain the effort needed to provide regular, consistent, good-quality services to clients. Recent research studies have identified many important and problematic issues arising out of the changing position of British voluntary organisations, including questions to do with accountability and democracy, governance and professionalism, consensus and advocacy (Nicholls 1997; Russell, Scott and Wilding 1996).

This picture is further complicated by the pluralist nature of British society, especially its cultural and ethnic diversity. The vast majority of national and local voluntary welfare organisations overwhelmingly represent and respond to white people as their primary constituents. Even the most recent literature examining the current position of the voluntary sector ignores or makes only the briefest references to black and ethnic minority non-governmental organisations and volunteers. Good coverage tends to consist of comments on the paucity of information about them and calls for 'more research' – a response reiterated so often by white researchers that it drives many black community groups and agencies (who generally have a good understanding of the needs of their own community members) to near despair!

It is becoming clear from recent studies that the concept of 'partnership' between statutory and voluntary welfare agencies is flawed by fundamental inequalities of power in the relationship. By and large, the state bodies have the upper hand, as they sponsor and guarantee the public funding allocated to voluntary bodies, determine the levels of accountability required for their continued support and financially squeeze voluntary sector providers over contracts for community care services. Additionally, there are real problems for organisations run by women and/or by black people, who described to Russell, Scott and Wilding (1996) how the 'old boys' network' marginalised them in relation to 'the places where decisions were made about the allocation of local authority grants and contracts'. Thus smaller and newer community groups which, by their very nature, often represent less 'popular' minority needs are placed at a particular disadvantage.

It is clear that in the new economic environment of competition and quality control, all voluntary organisations experience high costs in order to meet the rigorous targets, keep the detailed records and regularly produce the complex reports required by many service contracts and Nicholls (1997) draws attention to the complaints of white mainstream Mind groups about 'Purchasers [having] . . . high expectations of providers, for example skills and experience in budgeting, drawing up proposals and monitoring'. However, two black project managers have recently privately expressed the view to us that their organisations are subjected to particularly demanding targets, checks and balances, compared to established white organisations. Russell, Scott and Wilding (1996) suggest that black service providers do experience greater extremes in public authority responses to them. They cite one example of an African Caribbean voluntary day centre for older people being subjected to accusations of maladministration and corruption and a formal investigation, followed shortly afterwards by a substantial increase in their funding. This example of publicly 'shaming' a Black organisation with such serious charges, which are subsequently disproved, is not unique and we are concerned that persistent racist stereotypes may still play a part in shaping the reponses of some statutory agency managers to Black-led and managed voluntary organisations.

Recent studies on health and welfare issues conducted by the Centre for Research in Ethnic Relations at the University of Warwick (Johnson and Powell 1997) show that almost all the services identified as specifically aiming to be accessible and acceptable to Black, Asian and other minority ethnic populations are one-off projects, organised on shoestring budgets. On the other hand, however, it must also be acknowledged that the development of local authorities contracts to deliver community care services is providing opportunities for many black and minority ethnic groups to bolster their income and develop their role in the community.

African Caribbean respondents in our study of the needs of carers in Black families (Powell, Taylor and Johnson 1996) revealed a range of reactions to the mainstream agencies with whom they had had contact. These ranged from satisfaction with some practical services, through doubts about statutory agencies' ability to provide appropriate, culturally relevant support services, to active distrust and cynicism about the nature of white-dominated institutions' commitment to black people's welfare. These reactions were instrumental in the recent establishment of a new community-based service to provide support services specifically for African Caribbean carers. We are now in a situation where most non-governmental organisations are being diverted from their previous campaigning and advocacy role. They are becoming the providers of essential health and social services, under contract to the local state, because of their ability to give 'value for money' through using volunteer labour and operating on a non-profit-making basis. Government grants and community care contracts mean also that they are increasingly being drawn into the orbit of state control. This has obvious implications for everybody, but is particularly problematic for minority ethnic groups, which depend heavily on community groups to confront the societal racial inequalities which underpin the racial inequalities still to be found in British health and welfare provision. It is also a worry for those activists who believe that voluntary organisations can uniquely serve society by acting as independent watchdogs, identifying the gaps, inconsistencies and failings in social policies and campaigning for change – a critical role that is rarely encouraged by government!

Relationships between statutory and voluntary organisations are strongly shaped by the contrasting and sometimes apparently incompatible values of qualified professionals and unqualified community carers. Their relative strengths are often polarised as 'objective professionalism' versus 'subjective compassion', failing to acknowledge the fact that the best professionals are able to bring real care and concern to their work, while the best community carers readily accept the boundaries of confidentiality and self-determination. It is, however, crucially important to many minority ethnic service users, most of whom have experience of insensitive treatment by officials and professionals, that they can rely on easy communication with and unequivocal acceptance by their own community members when they need help.

Community organisations have been and remain a vital component in the lives of most minority ethnic people. They were originally formed to provide practical and spiritual support to migrants. Many came to have important political voices, campaigning against racial inequalities and representing minority ethnic concerns to the wider community. Gradually their functions have been extended to provide alternative but essential services to members of their communities whose welfare needs are not met by the mainstream agencies. They have demonstrated their ability to survive under the most difficult circumstances, displaying an extremely impressive level of collective compassion and determination.

Although many national and local agencies, both statutory and voluntary, separately and in partnership, are now aware of the need to develop their provision to address the welfare needs of black and minority ethnic groups, it must be said, as was argued about Social Services Departments in 1976, that the overall picture remains 'patchy, piecemeal and lacking in strategy' (ADSS/CRE 1978). The services provided for and by members of minority ethnic community groups themselves do still provide many of the best models of good, ethnically sensitive and culturally relevant welfare practice in Britain today.

GERMANY

Immigration and citizenship

Despite superficial similarities, the legal position and social experiences of migrants to Germany after the Second World War significantly differ from those of immigrants to Britain. Today the German minority ethnic voluntary welfare sector reflects such differences, although we feel there are some interesting resonances with aspects of the British situation. The most fundamental differences arise from the legal status of immigrants in each country and the similarities from mutual experiences of racial discrimination, which have thrown them back onto their own resources and community action to tackle welfare problems.

From 1945 to 1991 Germany was divided. West Germany was known as the Federal Republic of Germany (FRG) and East Germany as the German Democratic Republic (GDR). The FRG was not only much larger in area and population than the GDR but also much more highly industrialised. As in Britain, immigration was encouraged to ameliorate the post-war labour shortages in both Germanies. Despite measures to incorporate most women of working age into the workforce and to recruit immigrant labour from 'socialist friendly' countries such as Vietnam, Angola and Mozambique, the GDR never solved its labour shortage problem. The population in the FRG was greatly increased by the post-war migration of ethnic Germans from eastern Germany, from Poland, Hungary and the USSR and the economy was kick-started by redevelopment aid from the USA under the Marshall Plan.

From the 1950s, however, the FRG's industrial reconstruction required ever more labour and, having no ex-colonies to call upon, the government offered opportunities to people from Spain, Portugal, Italy, Greece, the former Yugoslavia and most significantly Turkey to become 'guest-workers' (*Gastarbeitern*). The FRG made formal agreements with these countries to admit their nationals as 'guest-workers' for only as long as the German economy needed them. Permanent settlement and entitlement to full citizen status was never on the FRG agenda and, unlike Britain's Commonwealth immigrants, they were legally excluded from mainstream German political, economic and social life.

In 1974 contractions in the German economy led to the introduction of legislation (known as the *Ausländerstopp*) which virtually ended this immigration although some dependants were still allowed to join their families, reflecting British measures similarly to restrict immigration in 1971. The ending of the *Gastarbeitern* policy was not the end of migration to the FRG, however, as its post-war constitution allowed easier entry for asylum seekers than was permitted by most other Western nations. Large numbers of Turks also continued to enter, seeking asylum from the oppressive regime in Turkey. The FRG had always reiterated that it was not a country of immigration (MacEwen 1995) – indeed German language usage has no equivalent for 'immigrant' or 'ethnic minority' – and the 'guest-worker' concept for overseas-born workers was deemed sufficient. However, it has become increasingly clear that many immigrant workers have become settled. From the mid-1970s the term '*Ausländer*' (foreigner) or '*Asyland*' (asylum seeker) became widely applied to those perceived as having an unfamiliar ethnic origin.

Both Germanies adopted laws outlawing incitement to racial hatred, although, despite strongly enforcing it, the GDR never publicised this legal provision. In 1993, research conducted in Berlin found that such activity had been heavily punished in the GDR, but that the victims of racial attacks and insults were bewildered by the state's insistence on keeping the events and the punishment secret (Hirsch and Katalikawe 1995). Conversely, in the FRG there seems to have been little commitment to punish incitements to hatred or racial attacks despite the legal framework.

Immigration and social policy since German unification

A new Aliens Act in 1991 gave some 'foreigners' improved rights of abode and greater hope of naturalisation, but in 1993, a huge increase in asylum seekers (around half a million) to the now reunited Germany led to constitutional changes enabling restrictions to be applied to asylum seekers and economic migrants. The current legal position is that unless an old 'guest-worker' agreement is still in place, a foreigner can only fill a job vacancy if no German citizen is available. The foreigner cannot apply for German nationality, which is based on the concept of *ius sanguini* (literally 'of blood') unless they can convincingly claim that 'they have German blood in their veins'. There is no right to nationality from being born in Germany (*ius soli*) so that even second and third generations of Turkish and other descent are generally not entitled to German nationality.

A unified Germany, except in the most general formulation of the constitution, has no specific anti-discrimination law and in most areas of life it is not illegal to discriminate against people on grounds of racial or ethnic identity This lack of official protection is largely justified on the grounds that 'foreigners', despite paying their taxes, are not entitled to the same housing, education, employment, social security, health or welfare rights as German citizens, simply because of their temporary status. There has been an increase in racial violence since unification, with some horrifying deaths receiving widespread publicity internally and externally. The allegation that such violence is largely a feature of the eastern provinces is, however, strongly disputed.

Although the post-war reconstruction of German cities means that there is not really an equivalent to British 'inner-city deprivation', many migrants do find themselves living in the remaining run-down, pre-war inner-city housing stock. Some special temporary housing provision has been made over the years, with many 'guest-workers' and other migrants living in special hostels. The scale of population movements into Germany in the 1990s also led to the establishment of large temporary camps, such as those on the eastern outskirts of Berlin. Many immigrants and their families are trapped in a cycle of disadvantage which is directly linked to their precarious legal status and in consequence to their racial or ethnic identity and certainly there is no legal remedy for such discrimination. For example, until the 1980s there was a complete absence of programmes specifically designed to meet the needs of Turkish children, reflecting the insistence of German federal and provincial governments that the place for the children and dependants of 'foreign' workers is back in Turkey. Even today, provision remains patchy and the German government makes no bones about the fact that meeting the health, welfare and educational needs of 'foreigners' is far less important than meeting the needs of the former ethnic Germans from Eastern Europe.

Thus Germany still simply takes the view that 'foreigners' are merely workers whose dependants have little claim on the state. However, although the 'myth of return' is still strong for many Turks in Germany (that is, the belief that one day they will return to their original homeland for good), the reality is that immigration restrictions, plus the growth of second- and third-generation families, have greatly increased the desire for permanent, legal settlement. What was originally expected to be a temporary migration has turned out, in practice, to be a resettlement – a pattern found in countries all over the world, including Britain. The contrast lies in the more secure legal position of most migrants and their descendants in Britain and in the widespread social and political consensus that minority ethnic groups are entitled to enjoy equality of opportunity combined with respect for their ethnic and cultural diversity.

Social welfare and community care before and since unification

The post-war constitution of the FRG, now the constitution of unified Germany, enjoined a welfare state upon Germany, but a welfare state of a fairly residual nature (Ginsburg 1992). The place of the state as provider of welfare services other than social security and related benefits has always been assumed to be that of last resort. Most social welfare provision in the FRG was organised through and by large voluntary organisations, most particularly the Catholic and Protestant churches. Surprisingly, according to Lorenz (1993), the church also played a crucial role in East Germany: 'the Protestant Church of the GDR had much greater direct influence over its social services, which often operated in opposition to communism, than it did after unification.'

German society does not consider itself to be a multi-ethnic society in the way this is understood in Britain. While the majority of migrants to Britain were and are legally entitled to access the social security, health and welfare systems at times of need, this was never the case for the FRG 'guest-workers', unless their national government of origin had made a special agreement with the German government or the migrants were members of a trade union offering such services. 'Guest-workers' were not expected to become a charge on the state if they became too old or too ill to work, or to have children. By contrast, many foreign workers in the old GDR were entitled to take up such services, but these were provided in such a way that the foreigner would not feel integrated into the wider society. For example, in the GDR separate housing complexes were provided for foreigners.

After unification, when West German institutions supplanted those of East Germany, the Vietnamese, Angolans and other 'guest-workers' in the GDR were treated as unlegalised foreigners in the new state, so many people lost their access to jobs, health and welfare services unless they could access some of these benefits through their membership of a trade union. German trade unions play an important role in defending 'guest-workers' against job discrimination and this is one reason why 'guest-worker' membership of and participation in certain unions was and remains consistently high.

Interpersonal social work and community care services in both German states were mainly located in the large voluntary sector. In the FRG this was organised by the churches and in the GDR by a 'citizen solidarity movement', which strongly encouraged all sections of the population to participate as volunteers. In the GDR even the adoption of children was arranged by such 'amateurs' drawn from professions such as teaching and medicine. The FRG has a stronger base of trained and paid workers. In fact Lorenz notes that in Poland in 1983, some 44,000 volunteers undertook 'face-to-face social work' compared with around 9,500 paid workers, of whom only about 30 per cent were professionally trained, which largely reflects the pattern of social work in the GDR until unification.

In West Germany, the left-wing Social Democratic Party lost power in the later 1970s to the conservative Christian Democratic Union Party under Chancellor Kohl, which continues to hold power in the new unified German state. There have been social policy developments similar to those in Britain, with a move towards greater market involvement with welfare provision and an even greater emphasis upon the involvement of the voluntary sector. A policy of saving state expenditure and policing the take-up of state benefits has been driven by a rapidly expanding rate of unemployment since unification, ascribed to several factors: the arrival of several million 'new Germans' (ethnic Germans from Eastern Europe); the arrival of very large numbers of 'new foreigners' in the FRG in the 1980s and early '90s; and the closing down of GDR state businesses. The situation has been further complicated, as in most Western nations, by demographic changes leading to a rapid growth in the proportion of older people in the population.

The role of the voluntary sector continues to be paramount in the modern German state, although, as Lorenz also points out, the activities of voluntary organisations have to conform to a 'host of laws and regulations' which 'have a restricting effect' on their service provision. Many smaller organisations in the united Germany have had to seek patronage or even incorporation from the larger voluntary organisations to remain viable. Mainstream organisations have not entirely ignored the needs of 'foreigners' and efforts have been made to recognise and respond to some migrant communities. However, the leading roles in projects aiming to help 'foreigners' which are sponsored by the FRG's mainstream voluntary sector were invariably held by what Krojzl (1987) calls 'white Germans'. The prevailing view has been (and tends to persist) that German nationals know what is best for 'foreigners'.

A similar pattern pertained in Britain for many years, but today major British welfare organisations regard this approach as racist and patronising and seek to appoint minority ethnic staff to run culturally specific welfare services. However, there is a striking similarity between Britain and Germany in the funding of minority ethnic services. Self-help groups set up by 'migrant' communities in each country may be autonomous in that they organise their own activities and choose their methods of work, but they are frequently dependent on ethnic majority money, which requires them to adopt priorities, aims, objectives and management systems that are acceptable and accountable to those funders.

Social welfare organisations and minority ethnic groups

In common with many other Western European countries in the 1980s, the FRG saw a large increase in the number of voluntary organisations, particularly self-help initiatives providing localised contact and information services (Lorenz 1993). However, although volunteers were a major part of the labour force in state sponsored social services, the states of Eastern Europe, including the GDR, had sought to suppress that aspect of civil society which gave rise to independent voluntary organisations. It was assumed that state provision would meet all needs and that alternatives might be a threat to the state, a situation which made the continuation of church-based welfare work all the more remarkable.

The development of various new social movements in the FRG in the 1980s challenged the dominant position of the more traditional large social and political organisations and the politics of state institutions. These included the green environmentalist movement, which for some time gained seats in the Bundestag, the peace movement, the women's movement and the squatters' movement, which gained greater influence, both philosophically and politically, than any equivalent movements in Britain. Not only did they, albeit temporarily, offer challenges to conventional and traditional ideas of politics in Germany, but they encouraged alternative life-styles and prefigurative models for services and organisations. These *Alternativen* provided a platform for anti-racist campaigns and created a climate in which some new Yugoslavian, Turkish, Spanish and Greek community organisations could emerge in the 1980s.

Institutional provisions to ease the social settlement of 'foreigners' are limited to a very few educational projects in a very few 'Turkish' areas, such as Kreuzberg in Berlin; a little mother-tongue teaching in a very few schools and a few multicultural programmes where radicalised teachers really pushed the local state towards 'concessions'. In the 1980s, sections of the teaching profession became radicalised, even though they were officially civil servants and subject to the policing of left-wing ideas through the law of *Berufsverbot*. Some of these teachers, for example, responded to Spanish and Greek parents' groups who were pressing for certain improvements in the education of their children, enabling the establishment of Saturday Schools.

The Turkish government has itself insisted that Germany should allow them to organise a Turkish education for young German-based Turks. Additionally, some Islamic groups active in vying for the allegiance of the Turkish population in Germany have set up Islamic supplementary classes. However, the formality and ideologies of these various sources of additional education have not always endeared them to the young German-based Turks, despite strong parental pressure to participate.

As Lorenz pointed out, because integration, rather than multicultural or anti-racist approaches, has been the only alternative official policy to deportation and refusal of re-entry, teachers and youth workers were being trained to 'deal with problems of integration, an approach which in fact problematised the pupil rather than the school'. He suggested that this approach implies that 'it is the alien who has to make the efforts to adjust' and that assistance primarily needs to address the deficits the ethnic group has in relation to the indigenous population.

Partly as a result of this kind of assumption, the main springboard for setting up minority ethnic community organisations has been to provide social and cultural services, but there are also projects which focus on providing ethnically sensitive advice and support services.

Some of the projects and programmes for minorities run by 'white German' organisations have been aimed at women and girls. This is partly because of the strength of the women's movement in Germany, but also because of the German view that women and girls have only very limited autonomy in some 'foreigner' groups (Krojzl 1987). However, as in Britain, the ethnocentric nature of this perception has become more widely acknowledged in recent years. Many self-help groups are primarily organised for and by women and the role of migrant women as community activists and welfare workers is also very important in both countries.

Some provincial governments have set up Commissions for Foreigners and these bodies are probably the nearest German equivalent to the British Racial Equality Councils, but the German bodies have less foundation in the national legal and administrative framework.

The 'foreigner' populations of the eastern *Länder* (states), who lost their original status at the time of reunification, were usually forced to move to asylum seekers' centres or camps, on the outskirts of Berlin and other large towns. Some official voluntary organisations were created to provide them with welfare advice and other information and a number of East Germans displaced from their jobs after unification were allocated to temporary 'training' posts to work with these bewildered and uncertain people.

Community action, self-help and 'foreigner' organisations

The position of 'foreign' minorities in Germany is affected by the predominant position of the Turks, who are by far the largest single minority group. Yet they themselves are not a united group in any way. National, ethnic, political and religious divisions are highly significant among this population. For example, one important and distinctive group is the Turkish Kurds, who have a separate language and different customs from other Turks. In addition to this and other 'minorities within minorities', there are serious religious divisions within the Turkish community in Germany, between different Muslim groupings, including fundamentalist groups. A strong secularist group also exists. It is clear, therefore, that voluntary and self-help organisations are inevitably also diverse, coming together on the basis of ethnic, language, religious and political allegiances.

Thus 'foreigners' organising politically as pressure groups or as welfare providers have to take into account three problems: many differences of identity, the lack of anti-discrimination law to support their work and struggles, and the continued insecurity of their settlement in Germany, even after three generations. Most significantly they are generally denied the right to vote in elections and it is this exclusion from the German democratic process which shapes the *raison d'être* of many minority ethnic community organisations.

The divided nature of the large Turkish population delayed the development of any co-ordinated Turkish political pressure for some time. Although some umbrella organisations do now exist, most minority ethnic community groups in Germany have been set up by and for very specific ethnic and religious groups. As in Britain, minority ethnic organisations in Germany often started as cultural projects, conserving and transmitting the culture and heritage of the homeland, but have subsequently found it necessary to add counselling, information and advice work to their original remit. They also undertake much literacy work, both in German and in mother tongue languages. Workers routinely spend a large percentage of their time accompanying clients to fill up the many and repeated official forms through which the German state controls its 'foreigner' population (Hirsch and Katalikawe 1995). These visits are frequent and take a very long time, as staffing levels in government offices are low and also because interpreting is needed by a proportion of the clients.

Case notes on three typical 'foreigner' organisations in Germany

Research was carried out in Berlin in 1993 (Hirsch and Katalikawe 1995) with sixteen organisations which were either set up by the local state, staffed by 'white German' or minority ethnic workers, to provide a variety of services to a particular group, or were set up by minority groups themselves staffed by their own members, sometimes as paid workers and sometimes as volunteers. Follow-up contact in 1997 found little change in the fundamental situations described below.

A statutory organisation

The Oase pankow – an 'oasis' for 'foreigners' to meet and obtain help – was set up by the German authorities just after unification, to assist a variety of minorities in the eastern part of Berlin. Most of the workers were 'white Germans' who had lost their jobs at the time of unification and were assigned to government work schemes. The small number of ethnic minority or 'foreigner' workers on the staff were there solely to interpret and translate, as assistants to the German workers. Considerable criticism was voiced by the staff about the limited resources made available to help 'foreigners' and in general they seemed to be quite sympathetic to the groups they were trying to help. However, there was a feeling that it would be better to provide aid and development programmes in the countries of origin than to help people to settle in Germany.

Two particular endeavours were evident at the Oase pankow: individual case-work with 'foreigners' (some newly arrived) and setting up multicultural education and events for local schools and the population at large. Arrangements were made for individuals such as Turks, Vietnamese and Bosnians to go into local schools to explain their culture to pupils and teachers and discuss how it was surviving in Germany. Lunches offering different cuisines on different days were offered in the Oase Centre and cultural evenings, Turkish dance classes and similar activities were held regularly, as part of an attempt to combat racism, which was understood to have its origins in German ignorance of other cultures. However, the preponderance of Romanians and Poles arriving at the Centre for advice was not reflected in the 'cultural understanding' work, which was concerned with minorities of longer standing.

This kind of educational work did not have a generic title such as 'multicultural' education. Educating the native population about other cultures was assumed to be a short-term activity, needed to stem a tide of racist attacks by Germans on 'foreigners'. Both the advice work and the cultural work had the character of fire-fighting exercises and were often undertaken by people who knew very little more than the recipients. The non-Germans involved in the cultural education work were nearly always unpaid. It was assumed that they would be glad to tell Germans about their culture on a voluntary basis, ultimately creating a more accepting and safer environment for themselves.

Oase pankow was financed through joint funding from the Berlin local state authority, the Berlin Commissioner for Foreigners Office and the national Job Creation scheme. It was still functioning on this financial basis in late 1997.

A minority ethnic self-help project

The Union of Turkish Women is run by women of Turkish origin and is unaligned to any religious or statutory body. It was set up with the aim of making cultural, leisure and educational opportunities available to women and girls of Turkish origin without repressing women's aspirations, which some of the more traditional Turkish and fundamentalist mosques can do. Nor is it under the control of 'white German' women who also might impose a separate agenda. The staff, two of whom are paid and full-time, are all of Turkish origin. The Union is funded partly by the Berlin Commissioner for Foreigners Office and partly by the Berlin Senat.

The organisation carries out case-work with individuals and undertakes 'inter-ethnic understanding' work. Advice work is also an important function – for example about pensions and income for older people in both Turkey and Germany. It is still quite common for women to join their husbands in Germany and their position for the following three years is equivocal, as their right to be in Germany depends on how their status is given on their husband's visa. If a marriage fails for any reason, the wife usually faces deportation. There are no refuges specifically for Turkish women yet and even if there were this would not necessarily offer protection from deportation.

The South East Centre

This was originally a cultural organisation, trying to provide a place for ex-Yugoslavs to meet, with the hope of fostering understanding between the various national and ethnic groups of the old Yugoslavia. During the research visits in 1993 (Hirsch and Katalikawe 1995) the Centre employed adults from various Yugoslav ethnic backgrounds, to teach children art and theatre skills in the languages of the old country. There were also parties, talks and dances, all aimed at keeping the cultures from the region alive and preserving some feeling of unity.

There were four paid workers, one of them part-time, funded by the federal state job placement scheme and a grant from the Office of the Berlin Commissioner for Foreigners. The Centre was forced to start offering individual help – both advice and continuing counselling – in response to the needs of people suffering directly or indirectly from the war in the former Yugoslavia. Perhaps because the main workers were women, the difficulties of women affected by the war had become a particular concern. There were 32,000 people of Yugoslavian origin in Berlin when the conflict began, but the numbers were still growing rapidly in 1993. The Centre offered help to all newcomers whatever their ethnic origin, providing housing, income, legal and immigration advice. However, encouraging cultural exchange remained their main philosophy.

The role and position of minority ethnic organisations in Germany

These three organisations have been mentioned only to give a flavour of the variety of organisations for and of 'foreigners' in Germany, Berlin in particular, in 1993. These three are quite typical in that they were usually trying to fulfil a wide variety of objectives. One major objective was to stimulate and conserve the culture of minority ethnic groups and to hand it on to new generations born and brought up in Germany, often with the idea that this would help them on their eventual return to their country of origin. Some of them were also expected to carry out 'multicultural understanding' work with German nationals, mainly as an 'anti-racist fire-fighting' exercise.

A second main objective was to offer support to individual members of such communities in their dealings with the German state and society. Most organisations were concerned with very specific ethnic groups living in the locality. Some groups, particularly those with women and girls as their focal point, to some extent offered support in the face of traditional and male cultural influences.

It has been suggested that, in Berlin at least, Turkish organisations have provided models for others, despite the fact that in Turkish traditional rural life there was no place for voluntary organisations. Women's and girls' groups have been particularly successful and are considered partly responsible for the fact that younger women are more integrated and achieving greater advancement in some German institutions than are men (Krojzl 1987). These organisations show greater informality and less of a hierarchy of 'helper' and 'client' than other organisations.

The organisations survive with low staffing ratios and need volunteer involvement to function. There are now trained social workers of 'foreigner' origin, who are always employed for their ethnic background rather than because they are trained social workers (Lutz 1993). However, most workers in these community organisations are still concerned lay people with no professional training in this sort of work. Indeed, there is little evidence of a yearning for professionalisation.

The importance of local state funding and funding by the Commissioners for Foreigners means that organisations must take care that their activities do not cause concern by being seen as too radical in any way. Although the level of funding was quite low, it was fairly secure, so that the organisations did not have to spend their time fundraising for core activities, as is so common in Britain. One umbrella organisation, the Union of Turkish Migrants' Organisations, had built up good relationships with the Commissioner for Foreigners in Berlin, but was subjected to attacks by the police through the media, for being 'over-ambitious' for Turkish civil rights. They were aware that the Berlin Commissioner was herself also attacked for being 'radical' in the field of foreigner relations, by the Berlin Senat and by the CDU Party (of which she was a member).

SOME COMPARISONS BETWEEN GERMANY AND BRITAIN

British governments over the years have funded many projects to tackle inner-city deprivation in general, which include specific objectives in relation to relieving racial disadvantage in particular. German governments have not developed such programmes for two main reasons: first, the rebuilding of so many German cities after the war (using Marshall Aid from the USA) and the consequent success of the post-war economy of the FRG, made it largely unnecessary to have any general redevelopment plans for inner-city areas as immigration began in earnest. Second, because minority ethnic groups were only allowed into Germany as temporary 'guest-workers' with few claims on the German state, there was almost no idea that the social or welfare needs of 'foreigner' minorities should be met at all. Acceptance of the fact of permanent settlement by Turks and others is still resisted by the German state.

Despite the British Conservative government assertions in the 1990s, that business support was the way forward for all voluntary organisations, there is little evidence that commercial companies themselves believe this to be appropriate, except where charitable grants attract tax concessions. Even where they do make grants, these are almost always to white mainstream bodies, rarely to minority ethnic groups. Similarly, financial involvement by German businesses in support of 'foreigner' organisations is virtually non-existent.

Although there are now many Turkish businesses in Germany, particularly in the Kreuzberg area of Berlin, they have not yet provided funding for minority welfare organisations. In Britain, there is a longer history of successful minority ethnic business enterprise, but our work in the Midlands suggests that where financial support is available from such businesses, it tends to be channelled to and through religious rather than welfare bodies.

Some grant aid is made available to a number of groups by German and British local government authorities. However, where these are controlled by the minority ethnic groups themselves, there tends to be strong central control by government representatives. In Germany these people are motivated by the belief that assimilation is a more desirable goal than are long-term multicultural or anti-racist aims. In Britain negative stereotypes about minority ethnic groups means that they are generally not trusted to manage either public monies or their internal affairs in an efficient manner. In both countries there is a widespread view in majority ethnic circles, that the increasing acculturation of British or German-born minorities means that ethnically specific services will be needed only for a finite period, so there is little commitment to incorporate such provision into the mainstream. However, there is a wide gap between the official British view that it is desirable and possible to build a multicultural society of British citizens, which enjoys respectful and equitable social relations between all its ethnic groups, and the German approach, which continues to differentiate legally between 'white German' nationals and everyone else, whatever their origin or history.

In both countries, too, the better funded, larger voluntary organisations, as well as most statutory bodies, are usually run by men and almost always by members of the ethnic majority. Organisations run by 'foreigners' in Germany are also similar to minority ethnic welfare organisations in Britain, in that they are small, very local and offer specific kinds of services – income and legal rights advice, together with counselling and support work are typical. They are much more likely to be led and staffed by women. Their income is small and insecure enough to mean that they can have difficulties in recruiting and keeping suitable managers and workers. This is due to a variety of factors. In Britain, for example, their small size and their remit to help minority groups means they are marginalised even in the voluntary sector and project leaders and staff gain experience and skills which often enable them to obtain better paid work or to access adult education schemes. Such voluntary work has long been a springboard for black, minority ethnic and white working-class politicians, especially in local government; it has also given significant opportunities to black and white women and working-class people to access further and higher education – for example, over the past fifteen years, we have worked with a growing number of social work students drawn from such backgrounds.

The German *Alternativen* groups offer a variety of local advice, drop-in, women's social and discussion groups, literacy classes, German language classes and so on, in contrast with the more official, centralised organisations controlled by 'white Germans'. The British voluntary work sector has always been very varied and throughout this century has provided a home for community action by many small radical groups. Nevertheless, the work of minority ethnic voluntary groups is still frequently overlooked and marginalised, so that the ethnic majority remains largely ignorant of the range, quality and sheer quantity of vital welfare work undertaken in the various communities. Few minority ethnic organisations in either Berlin or the British West Midlands are represented in large umbrella organisations and networks of mainstream voluntary and statutory organisations. This inevitably means that they are often not aware of the important fund-seeking, advice work and other training courses which are available (Caglar 1995). It also continually reinforces the idea amongst white welfare managers that there are very few viable black welfare groups with whom to consult and collaborate. In Britain there is also a distinct lack of training designed for Black and Asian volunteers and community leaders (Billis and Harris 1996).

Germany's 'foreigner' minorities do not have the right to vote in most elections, so are usually excluded from local political networks; hence they do not pick up on developments until much later than do German citizens' groups and organisations. It is only through trade union networks that Turks and others have been able to become politically active, but trade unions are not usually connected up to those networks that are important for developing work in localities. This is true to some extent in Britain too, where community projects are usually organised by and for those who spend most of their time in the neighbourhood where they live – people with young children, especially mothers, disabled people, older people and unemployed people – all sectors of society unlikely to be found in the informal corridors of power, where many decisions about local government policy and resource allocation are really made. However, the gradual increase in the number of black professionals and managers and the growing influence of black political activists and elected black politicians, particularly at local government level, is beginning to have a discernible impact on the ability of black groups to access resources and facilities. Black national networks and umbrella organisations do now exist in Britain, offering guidance and support to local welfare groups. For example, the nationally produced Black Carers' Charter provided an influential guide to good practice for a carer support project recently established in the West Midlands (Powell *et al.* 1996).

The much more secure settlement situation of ethnic minorities in Britain has meant that statutory bodies, including the professional training agencies, have been forced to develop responses to the presence and needs of minorities. The inclusive nature of the professional code of ethics for social work has also provided a valuable springboard for the articulation and implementation of anti-racist values, policies and codes of practice. Trained Black and Asian workers are a small but growing minority in the profession and are moving up the British social welfare hierarchies. The few 'foreigner' social workers and youth workers who exist in Germany are still confined to the grass roots, often as interpreters and aides to white German workers as they interface with 'foreigner' clients. Efforts in Britain to include minority ethnic groups in joint endeavours have not been particularly successful, but this should not mean that such efforts should be abandoned but rather that they must be more imaginative, consistent and continuous, carried out with more consultation and ultimately deliver greater self-determination and control to the minority groups themselves. In Germany there is still little idea that 'foreign' minorities should ever see their needs met by German statutory agencies, while the large voluntary agencies concentrate on a few well-defined concerns, such as tackling racist attacks and harassment – a social problem which has, of course, a peculiar resonance for the German people. Unlike Britain, Germany has no supporting anti-discrimination legislation and, until minorities achieve civil and political rights, it is difficult to see how such legislation might be framed.

It is clear that it is impossible adequately to meet the welfare needs of minority ethnic groups in either country solely through separate, ethnically specific provisions, except in a very few areas where there is a big enough concentration of one minority population. Even then, an outwardly united group is likely to contain significant numbers of people who speak different languages, follow different religions, hail from regions hundreds of miles apart and belong to different social classes.

CONCLUSIONS

The multiplicity of ethnic groups now resident in each country means that an effective equality of service will probably only be achieved through the development of non-racist, multicultural services located within the mainstream statutory and voluntary welfare sectors. The current British trend of contracting out ethnically specific local services to community projects has many benefits, but it can lead to some individuals not getting the specialised help they need, such as mental health support. It also places a considerable administrative burden on small groups and can result in tying them in so closely with targeted funding and keeping them so busy with routine chores that they can no longer tackle controversial political issues or respond to new needs in the community. A much better balance has yet to be achieved, between informal support systems, ethnic sensitivity and high-quality professional care.

Although British social workers are required to develop their sensitivity to racism and cultural diversity in their professional training, German social workers, particularly in the youth services, not only have to come to terms with and face their country's recent racist past, but also have to learn the hard way, on the job as it were, how to challenge the groups of German youths who are actively sympathetic to neo-Nazi ideas (Lorenz 1993). In this area of work, there is a large body of experience in Germany which could usefully be shared with British youth and community workers.

We have noted that racist stereotypes constantly influence transactions between majority and minority groups in both countries, which undermines the effectiveness, confidence and independence of minority ethnic workers and community-based services in a variety of ways. Despite their commitment, tenacity and originality, it is clear that, unless a very real effort is made to overcome these prejudices, minority ethnic voluntary organisations will never be able to meet all the welfare problems of their own communities. It is also clear that they could offer the wider societies some alternative and imaginative approaches to social care, but the effort needed to sustain their efforts at local level also constantly militates against this.

Finally, minority ethnic voluntary organisations are the main source of ethnically specific welfare provision for discrete minority communities in both Germany and Britain. If they are to deliver ever more efficient and effective services, then certain points need to be taken into account by the mainstream funding bodies, welfare agencies and community social workers:

- All community-based services benefit from funding arrangements which are secure over several years and do not impose excessive surveillance and control by funding agencies;
- Minority ethnic voluntary organisations must be fully independent and free to undertake advocacy work and campaigns on behalf of their constituents;
- Regular non-patronising consultation between mainstream and minority agencies and managers is essential for the development of equal opportunities and a high standard of service in both sectors;
- Minority ethnic workers and service users are themselves the best experts on their own needs and how to meet them effectively;
- Minority ethnic groups are best helped by appropriately trained paid or voluntary welfare workers from the same background.

BIBLIOGRAPHY

Association of Community Workers (1978–81) The Community Work Series. Routledge and Kegan Paul, London.

Association of Directors of Social Service/Commission for Racial Equality (1978) *Multi-Racial Britain: The Social Services Response*. CRE, London.

Atkin, K. and Rollings, J. (1993) Community Care and Voluntary Provision: a review of the literature. *New Community* 19 (4), 659–67. July 1993.

Behrend, H. (ed.) (1995) *German Unification: The Destruction of an Economy*. Pluto Press, London.

Ben-Tovim, and Gabriel, (1982) The politics of race in Britain, 1962–79, in C. Husband (ed.) *Race in Britain: Continuity and Change*. Hutchinson University Library, London.

Billis, D. and Harris, M. (eds) (1996) *Voluntary Agencies: Challenges of Organisation and Management*. Macmillan, London.

Bort, E. (1997) German Identity after Reunification. Paper to Questions of Identity Conference, Queen Mary and Westfield College, March 1997.

Caglar, A. S. (1995) German Turks in Berlin: social exclusion and strategies for social mobility. *New Community* 21 (3) July 1995.

Cheetham, J., James, W., Loney, M., Mayor, B. and Prescott, W. (eds) (1981) *Social and Community Work in a Multi-racial Society*. Harper and Row/Open University Press, London.

Cochrane, A. and Clarke, J. (eds) (1995) The German Welfare State: a conservative regime in crisis, in *Comparing Welfare States: Britain in an International Context*. Sage with Open University, London.

Cross, M. and Smith, D. I. (eds) (1990) *Black Youth and YTS: Opportunity or Inequality?* National Youth Bureau, Leicester.

Davis Smith, J., Rochester, C. and Hedley, R. (1995) *An Introduction to the Voluntary Sector*. Routledge, London.

Edwards, J. and Batley, R. (1978) *The Politics of Positive Discrimination*. Tavistock, London.

Faist, T. (1995) *Social Citizenship for Whom?* Avebury. Aldershot.

—— (1997) Immigration, Citizenship and Nationalism. Internal internationalization in Germany and Europe, in M. Roche and R. Van Berkel (eds) *European Citizenship and Social Exclusion*. Ashgate, Aldershot.

Farleigh, A. (1990) Invisible Communities. *Community Care* 22 March.

Fryer, P. (1984) *Staying Power: The History of Black People in Britain*. Pluto Press, London.

Harlesdon Community Project (1980) *Community Work and Caring for Children*. Owen Wells, Ilkley.

Ginsburg, N. (1992) *Divisions of Welfare: A Critical Introduction to Comparative Social Policy*. Sage, London.

Harris, M. (1997) *The Jewish Voluntary Sector in the United Kingdom: Its Role and its Future*. Policy Paper No. 5. Institute for Jewish Policy Research, London.

Hirsch, M. M. and Katalikawe, J. (1995) Sources of Redress for Ethnic Minorities in European Union Countries: notes from a comparative study. *Studies in/Equality* 1 (2). Summer 1995. Coventry University.

Husband, C. (ed.) (1982) *Race in Britain: Continuity and Change*. Hutchinson University Library, London.

Johnson, M., Cox, B. and Cross, M. (1989) Paying for Change? Section 11 and local authority social services. *New Community* 15 (3). April 1989.

Johnson, M. and Powell, D. (1997) *The Coventry and Warwickshire Alcohol Advisory Service and the African Caribbean Community*. CRER, University of Warwick.

Johnson, M., Powell, D. and Tomlins, R. (forthcoming) *Minority Housing and Social Care Needs in Warwickshire*. CRER, University of Warwick.

Jones, Trevor (1996) *Britain's Ethnic Minorities: An Analysis of the Labour Force Survey*. Policy Studies Institute, London.

Krojzl, C. (1987) The Social Institutions of Turkish Migrants in West Berlin. D.Phil. thesis, Oxford University.

Langen, M. (1990) Community Care in the 1990s: the Community Care White Paper 'Caring for People'. *Critical Social Policy* 10 (2).

Littlechild, R. (1996) *Investigating the Mental Health Needs of the South Asian Community in the Small Heath Constituency of Birmingham*. Social Services Research Paper No. 3. University of Birmingham.

Lorenz, W. (1993) *Social Work in a Changing Europe*. Routledge, London.

Lutz, H. (1993) In Between or Bridging Cultural Gaps? Migrant women from Turkey as mediators. *New Community* 19 (3). April 1993.

MacEwen, M. (1995) *Tackling Racism in Europe: An Examination of Anti-Discrimination Law in Practice*. Berg, Oxford.

Marshall, T. F. (1996) Can We Define the Voluntary Sector? in D. Billis and M. Harris (eds) *Voluntary Agencies: Challenges of Organisation and Management*. Macmillan, London.

Nicholls, V. (1997) Contracting and the Voluntary Sector. *Critical Social Policy* 17 (2). May 1997, London.

Phaure, S. (1991) *Who Really Cares? Models of Voluntary Sector Community Care and Black Communities*. London Voluntary Service Council, London.

Powell, D., Taylor, P. and Johnson, M. (1996) *The Needs of Carers in African Caribbean Families in Coventry*. CRER, University of Warwick.

Rathzel, N. (1991) Germany: one race one nation. *Race and Class* 32 (3), 31–48.

Reading, P. (1994) *Community Care and the Voluntary Sector*. Venture Press, Birmingham.

Rex, J., Joly, D. and Wilpert, C. (eds) (1987) *Immigrant Associations in Europe*. Gower, Aldershot.

Rex, J. and Tomlinson, S. (1979) *Colonial Immigrants in a British City*. Routledge and Kegan Paul, London.

Roche, M. and Van Berkel, R. (eds) *European Citizenship and Social Exclusion*. Ashgate, Aldershot.

Russell, L., Scott, D. and Wilding, P. (1996) The Funding of Local Voluntary Organisations. *Policy and Politics* 24 (4). October 1996.

Scarman, Rt Hon. The Lord (1981) *The Brixton Disorders 10–12 April 1981*. Cmd. 8427, HMSO, London.

Siddall, R. (1995) Journey's End. *Community Care*, 6–12 July 1995.

Smith, D. and Wistrich, E. (1997) Citizenship and Social Exclusion in the European Union, in M. Roche and R. Van Berkel (eds) *European Citizenship and Social Exclusion*, Ashgate, Aldershot.

Smith, D. (1977) *Racial Disadvantage in Britain*. Penguin, Harmondsworth.

Taylor, P., Powell, D. and Wrench, J. (1997) *The Evaluation of Anti-Discrimination Training Activities*. International Labour Office, Geneva.

Titmuss, R. (1973) *The Gift Relationship*. Penguin, Harmondsworth.

Chapter 8

Child welfare in wartime and under post-war conditions

The Bosnian case as a point of departure for reflections on social work with refugees

Sven Hessle and Marie Hessle

INTRODUCTION

An analysis of the activities described in this chapter confirms the somewhat foregone conclusion that psychosocial work under conditions of war and post-war differs from psychosocial work in times of peace. And of course the conditions for organising and implementing social work in a country at war differ from the conditions existing in the country or countries of exile. To articulate these differences more fully, we conclude the chapter by introducing an exploratory model, based on our experiences, in which some of the prerequisites for doing social work with people fleeing from war or post-war conditions are delineated. The refugee's journey from a war-torn country, such as former Yugoslavia, to a country of exile, such as Sweden, and back home again upon the restoration of peace is a very complex and tortuous one, particularly if we take into account the continual outbreak of ethnic group conflict and the differences between the two countries' welfare systems and ways of organising social work.

BACKGROUND

The war in former Yugoslavia has resulted in the forced migration of nearly half of the inhabitants of the now divided nation. Thousands of children have been orphaned, made homeless or sent away to a place of refuge in other countries. In this chapter we will describe the efforts to devise tools for doing psychosocial work with war-traumatised children and their parents and relatives who came to Sweden as refugees during the war. We have also participated in setting up similar projects in Bosnia since 1996 during the peace process under the Dayton Agreement. With support from UNICEF, the schools of social work at the universities of Stockholm and Sarajevo have been engaged in training social workers in the field to organise and evaluate the placement of around 3,000 unaccompanied minors in Bosnia.

There are three basic principles that have guided the conduct: the principles of family continuity, closeness and affirmation. These principles can be derived from knowledge accumulated in the field of child welfare throughout the twentieth century, the so-called 'Century of the Child' (see Hessle 1997). The *principle of family continuity* is concerned with the child's need of family connectedness throughout his or her entire childhood and into adult life. In this context, and working with persons from different ethnic backgrounds, we have broadened our theoretical frame of reference to include the underlying cultural discourse on forced migration as a complication that child welfare authorities must come to terms with. The *principle of closeness* focuses on the child's need to feel close to trustworthy adults who can provide protection and help him or her to understand phenomena in the surrounding world at his or her level of development, in particular when the child's experiences surpass the realm of normality. The *principle of affirmation* we find to be especially important because children need to be understood and valued from their own perspective and as partners in a dialogue. The child's need of affirmation compels adults to engage in dialogue with children on terms of equality. Aspects of these principles are codified in the UN Convention on the Rights of the Child (1991). We have endeavoured to relate them to practice and to point at some of the complications that arise when one is attempting to apply these principles in situations of ethnic conflict.

FAMILY CONTINUITY, CLOSENESS AND AFFIRMATION AS GENERAL PRINCIPLES IN CHILD WELFARE

The *principle of family continuity* means establishing a praxis for strengthening the child's network of family and friends, and above all incorporating a lifelong perspective into our understanding of family continuity. 'This [family continuity] approach recognizes that a child's identity is formed within a web of family relationships in extended and augmented kinship networks, which are a part of a culture and embedded in the community' (McFadden and Downs 1995:40). Towards the end of the 1980s, a movement got under way in the USA that has been called alternately 'the family support model', 'the family empowerment movement' and 'the family preservation movement' (see, e.g., Kagan and Weissbourd 1994).

Ecological thinking, in combination with increasingly successful pedagogical approaches to working with families in their own environments, has paved the way for reintroducing the practice of social mobilisation of residents in the local community. This trend has been observed not only in the USA but in the international arena as well. The Family Group Conference (FGC) model, incorporated into the New Zealand social welfare legislation of 1989, is based on a similar line of thought.

The thinking on family continuity in child and family welfare has been broadened to include a life-course perspective. The goal today is to identify, support and enhance vital lifelong relationships, particularly family relationships, as these are a vital part of the child's sense of continuity in an otherwise overloaded network of short-term, unpredictable and repeatedly broken contacts in care. The family is always a factor, for better or worse, and figures in cultural rituals and other events which call for the gathering together of the extended family. A basic tenet of permanency planning is that, wherever children are placed, they are to continue to have access to an extended or augmented network of family relationships, that this network constitutes the child's permanent base and is essentially a supportive platform. It should no longer be necessary to plan placement alternatives on a sliding scale: first a public institution; if that does not work then a foster home; and if that fails then adoption; and so on. Instead, with an extended or augmented family relationship network as the basis, it should be possible to determine which alternative is really best for the child, for how long a period of time, and in relation to the current problem situation. In the past ten years an advanced social methodology has been developed in the USA for strengthening families who are in danger of falling apart under external and internal pressures.

In conditions of war and other catastrophes, the life-course perspective in family continuity is essential when placement possibilities for unaccompanied minors are being investigated. It is urgent that these children be identified and that placements be found for them among close relatives rather than in institutions.

The *principle of closeness* in psychosocial work with families and children has been derived basically from studies undertaken decades ago showing a retardation in the development of children placed in large institutions. Following upon these studies, most of the larger public institutions for children have been disbanded. The principle of closeness can also be traced to the work of attachment theorists like Bowlby (1969) and Ainsworth (1983), and ecologists like Bronfenbrenner (1979) and Garbarino (1992), all of whom put stress on the interplay between the child and the contextual social and physical environment.

Closeness as a general principle in child welfare means, first of all, that children have to be able to count on being protected by those upon whom they are dependent. Second, children need close bonds with specific individuals if they are to have a favourable emotional and social development. It is, for example, from the protected position within a close relationship with a significant other that a child develops the self-confidence needed to embark on an exploration of the surrounding world. Third, the capacity to establish close relationships in adulthood is likely to be related to a person's initial experiences of closeness with significant others during childhood.

In accordance with this line of thinking, it has been found that children are more able to recover from the trauma of war if they have remained together with their families throughout instead of having been separated from them and evacuated to a protected area (Garbarino 1992). Moreover, children may find it easier to cope psychologically with violent environments if they can find a subjective meaning to their experiences (ibid.). It may, for instance, be less traumatising for a child in Bosnia to experience the violence of war in the company of his or her family than it is for a child in Chicago to be forced to take a detour to school every day to avoid rival drug gangs.

Asserting *affirmation* as a general principle in child welfare entails becoming cognisant of the current discourse in child psychology which questions the assumptions of Freud and Piaget that the child at birth is an egocentric, autistic bundle of reflexes, an animal steered by its instincts that has to be tamed through socialisation. A paradigmatic shift is currently taking place in which children are conceptualised as subjects engaged in a dialogue with their life-world instead of as hapless victims of the machinations of the adult world (Bråthen 1996).

Affirmation as a communicative concept in dialogue between people has a far more profound meaning than the decoding of information in, for example, information technology. Affirmation has to do not only with responding to a communication from the other, but also with discovering the unique qualities of the other. For a dialogue to take place, both parties must be subjects, but also each must perceive the other as a subject and not as a passive receiver or recorder of information. Somewhat simplified, one has both to perceive the other person from one's own vantage point and to perceive oneself from the vantage point of the other. Mead's theory (1934) comes closest to this standpoint, but falls short where dialogue with children is concerned. This paradigmatic breakthrough, which offers us a new way of relating to children in a subject–subject relationship, has begun in the last decade to win acceptance in child welfare and child protection work. Dialogue with abused or neglected children can be given a new rehabilitative meaning compared with the diagnostic and procedural orientation that has characterised social work up to the present.

Until recently children were not thought to be affected by traumatic events (such as war and other disasters) in the same way and to the same extent as adults. Today we know better. The most important diagnostic category to be developed in connection with natural stress reactions to unnatural events – Post Traumatic Stress Disorders (PTSD) – is now available as a tool for ascertaining children's need for special attention when war or other disasters intrudes upon their life-world. Children as well as adults react to overwhelming stress, but this has seldom been taken note of because adults are often less interested in affirming children in a subject–subject relationship than they are in dealing with their own traumatic experiences.

The important diagnostic process and rehabilitation through dialogue with children afflicted by war has won appreciable ground during the last few years, not least because of the war in former Yugoslavia.

THE UN CONVENTION ON THE RIGHTS OF THE CHILD

The UN Convention from 1989, ratified by 177 countries so far, can be said to contain the fundamentals of the principles for child welfare described above (see Hessle 1997). It is referred to repeatedly by child welfare social workers and others who advocate the rights of children. As for social work in connection with persons forced to migrate because of war, the Convention becomes even more urgent because the rights of children are so blatantly abused in war.

SOCIAL WORK WITH FAMILIES AND CHILDREN IN FORMER YUGOSLAVIA UNDER WAR AND POST-WAR CONDITIONS

Before the outbreak of war in former Yugoslavia, the country had a relatively advanced institutionalised welfare state system. Most of the activities in social work were and are organised from about one hundred centres for social work located throughout the country. These centres are generally run along similar principles of organisation and serve as the public local social service organisation for individuals and families in every phase of life. Permanent staff at the centres include a number of social workers, a psychologist, a defectologist (an expert on children with handicaps), a lawyer (mainly for marriage and divorce counselling) and a medical doctor. About 3,500 social workers have received their training at the University of Sarajevo, whose School of Social Work within the political science faculty was and still is the educational centre for social work in former Yugoslavia. (Other schools of social work in former Yugoslavia are located in Zagreb, Ljubiljana and Belgrade.) During the war about 50 per cent of the staff left the centres and either became refugees in other countries, were displaced within the region or left voluntarily to live in an ethnically homogeneous territory. This has meant that some centres had to close down. Nevertheless, most of the centres were able to make important contributions to aid the survival of people who remained in the country. The centres for social work distributed material aid (food, clothing and other basics) and provided important local psychological support for families traumatised by war. Of special importance were the activities in the eight out of ten centres that remained in operation during the siege of Sarajevo. During the isolation of the city, social workers distributed material aid (including food) to the most vulnerable families in the district. One of the leading professors at the School of Social Work headed the distribution of all necessities in Sarajevo during the siege.

The centres of social work have thus been essential to the survival of many people during the war. They were at the core of the local community, just as they were in peacetime. Staff members were known to have walked miles under bombing attacks to get to their unpaid jobs at the centre.

After the Dayton Agreement was signed at the end of 1995, reconstruction work was initiated in the whole of former Yugoslavia, but most intensively in the Federation of Bosnia and Hercegovina, with Sarajevo, the capital city of the region. It is not possible in this context to give a systematic description of how the reconstruction phase in the devastated society of former Yugoslavia was initiated. The whole nation was in a state of trauma. Moreoever, lingering tension among ethnic groups in the region and the rise of new organisational bodies in the political entities of the Federation of Bosnia-Hercegovina and the Republic of Srpska have added to the chaos out of which a new civil society is struggling to emerge. In addition, several hundred NGOs (non-governmental organisations) from all over the world (as well as international bodies like the UN) have been on the spot to lend their particular forms of support to the peace process. Considering the complexity of the situation, our aim here is merely to give a glimpse of how the work to place unaccompanied minors was envisioned by social workers in Bosnia who took part in a bilateral further training course in social work.

At the initiative of UNICEF, the Schools of Social Work at the universities of Stockholm and Sarajevo entered into a partnership that resulted in the development of three courses for further education of persons engaged in child welfare work in former Yugoslavia. One course was designed for supervisors of children's institutions, a second for social workers employed by the social work centres, and a third was designed as a specialist course for child welfare social workers. The participants were recruited from the whole territory of B-H[1] and included all levels from field staff to government representatives. The authors of this chapter were commissioned to conduct a specialist course for fifty child welfare social workers. Muslims, Croats and Serbs were represented, with Muslims in the majority. The participants had no difficulty developing an attitude of conciliation throughout the course. They attended all three of the five-day workshops, spread out over a six-month period, sometimes travelling from an appreciable distance (12 hours by car) and even though the continued outbreak of ethnic conflicts made travelling dangerous. The main object of the course was to increase the participants' competence in placing unaccompanied minors in foster care. The course focused on the recruitment, support and supervision of foster families and the organisation of child welfare based on a holistic view of the child's total situation.

There are three outcomes of the training programme that are particularly interesting to take note of here. First, the programme led to the establishing of a network of child welfare experts which is convened on a regular basis to attend to the needs of children in Bosnia and Hercegovina, in particular the most vulnerable children (i.e., unaccompanied minors and physically or mentally handicapped children). The network will continue to look after the interests of children during the repatriation process.

Second, an important measure in the course was to introduce the use of dialogue with the child as an important instrument for placing children and evaluating foster homes. This was the first opportunity the participants had to engage in a professional dialogue with the children they worked with, and they were surprised to discover that affirming the child in this way had a profound effect on their attitude to placements (some of the children were subsequently moved to another placement) and to the situation of children in general.

Third, lecturing about the international experience on family continuity as a principle for child welfare decisions proved to be superfluous, since it was already common practice among the social workers to place unaccompanied minors with relatives. Foster families were found for two-thirds of the nearly 3,000 children requiring placement through informal networking and most of them were placed with families who were already known to them. There was some concern among social workers about foster parents who were of the age of elderly grandparents. But generally the social workers had good control over most of the placements, which is quite remarkable considering the wartime and post-war conditions. The fact that most of the foster parents were receiving temporary subsidies from the World Bank was a major topic of discussion in the course. As most of former Yugoslavia was on the verge of total bankruptcy, the participants were concerned about the fate of the children in foster care when the flow of money from the World Bank dried up.

To conclude, the child welfare workers we came into contact with through our work in these projects in former Yugoslavia appear to have good control over the placement of unaccompanied minors. The way of placing children that seemed most natural to them coincides with the family continuity principle that we in the rest of the Western world have taken decades to (re)discover. Many of the hundreds of NGOs from all over the world in place in Bosnia during the war and post-war years were competing with one another to train social workers and others engaged in promoting child welfare. The underlying message behind this worldwide commitment to child welfare in former Yugoslavia seemed to be that social workers needed to change their way of working with placements. Did we fall into the same trap? We think not. What is unique about our training programme is that it was designed in partnership with colleagues at Sarajevo University. When the international staff of NGOs leave former Yugoslavia for new disaster areas in other parts of the world, this partnership will still be in effect, working towards developing new long-term programmes.

The involvement of foreign NGOs in the social reconstruction of former Yugoslavia, or of any country for that matter, is of course a mixed blessing. We should not make the mistake, however, of negating the potential of NGOs to exert a positive influence on the understanding and practice of social work in the country receiving aid. In the Federation of Bosnia-Hercegovina, for example, especially vulnerable children, e.g. the mentally retarded, are by tradition placed mainly in institutions, ten of which are rather large, with over 100 children each. Although these institutions are supervised by experts (*defectologists*) affiliated with a centre of social work, in several of them children are housed together with mentally retarded adults. Here the social welfare authorities have something to learn from the international experience.

PSYCHOSOCIAL WORK WITH BOSNIAN REFUGEES IN SWEDEN DURING THE WAR AND POST-WAR YEARS IN BOSNIA

When the war broke out in former Yugoslavia in 1992, refugees soon started to arrive in Sweden. The Swedish organisation for receiving persons seeking asylum was forced to adjust its routines to cope with a greater number of refugees than ever before. The over 80,000 refugees from former Yugoslavia represented the largest single group of refugees to Sweden from one and the same country. In June 1993 the Swedish government made a decision in principle to grant most of the refugees from former Yugoslavia permanent permission to stay in Sweden. The Bosnian group was specially noted because of its size and the traumatising war experiences of its members. The Swedish refugee policy with respect to the Bosnian group differed from the policies of many other countries. In Norway, for example, the Bosnian refugees were granted temporary permission to stay, which meant that they were expected to return home as soon as conditions allowed. Germany, the country in Europe that accepted the largest number of Bosnians, around 300,000, and granted them temporary permission to stay, is now the country pushing hardest for the repatriation of the Bosnian group.

A large number of projects were initiated throughout Sweden, entailing economic investment in extraordinary measures for the Bosnian group. Most of the resources were distributed to centres with special knowledge in the field of trauma and torture treatment. Sweden, with its in-migration policy, has wide experience of treating trauma among large numbers of refugees coming from countries like Chile, Argentina, Uruguay, Iran, Iraq, Somalia and Afghanistan. Sweden has shifted emphasis from a labour migration policy to a refugee policy in the last twenty years. It has been estimated that a fifth of the children in Sweden have their roots of origin in other countries (Children's Ombudsman 1996). But knowledge of trauma treatment among professionals is still fairly general and there is a continuing need for specific knowledge acquired through dialogue with traumatised people. In Sweden there seems to be a watertight bulkhead between specialists on war trauma treatment and generalists (mainly social workers) at the social service centres. The service centres seem to be uninterested in developing the methods needed for working with this fairly new group of refugees.

Case 1

The following example is a case in point. Emir and Amira arrived in Sweden in 1994 with their two children, aged 6 and 8. The family came from a small town in Bosnia which had experienced the horrors of war at close quarters. The father had been a soldier and had been incarcerated for a time in a concentration camp. The parents were united with the help of the Red Cross after one and a half years of separation and were finally evacuated to Sweden. Everyone in the family had experienced severe trauma. The father had been tortured in the concentration camp. The mother had been raped in front of the children. All of them had witnessed killings and maiming. The grand-parents were killed in the war, as were many close relatives. After about a year in Sweden the family was reported to the Social Service Centre as suspected of child abuse. The father had told the interpreter in confidence that he had beaten the older child three times to teach him/her a lesson. The family was immediately placed in an institution specialising in family investigations; the overriding question was whether or not to take the children into public care. Unfortunately, the institution's staff had no prior experience of non-Swedish families, particularly not of families traumatised by war, and they were unable to carry out the investigation. The parents felt humiliated and contacted a specialist who obtained the family's release in a very short time and helped them to find relief from their PTSD symptoms. In a follow-up control some time later, social workers were able to report that the children were well cared for by their parents.

Because Bosnian refugees to Sweden have been granted permanent residence permits, they are in a position to make long-term plans. They are accorded the same rights as ordinary Swedish citizens and are free to look for housing accommodation anywhere in the country. Many of the adults attend classes in Swedish and thereby become eligible for social assistance, and their children are in school. But the economic recession and high unemployment rate means that the job market is much less accessible to Bosnian refugees and Swedes alike.

Another complication affecting the refugees' adaptation to their new country is that the ethnic conflicts that figured so tragically in the war in former Yugoslavia are sometimes replayed in Sweden. The interpreters' home of origin remains an important issue and different associations have been set up that underline ethnic affiliation. A reconstruction of a multicultural society that was part of the spirit of the Dayton Agreement seems a near impossibility in Sweden as well as in former Yugoslavia.

The strategies for spreading knowledge about how traumatic experiences affect a person's entire life have generally taken two directions:

1 General information about trauma experiences and their consequences is being spread to all welfare agencies that encounter refugees with trauma experiences.
2 Strategies are being developed to help traumatised adults and children, individually, in their families or in groups:
   - to work through their traumatic experiences,
   - to cope with their situation in school and at work.
   - to help both adults and children to make sense of their everyday life in Sweden
   - to help them obtain information about relatives and friends back home.

The specialists on trauma treatment have developed supervisory methods to help schoolteachers and pre-school staff to identify children who are in need of immediate short-term treatment. These are children who suffer from 'flashbacks' while at school or who are persistently plagued by nightmares. The children are usually treated in groups, with attention given to each child's personal trauma. Nearly all the Bosnian children in the Stockholm area have been offered group treatment for their war traumas. Trauma specialists, however, are unevenly distributed throughout Sweden and it is unlikely that many children and adults outside these areas have received help to resolve their traumatic stress.

When the question of repatriation was brought to the fore because of the peace process in Bosnia, social workers in Sweden found themselves without guidelines for action. There is no tradition or praxis to fall back on when it comes to helping refugees to decide whether to return home. We grope for a strategy, perhaps because we fail to understand that most of the refugees who seek asylum in Sweden at heart long to return home. Perhaps it is difficult to understand that a person could want to leave the 'paradise' of Sweden for a totally bankrupt, devastated and disrupted country. This is the kind of problem that social workers face today in Sweden. In Case 2 it should be noted, first of all, that this young girl had been raised in a multiproblem family, i.e. her life before the outbreak of war was already troubled. The problems became more acute because of the war. This diagnostic assessment is

Case 2

The following case will serve as an example. Anna was only 9 years old when she came to Sweden from a little town near the border of Srpska. She had lived with her two younger siblings and her mother, an alcoholic who subjected Anna to repeated abuse. The parents had been divorced for many years but Anna had maintained regular contact with her father. Then came the war. The father, a Croat, fled to Sweden in 1992. Here he met a woman from his home country and set up household with her and her 10-year-old son. When Anna came to Sweden in 1994, she joined the family. Her situation was very complicated. She had a troubled background, her family situation at home was difficult, and her new family in Sweden was unknown to her. Anna felt that her father had become a stranger and that she herself was a stranger in Sweden. At the same time she worried about her mother and siblings at home. When the war was in progress, she feared that they would be killed. After the war ended she began to fear that her mother was abusing her siblings. 'I was always the one who took care of the smaller children.' Anna did not do well in school and she failed to learn Swedish. Eighteen months after her arrival in Sweden, she was found lying in a ditch not far from her home. She had taken an overdose of sleeping pills. When she woke up at the hospital, her first words were: 'I want to go home to my mother.'

important as it indicates that short-term treatment would not be effective in Anna's case. Most of the clinical cases treated in Sweden concern war traumas that can be treated with short-term measures. Moreover, in sending Anna to her father, the mother was doing what she thought was best for her daughter. The main question facing the social worker in this case is whether the child's refusal to remain with her family in Sweden is reason enough to place her in foster care. And if so, what kind of foster home? With a Serbian family? A Croatian family? A mixed family? In Sweden, or should Anna be sent back to Srpska with the support of their Serbian social workers? Is the father intending to return to Croatia? Would Srpska be too dangerous for him? Questions like these complicate child welfare issues because they add a migration (refugee) perspective (e.g. with reference to repatriation) to the visible problems. The question is whether social workers have this perspective or not.

A MODEL FOR ANALYSING CONDITIONS FOR DOING SOCIAL WORK WITH REFUGEES UNDER WAR AND POST-WAR CONDITIONS

In Figure 8.1 we have listed four different sets of circumstances for doing social work with refugees: (1) social work undertaken during the war in the country of origin; (2) social work praxis in the exile country; (3) social work undertaken with refugees in the exile country as post-war conditions develop in the country of origin; and (4) social work initiated and developed in the country of origin under post-war conditions.

Obviously, the conditions for doing social work in countries at war or under post-war conditions and in countries at peace differ markedly. Persons who have been forced to leave their home and country because of war escape from a situation that imperils their personal welfare and the welfare of their families more or less temporarily and more or less acutely, and they migrate to a country that has greater or lesser experience of receiving refugees seeking asylum. If anything in general is to be said about these two sets of conditions for doing social work, it would be that social work in connection with refugees in a war-torn country is directed towards survival and social work in connection with refugees in the exile country is directed towards integration, assuming of course that the refugees have been granted permanent permission to stay.

Refugees seeking asylum live in a state of limbo, anxiously waiting for official permission to reside permanently in their new country, permission that will make it possible for them to plan for a new life in exile. Of course, social work may be better or less well developed as a system of action in both the country at war and the country of exile (see Chapter 2). And even a highly developed system of social welfare in the country of exile may prove to be inadequately equipped for dealing with the kinds of problems forced migration entails.

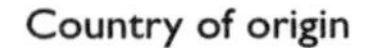

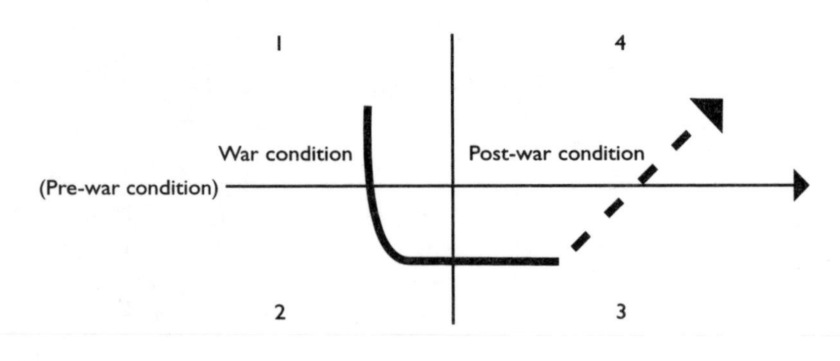

Country of exile

Movement of refugees from country of origin to country of exile and presumable return to country of origin during post-war conditions

Figure 8.1 Model for analysis of different circumstances for social work with refugees in wartime and post-war conditions

By following the arrows in the figure, we can perhaps better understand the kinds of conditions refugees encounter as they flee from their country of origin to a country of exile, a flight marked by traumatic experiences of war, separation from close relatives and friends, and the uncertainty of finding at least a temporary haven in a strange society. The length of stay in the country of exile varies, of course, depending on how conditions develop in the country of origin, but also depending on the attracting and repelling forces ('push-and-pull', see Chapter 2) at play in the country of origin and the country of exile.

The conditions for doing social work in a war-stricken country hinge upon the degree to which the country had evolved into a welfare state prior to the war (Spicker 1988). Countries with poorly organised welfare systems may find themselves totally at the mercy of external foreign aid policies in the war for survival. The current situation in some African states is a case in point: Rwanda and former Zaire are examples of countries at war that have become totally dependent on external aid. But even advanced welfare states may have failed to develop organisations that are prepared to deal with war conditions or other catastrophes (Castenfors 1994; Ioka 1996). Networks of local NGOs that can be activated in times of disaster could, for example, serve as a complement to a country's formal public welfare organisations (Ioka 1996; Mujan 1996).

The following is a presentation of our findings, summarised in Figure 8.1, as they pertain to the problem of doing social work under the divergent conditions of war, post-war and peace:

1 *Social work during wartime in the country of origin*. One of the conditions for doing social work in a country at war concerns the country's loss of human resources and the disruption of ordinary social networks. Usually, war means that a considerable part of the population becomes displaced throughout the country, particularly when ethnic conflicts are one of the causes of the war, as in the cases of Rwanda and former Yugoslavia. Ethnic groups are forced to leave their homes and seek refuge with relatives or others of the same ethnic affiliation. A pressing task in times of war is survival work, and here social workers could play a major role in distributing material aid (e.g. food and clothing), in providing psychological support, and in identifying displaced persons. Both adults and children are traumatised by war, and providing treatment for PTSD is an essential part of psychosocial work. Unattended children must also be identified and placements found for them, preferably with foster families with whom they are well acquainted.

2 *Social work praxis in the exile country*. Refugees from a country at war have usually been forced into exile, which means that they can seldom choose in which country to seek refuge for the duration of the war. This is even more true of the children. It is always the adults who figure in the decision to evacuate a family to a particular country of exile. The children have no choice but to follow the grown-ups. And the flight to the country of exile may be

even more traumatising for the children than the war itself. Refugees are understandably more preoccupied with grieving over the death of family and friends, worrying about the family members they left behind and struggling to find relief from their war traumas than they are with finding out about the country to which they have just arrived. The conditions for social work focusing on forced migration issues vary with the refugees' status in the country of exile. Have they been granted temporary or permanent permission to stay? The unpredictable time frame poses a special challenge for psychosocial work in that methods have to be devised for supporting people whose whole life situation is shrouded in uncertainty. The social welfare legislation of the country of exile may or may not include refugees in the categories of people who are eligible for material assistance. In Sweden social welfare legislation pertains to everyone residing within the country's borders, which means that all children and refugees with permanent residence permits have the same rights as everyone else. It also means, however, that refugees are judged according to Swedish legislation whenever questions of child abuse and neglect arise.

3 *Social work with refugees in the exile country as post-war conditions develop in the country of origin*. The war has finally come to an end in the refugee's country of origin. Information about the fate of relatives may now be easier to obtain and there is some relief from the strain of uncertainty. But it may still be unsafe or even impossible for refugees to return home despite the declaration of peace. Continued ethnic conflicts may impede repatriation and refugees may be unable to return to their home towns. Mixed marriages between ethnic groups may be unacceptable in the refugees' home community. Other families may have moved into their homes, or their homes may have been destroyed during the war, and so on.

At the same time, the country of origin may be sending out a strong signal that it requires the refugees' return from exile to help in the reconstruction of the country. The country of Bosnia, for example, wants its human resources back, but is also prepared to pass the harsh judgement of desertion on those who do not return soon. In some cases, if the refugees wait for their own country to be rebuilt before deciding to return home, there is a great risk that they will no longer be welcome.

So, the time frame is important here. The longer the refugee remains in exile, the more difficult becomes the decision to return home. To add to the dilemma, circumstances in the country of exile may constitute an attracting force; the children may have adjusted to their new country; they attend school and have probably learned to speak the language; they may have acquired new friends. And if the country of exile is like Sweden, it has a generous welfare system which provides economic assistance and decent housing and offers some compensation for the lack of job opportunities in a strained labour market. Differences in the level of welfare between the country of origin and the country of exile may thus create a whole new set of problems for war refugees. With the experiences of refugees from Chile in mind, the concept of 'assistensialism' has been suggested to give a name to the protracted dependency on state welfare in the country of exile that obstructs the individual's development of self-reliance upon his or her return from exile (Hessle and Hessle 1993). Apparently very little systematic knowledge has been accumulated to date addressing the issue of social work focusing on repatriation.

4 *Social work in the country of origin under post-war conditions.* At what point can persons in exile be said to enter into a life characterised by post-war conditions? When they first make the decision to return home? When they begin the process of physical relocation? When they start reconstruction work on their houses? When they can register a feeling of relief? When they begin to think about the future without fear? The questions are many and there are no easy answers to the problem of describing a post-war condition. We know that many refugees will choose to remain in exile and try to adapt to their new country. Many will be unable to return to their homes and villages. And perhaps many of them, persons for whom the war has created an even deeper chasm between ethnic groups, will never find relief. Individual circumstances require individual answers. A society undergoes a reconstruction process by the progress of many small links all working in the same direction.

'The war has destroyed the civil society,' Bosnian social workers have commented, 'and we are the ones who have to take responsibility for the work of reconstruction.' And of course there is much for social workers to do. We can add a few items of our own to the list above: scores of split families need counselling and support after the war to cope with traumas of separation, divorce and death. The number of single-parent families, known to social science as the most vulnerable household unit, will increase because of the war. Soldiers returning to their families are a special stress factor to consider, since many may have unresolved traumatic experiences of war and many face long-term unemployment. Children need a stable placement with frequent contacts with their relatives. Many elderly people displaced because of the war will have to be relocated. The list could be made much longer. Times will be difficult for refugees returning from exile, how difficult will depend on the time and circumstances of their return, and the time and circumstances of their emigration. Azem Mujan (1996:288) has predicted that returning refugees will undergo a process of alienation that will pose a serious challenge to their reacquiring a sense of belonging:

> Nothing will be the same as before. They [the refugees] will have changed and the communities to which they return will have changed. New variables will be introduced into their old communities: veterans returning from the war; friends and acquaintances will have changed as a consequence of their experiences; the attitudes of colleagues at work

will have changed; families will have been dispersed; state institutions will have changed.

CONCLUSIONS

The refugee's journey from a war-torn country, such as former Yugoslavia, to a country of exile, such as Sweden, and back home again upon the restoration of peace is a very complex and tortuous one, particularly if we take into account the continual outbreak of conflict among ethnic groups and the differences between the two countries' welfare systems and ways of organising social work.

This chapter has taken as point of departure the obvious differences in conditions for psychosocial work during war and in times of peace, the differences in conditions between countries of war and countries of exile. We have introduced an exploratory model to illuminate the experiences of working with refugees in Sweden in wartime and in the post-war period and of reconstructing social work in Bosnia-Hercegovina during peace under the Dayton Agreement.

- Some general principles of social work within child welfare have been found to be universal, such as the principles of family continuity, closeness and affirmation. The UN Convention of the Rights of the Child strongly supports the main part of these principles. But they might be difficult to implement within the field of psychosocial work with refugees, as some of our examples have shown.
- Different European nations have opposing strategies to handle the refugee situation within their particular models of welfare state, that contribute to create the conditions for psychosocial work with asylum-seeking refugees. In Sweden, with an institutional and universal welfare state model, the strategies have been shown to be difficult to change to meet the needs of new asylum-seeking groups. The refugees are forced into a static structure meant for other vulnerable categories in the society.
- Social work with refugees must, if possible, take into account both the need to feel safe in exile and the potentiality to return to the country of origin when it is possible as natural components of an integration policy. Time perspective is essential in the sense that the longer the refugee remains in exile, the more complicated becomes the decision to return home, especially when children are involved.

NOTE

1 Participants from the Republic of Srpska were not included in these courses for political reasons. But a course is planned together with UNICEF to take place in Srpska in the year from October 1997.

REFERENCES

Ainsworth, M. D. S. (1983) Patterns of infant–mother attachment as related to maternal care. Their early history and their contribution to continuity. In D. Magnusson and V. L. Allen (eds). *Human development. An interactional perspective.* London: Academic Press.

Bowlby, J. (1969) *Attachment and loss.* London: The Hogarth Press.

Bronfenbrenner, U. (1979) *The ecology of human development.* Cambridge, MA: Harvard University Press.

Bråthen, S. (1996) Videoanalyser av spedbarnet i samspill bidrar till å uppheve et modellmonopol (Video analysis of infants in interaction invalidate a monopoly model). In H. Holter and R. Kalleberg (eds). *Kvalitative metoder i samfundsforskning* (Qualitative methods in social research). Oslo: Universitetsforlaget (166–93).

Castenfors, K. (1994) Preparedness within the municipal social services in Sweden: planning for the home help service organization for elderly people in war and crises from two organizational perspectives. *Scandinavian Journal of Social Welfare,* 4:280–9.

Garbarino, J. (In collaboration with Dubrov, N., Kostelny, K. and Pardo, C.) (1992) *Children in danger coping with community violence.* San Francisco: Jossey-Bass Publishing Co.

Hessle, M. and Hessle, S. (1993) Återvändandets dilemma (The dilemma of returning). *Socionomen,* 2:38–43.

Hessle, S. (1997) *Child welfare and child protection on the eve of the 21st century – what the 20th century has taught us.* Stockholm Studies of Social Work, No. 12.

Ioka, B. (1996) Lessons on community social services from the great Hanshin earthquake. *Scandinavian Journal of Social Welfare,* 5:125–9.

Kagan, S. and Weissbourd, B. (eds) (1994) *Putting families first.* San Francisco: Jossey-Bass Publishing Co.

McFadden, E. J. and Downs, W. S. (1995) Family continuity: the new paradigm in permanency planning. *International Journal of Family Care,* 7, No. 1:39–59.

Mead, G. H. (1934) *Mind, self and society,* Chicago: University of Chicago Press.

Mujan, A. (1996) Psychological and social processes among refugees – the case of Bosnia and Hercegovina, *Scandinavian Journal of Social Welfare,* 5:286–9.

Spicker, P. (1988) *Principles of social welfare.* London: Routledge.

Chapter 9

Collective action in a refugee camp[1]

A case study

Eva Segerström

INTRODUCTION

Experiences from the developing countries of the so-called Third World are invaluable to the development of good community work practice in any context. This chapter provides a case study of a project implemented in Yemen with Somali refugees by the Swedish organisation Rädda Barnen (Save the Children). The chapter describes the processes of community- based forms of intervention within a refugee community organising to resolve its own problems and difficulties. The study illustrates that human potential and agency are the most important resources to development, which becomes particularly obvious in a country where few other resources are available. The starting point of this approach is that local communities can effectively organise to identify, direct and implement programmes that enhance their social and economic well-being if stimulated and supported appropriately to do so (Burkey 1993). Respect for persons, for their ability to be creative and to be motivated even in circumstances of crisis, such as the experience of being refugees, is the core of collective action strategies. This particular study also forcefully illustrates the major contribution of women in the development process (Van den Hombergh 1993) and the lesson to Western social work thinking 'we must do it our own way'. People's cultures have within them their own potential and their own solutions which should guide and direct the social work intervention.

BACKGROUND AND CONTEXT

Most of the Somali refugees who fled to Yemen during the spring and summer of 1992 crossed the Sea of Aden and ended up in Medinat Al Shaab

1 'Collective action in a refugee camp' is a revised version of a chapter with the title 'Contamination by war' in D. Tolfree (1996) *'Restoring Playfulness'. Different Approaches to Assisting Children who are Psychologically Affected by War or Displacement.* Stockholm: Rädda Barnen.

refugee camp in a sandy desert 10 km from the city of Aden. The camp environment had few facilities apart from a food distribution centre and a small health clinic.

Rädda Barnen (Swedish Save the Children) had been working in Yemen for the previous thirty years, mainly in the field of primary health, and, as one of the few NGOs working there, took the initiative to plan and start a primary school in the camp. It was immediately apparent that many of the children and their parents had experiences of violence and other traumatic events in Somalia which were compounded by the current stresses and absence of support in the refugee camp. Six months later, a survey was undertaken to assess the psychological well-being of refugee mothers, and to evaluate their competence to meet the needs of their children. As a result of this survey, ideas were formulated on ways to improve the mothers' sense of psychological well-being and parental competence by encouraging their active participation in a range of community development activities.

The initiation of the school and work with women in the camp were seen as the two main aspects of a strategy adopted by Rädda Barnen to promote the psychological recovery and social integration of Somali refugee children in Yemen. The aim of the school was not just to provide education in a traditional manner but also to provide training for teachers in order to enable them to assess the psychological needs of children, to provide social support to them through supportive conversations, and to encourage their participation in cultural activities such as music, dance and drama.

This case study examines these two aspects of Rädda Barnen's strategy to impact on the psychosocial well-being of the children. The implementation of the strategy was, however, impeded by two major factors.

First, the refugees experienced several moves, and the extreme disruption created by the outbreak of civil war in Yemen. After suffering further traumatising experiences through being caught up in this war and the need to flee the refugee camp, they were eventually resettled in Algahin, which is situated in a barren, rocky area two hours' drive from Aden.

Second, for various operational reasons apart from these disruptions, it was not possible for Rädda Barnen to provide the level and consistency of professional support which these programmes really needed. Although the school received good technical support in the form of various teacher training modules, it was not possible to provide social work input into the Women's Union. However, when in the spring of 1995 the writer, who was involved in setting up the programmes, was able to revisit the refugees in the new camp in Algahin, the information which emerged provided some interesting and unexpected findings, which will be described in this case study.

A description of the development of the school will be offered, along with a picture of what was encountered during the return visit in 1995. This will be followed by an account of the survey of women in the camp which was undertaken in 1993, and an explanation of the developments which occurred as a result of this. Following a section which discusses and analyses some of the main issues arising from the development of these two programmes, some conclusions will be drawn.

THE PLANNING AND DEVELOPMENT OF THE SCHOOL

The school started in November 1992 after one month's planning and preparation. The first step was to establish an Education Committee comprising refugees selected by the community. The committee eventually consisted of seven men and three women, chosen from different tribes (seen as vital in a society deeply divided along tribal lines) and from different zones in the camp. The planning of the school was based on a clear statement of community development principles, which included the following: the approach should be collective, within and with the refugee community; the community should define needs and objectives; resources should come from within the community, supported where needed by external ones; decision-making should be democratic (Brokensha and Hodge 1969). It was also decided that the approach should aim to meet the broader psychosocial needs of children.

The role of Rädda Barnen's community worker was to urge, motivate and assist in developing the refugees' own system of leadership and organisation, and create the necessary condition for participation in planning the school. The focal point for participation in community development processes is to give the refugees real responsibility, which means that who makes decisions and how they are made is crucial. This is a process in which the community worker is active in sharing views of problems, listening and asking questions about how people want to solve problems, helping them to understand, analyse, plan and carry out their ideas but not to do it for them. The community worker is important but has to be a facilitator not a leader.

Much of the planning was undertaken by the Education Committee, working largely without representation of Rädda Barnen staff. Rädda Barnen was, however, requested to take an active role in teacher selection to prevent suspicion of tribal preferences, though the final selection was made jointly. Rädda Barnen determined that only modest salaries should be paid. Only teachers who expressed a more altruistic motive were considered – i.e. those who wanted to work for children and not those motivated by material rewards or the need for 'something to do'. Another criterion was the capacity to deal with the children in difficult situations: only teachers who expressed a wish to understand the child, to avoid physical punishment and to find constructive approaches were appointed. When the school started, there was one head teacher, ten teachers and 450 children aged from six to nine years of age.

Early discussions with the Somali teachers revealed the general view that 'it is best for children not to talk about the bad experience they have gone through even though sometimes children want to talk about them'. This suggested the existence of a taboo against discussing painful issues, and from this it seemed that there was a need for knowledge and awareness of psychological concepts. It was therefore recommended that it was necessary to include, in the subjects for teachers' training, the knowledge and skills required for offering 'supportive talks' with children to give them help, advice and emotional support in their daily lives.

The school in Algahin, two years later

When the return visit was made in 1995, it was found that the camp consisted of nine huge hangars, one of which was used as the school and also used for food distribution. In spite of the extreme hardship the refugees had experienced prior to their resettlement in Algahin, the group of teachers had immediately re-established the school.

The school comprised a pre-school and primary school, with a total of sixteen teachers, including two female pre-school teachers, a headmaster and a deputy. Most had been involved in the school since its inception. There were 507 children enrolled, of whom 211 were girls. Owing to the civil war in Yemen, no textbooks were available.

First impressions suggested a traditional school with traditional methods – i.e. teachers operating in a 'top-down' relationship to the children and using a very formal and non-interactive approach, which included the use of repetition as a learning method. But in other respects the school was found to be most exceptional. The deputy headmaster made a very significant comment: 'The school is not just a school for education, it is a community school.'

The school had become the main social structure within the camp and the most important service available. The camp was found to lack an official and united camp committee – rather, a number of leaders represented different tribes within the community but did not speak with one voice on behalf of the whole community. However, mutual respect between the elders and the teachers' group was clearly seen to exist.

When the school started, the Education Committee had a central role, but by the time of the return visit in 1995 it was found to have been disbanded because of conflicts of interest. The head teacher and his staff formed a self-steering, independent unit which was considered by the teachers to be a clear strength.

During this return visit, a participatory review was undertaken with the school staff in order to provide a structured way of analysing the way in which the school had developed. The following are some of the key issues to emerge from this review:

- All teachers valued their involvement in discussions and decisions concerning the school. The teachers committed a great deal of time to discussing issues, and though the headmaster would make final decisions it was always on the basis of thorough discussion.
- Co-operation with parents was referred to as 'partnership'. Parents were actively involved in communication with the teachers regarding the children's progress and behaviour. Teachers knew the parents and the family background of the children. School staff were also involved with issues beyond the confines of the school. They were, for example, consulted in matters such as arranging celebrations and activities, dealing with interpersonal conflicts and so on. During the visit, a group of eight parents voluntarily assisted in the construction of a storehouse for the school, complete with furniture, working until late at night to complete their task.
- The teachers showed a great deal of interest and knowledge in recognising and assessing stress in children, including gender differences and the need to recognise the problems displayed by children who failed to attend school or who were sad and silent.
- Teachers' responses to children who were troubled by their difficult experiences included the following:

    they discussed the problem with parents;
    the children would be given extra attention in the class;
    teachers would encourage the children with hobbies and interests;
    other children would be encouraged to read the Koran and listen to music.

- It was significant that, contrary to what had been intended when the school was established, teachers remained generally reluctant to talk directly with the children about war experience, though some would have individual discussions with children when they themselves showed the desire to talk. However, it was clear that in activities such as singing, drama and free drawing, experiences of war and children's reactions to them were expressed.
- The teachers themselves adopted a number of strategies for dealing with their own difficult experiences. These included reciting the Koran and developing their faith, learning more through reading and listening to the radio and taking part in a range of different activities.
- Teachers had become involved in a wide range of activities within the wider community. Boy Scout and Girl Guide groups were established to teach good social values, social awareness, discipline and self-reliance, and to involve children as active participants in community development programmes. A 'Children's Corner' was established to provide a forum for various out-of-school activities – including story-telling, plays, singing, quizzes, etc. These took place at various times during the week, with parents also involved in two of the weekly sessions. One teacher

expressed a major function of the Children's Corner thus: 'Teachers will present different stories that touch on aspects of real life. – This will help the teachers to draw out the child's emotions of happiness and sadness.' Another important objective was to develop clear forms of communication with other children, with parents and within the wider community. Sports activities were also organised by the teachers, including football and volleyball teams.

- Teachers had also involved themselves in a number of other activities, which included: translating useful written material from English into Somali, evaluating the school's performance and reviewing the curriculum, undertaking case studies (e.g. on why there are fewer girls aged 12 to 15 than boys in the school, and on children who are affected by their experiences of war), and planning publications (including a school paper to include writings on various topics).

This wide range of activities illustrates both the enthusiasm and commitment of the teachers and their desire to be involved in the lives of the children, their families and in the wider community on a much broader basis than is typical of the traditional role of the teacher. The particular approach taken in responding to the needs of children, mentioned by some teachers as 'contaminated by war', i.e. psychologically affected by their experiences of war, will be discussed further below.

DESCRIPTION OF THE PROGRAMME PLANNED FOR WOMEN

Previous research

It is well known that mothers' emotional well-being is important for their children's psychological health and development. Recent research indicates that young children can cope well with the stress of social disasters like war if they retain strong attachment to their families, and if parents can continue to project a sense of stability (McCallin and Fozzard 1990:22; see also Hessle and Hessle, Chapter 8). In this sense, parents can enhance the resilience of their children by mediating between their difficult experiences and their sense of well-being. Research also suggests that, if mothers themselves received good social support, this is likely to reduce their levels of stress related to traumatic events. These findings were the basis for a survey of 198 mothers made in Medinat Al Shaab in May 1993 (Segerström 1994:12–13). The study sought to enquire into the Somali refugee mothers' psychological well-being and their feelings of competence in caring for their children. The study was conducted not just out of theoretical interest but in order to place emphasis on mothers and the central role they should have in any programmes planned in the camp.

The survey showed that the refugee mothers' psychological well-being was very poor. Half of the mothers interviewed expressed an extremely high degree of psychosomatic and emotional problems, while only 2 per cent had no, or very few, symptoms. A majority (85 per cent) suffered daily from different stress factors to an extreme degree. About 20 per cent of the mothers had been exposed to many traumatic events, half to some such events, with only 3.5 per cent having had little or no exposure to traumatic events. About 90 per cent of the mothers expressed feelings of helplessness about bringing up their children. A similar proportion considered themselves as being the most important person for the child. About 40 per cent of the mothers received support from their husbands, but most said that they had nobody giving emotional support.

Enhancing maternal support to children

All children, and especially those affected by war, need a daily structure and routine. The camp school provided an important part of this structure and became the first community service for children. But what could be done to increase the mothers' sense of competence to enable them to be more supportive to their children?

As a result of the survey, a strategy to empower women was devised. Some of the women had organised themselves into a Women's Union and they requested donor organisations to assist by providing a meeting centre for all women in the camp where they could discuss issues of interest and concern to themselves. This proposal was consistent with McCallin and Fozzard's conclusion (1990:40) that an effective means of support is to strengthen women's social networks, which can be seen as a protective factor, and increase their participation in the community. This in turn should result in a greater sense of control over their lives and a diminished sense of helplessness. The result is an increase in resilience both for women and for their children.

The Women's Union and subsequent developments

In the Medinat Al Shaab camp, a meeting place was duly provided and the women began to regain control of their lives through the dynamics and resilience of the Women's Union, which was becoming an important resource for women and children. Various interest groups were set up, education and child care, social and cultural activities and home economics, conflict resolution, and help to people in need. After the camp moved for the first time, the group again was provided with a place to meet, but the activities appear to have been limited to handicrafts and literacy classes. At the time of the follow-up visit to Algahin, the Women's Union had been re-established, but its apparent lack of impact on the life of women in the camp was disappointing. It had ceased to be a democratic organisation, leadership being concentrated in the hands of one very authoritarian person. Its lack of commitment to community development was illustrated by the demand that an institution should be opened for all the orphans currently cared for by their relatives. The Union had become little more than a place for women to meet and undertake a limited range of activities. The various subgroups no longer existed and the Union had lost its concern for child health, play, and the broader pursuit of women's issues in the community. Why was this, when the Women's Union seemed to have the potential for becoming an extremely important resource for women?

One reason appeared to be the lack of leadership which was needed for the Union to develop in a committed and imaginative manner. Many of the more influential female leaders in the camp left, and were replaced in the Women's Union by self-elected women who had more interest in financial benefits than the good of the whole community.

A second reason is probably that the women seem to associate and socialise mainly in small informal groups rather than in large, visible, well-structured organisations. At the time of the follow-up visit, it was noticeable that about half of the small businesses in the marketplace such as tea-shops, market stalls, were run by women. Moreover, the majority of mothers were spontaneously and informally meeting other mothers (especially those with small children) in small groups, or they were busily occupied in the traditional activity of running the home.

DISCUSSION AND ANALYSIS

The school was observed to be operating with an amazing level of enthusiasm and commitment, despite the experience of two wars, repeated displacement, the very poor physical environment of the camp and the lack of teaching materials. The teachers give much of the credit for this to the management and the leadership in the school, though the recruitment of effective and devoted teachers who had a high commitment to the children was also a very significant factor. Personality attributes were a more important selection criterion than experience of teaching. The approach to the planning of the school was also extremely important. The people themselves took responsibility for defining needs, taking decisions collectively and planning the school. Given the tribal nature of the conflict in Somalia, the recruitment of members of the Education Committee, and of the teachers themselves, from different tribal groups was significant. This enabled a participative ethos to develop in the school, in which all teachers felt themselves to be involved in decisions. This resulted in a strong sense of ownership of what they were doing, coupled with an equally strong sense of responsibility to the community as a whole.

Despite the fact that the teachers adopted the traditional educational methods which are typical of the culture, outside the classroom situation their role evolved in a flexible and non-conventional manner, extending their work and influence out into the community. This broadening of their role partly reflected the broad range of teacher training modules provided by Rädda Barnen.

Many factors are important in working to promote the psychological well-being of refugee children. Undoubtedly the most important factor for children is to belong to a family and a community, both of which can serve to rebuild a sense of stability and security and thereby enhance their resilience (see Chapter 8). A social environment of care and support promotes both health and psychological recovery, and this is just what the teachers' group shows in action. These teachers also demonstrate that it is possible not just to run a school but to do so in a way that makes the school the most influential and stable community resource.

It has to be admitted that the school was not consciously planned in quite this way, and the return visit in 1995 showed that all expectations of what the school could achieve had been exceeded. In the context of a refugee camp lacking a strong and united leadership structure, the teachers' group took this role, becoming respected leaders within the community. The sense of partnership with parents also helped to raise their status and enhance their role *vis-à-vis* families in the camp.

By way of contrast, the high hopes of an effective and dynamic Women's Union did not materialise. Just as the school became successful partly as a reflection of good leadership, the Women's Union failed partly because of the lack of good leadership, a problem which seems to have been compounded by the assumption that, once established, it would develop through its own internal resources. With hindsight, it seems that the women might have benefited from more facilitative support during the early implementation stage. Greater clarity of aims and a stronger sense of ownership by the women themselves probably required longer-term support by external personnel with sound knowledge and experience of community work practice and principles: this Rädda Barnen, for various reasons, could not provide.

But a second reason had also been suggested, that perhaps Somali women are more familiar with a pattern of social interaction that is more informal and occurs in small groups. With hindsight, perhaps the vision for the Women's Union was too ambitious. It might have been more appropriate to begin with the more immediate life-tasks facing Somali women such as giving birth, feeding and caring for children, looking after the home and perhaps engaging in modest business enterprises. Instead of trying to support the more formal leadership patterns required by a social organisation such as a Women's Union, it might have been more appropriate to work to identify the less visible patterns of informal leadership amongst the women in the camp, and find ways to support and strengthen these. Given the lack of the more formal, more visible patterns of leadership among the women in Algahin, the leadership of the Women's Union was likely to depend on a small number of powerful women, leaving the Union vulnerable to inappropriate and autocratic leadership.

Perhaps the most interesting issue to emerge from the follow-up visit was the manner in which the school teachers had approached the psychological needs of the children. The original intention was to introduce a substantial element of psychological knowledge into the training of teachers to enable them not only to recognise the symptoms of stress in children but to be able to respond to them through individual and group discussions about their experiences and the impact of them in their lives.

In the follow-up visit in 1995, it was revealed that the intended training in psychosocial needs had not been undertaken, for a variety of reasons. It was equally clear that the teachers' group had a very clear concept of children's psychosocial needs, though terms such as this were not actually used. But rather than pursuing the idea of group discussions in school about difficult experiences, and the idea of 'supportive conversations' with individual children, the school staff had evolved their own methods of working purposefully with the children. These methods emphasised patterns of communication and expression other than verbal interaction, which Western approaches tend to stress. They had placed particular emphasis on the importance of daily structure, adult support and play in promoting the psychosocial well-being of the children, and these were very evident in the various activities planned and implemented by the teachers. They had taken their role outside the school, first in promoting partnership with parents, and also in developing a wide range of out-of-school activities. Rather than seeing reactions to traumatic experiences as individual problems, they preferred rather to emphasise that everyone in the camp has experienced violence, war and displacement, and that the whole community is not only grieving together but also coping collectively.

Community-building is a way for adults to cope with difficult experiences, a collective coping strategy. The teachers expressed this by saying that they deal with difficult experiences by such means as 'taking part', 'creating', 'learning more' and by 'maintaining a strong belief in God'. To belong to a well-functioning community where there are strong ties between its members may be the most important coping strategy.

This group of Somali refugees had been not only traumatised by their experiences of war and displacement in their own country, but had to contend with a move to another site in Yemen and finally the experience of being caught up in a war in the country of refuge, and the consequent sense of retraumatisation and further displacement. Furthermore, the camp environment was far from satisfactory, located in a barren area with a harsh climate.

In the face of all these difficulties, and with only minimal external assistance, the school re-established itself, and at the time of the return visit offered a vibrant resource to the children and to the whole community. Morale was high among the school staff, reflecting various factors, including excellent leadership, the participative manner in which the school was first developed, and the support and training provided by Rädda Barnen. It was these very factors that produced so much success in the school project that were overlooked in the development of the Women's Union and thus ensured its failure. With hindsight, more should have been done to identify the less visible, small-scale leadership patterns already existing amongst the women of the camp, and support these rather than promoting a more formal style of leadership.

The modest level of professional social work input from Rädda Barnen was also probably a significant factor in the Women's Union not succeeding in fulfilling its promise. A social worker could have actively supported the women and assisted them to analyse the weak points at an early stage and encouraged presumptive female leaders to come forward. Interestingly, the school accepted and rose to the challenge to respond to the broader psychosocial needs of its pupils but, rather than uncritically accepting Rädda Barnen's concept of how this should be achieved, the teachers' group developed their own approach. In contrast to typical Western approaches, the school's strategy emphasised the collective nature both of the psychological problems being addressed and of the way in which they should be approached.

CONCLUSION

Good community work is based on a positive view of humanity: it sees refugees as being resourceful, creative and committed to the well-being of their own community. It avoids the negative and cynical perception of refugees as passive, dependent and exploitative. In this study, teachers demonstrated a natural understanding of the psychosocial needs of the children, an awareness of their own emotional needs, and a real desire to assist children who had been affected by their experiences. The school provided a sustainable environment in which the teachers could use their own, largely intuitive understanding, and help to provide a range of ways in which, collectively, people could cope with these difficult experiences in a culturally appropriate manner. The women of the community had directed their resources and mobilised action in areas of social life that were beneficial to them and their community.

Social development perspectives in social welfare are as yet significantly undertheorised (Midgley 1995) and command no universal acceptance. The term remains poorly defined and the literature highly fragmented. In some European countries this fragmentation is replicated in practice, with community development concerns being hived off from the traditional remit of social work to other professional groupings. Retreat into the individualistic, case-work orientation is all too common. Midgley suggests the field has been marked by much 'hortatory exhortation' rather than informed by the articulation of specific interventions (Midgley 1995:8). Lessons for the Western world can be gleaned from strategies and interventions emerging from the developing countries.

Summary

This chapter has highlighted the following points:

- People themselves as the resource for social change and development;
- The importance of the role of women and their informal social networks in the development process;
- The importance of traditional and culturally specific coping strategies;
- The importance of supportive adults and daily structure in the lives of refugee children;
- The importance of social work/community-based interventions being directed by the community itself.

REFERENCES

Brokensha, D. and Hodge, P. (1969) *Community Development: An Interpretation*. San Francisco and Los Angeles: Chandler.

Burkey, S. (1993) *People First: A Guide to Self Reliant, Participatory Rural Development*. London: Zed Books.

McCallin, M. and Fozzard, S. (1990) *The Impact of Traumatic Events on the Psychological Well-Being of Mozambican Women and Children*. Geneva: International Catholic Child Bureau.

Midgley, J. (1995) *Social Development*. London: Sage.

Segerström, E. (1994) *'From Exposed to Involved'. An Action-Oriented Study of Somali Refugee Mothers' Psychological Well-being and their Sense of Competence to Care for their Children*. Stockholm: Rädda Barnen.

Van den Hombergh, H. (1993) *Gender, Environment and Development: A Guide to the Literature*. Utrecht: International Books.

Chapter 10

Gypsies and social work in Sweden

Karl-Olov Arnstberg

WHAT DOES THIS CASE STUDY ILLUMINATE?

Since the Second World War social authorities in Sweden have been practising social engineering on different Gypsy groups. They have been offered housing, education, economic security, work training and employment of different kinds and through various programmes. The desire to help the Gypsies has been very strong – it is possible to talk about positive discrimination from the social authorities.

However, attempts to integrate Gypsies as self-supporting citizens, loyal to the state, have been unsuccessful. Today a majority among the Gypsies in Sweden are dependent on social welfare. Crimes and escalating drug-abuse are problematic traits. Nevertheless, the various Gypsy groups in Sweden are ethnically strong and successful in defending their ethnic identity.

INTRODUCTION

At the beginning of the 1950s Gypsies in Sweden were no longer able to finance a nomadic life-style. They settled down, first in camps and after a few years in modern apartments. Compared with Gypsy groups in other parts of Europe, these Gypsies were inclined towards assimilation. However, their international contacts increased, there was ethnic consolidation and Gypsies learnt how to handle the Swedish welfare system. The Swedes did not mind very much since there was a standing obligation to help the oppressed Gypsies.

The 1950s and 1960s were so-called decades of 'giving'. During the 1960s Sweden might well have been the most 'Gypsy-friendly' society in the world. Many Gypsies seized the opportunity, strengthened their Gypsy identity and chiselled out a minority status based on their hard fate. The picture changed during the next decade and the education of the Gypsies was seen as the most important question in social work. Soon the picture changed again and today the aim is to 'normalise' social work. A minimum of extra help and special treatment is to be given to Gypsies.

In the late 1960s and early 1970s large-scale housing-construction projects were carried out in Sweden. Today many of the resulting 'concrete suburbs' appear to be rigidly segregated. Mostly Gypsies live in such areas, among other migrant groups. Skilful social work is executed but when it comes to the more complicated questions concerning assimilation or at least an overall, peaceful integration, this seems to be beyond the reach of social welfare.

GYPSIES IN EUROPE

In Western Europe the Gypsy population is estimated at approximately one and a half million. In Eastern Europe there are more than twice as many. The numbers are uncertain, depending on how Gypsies are defined. Although Gypsy life-styles are normally concealed from the eyes of other groups and national authorities, Gypsies are often discussed and they are probably also the ethnic minority which has been most written about.

Gypsies have many words for defining non-gypsies: *gajé*, *gadjo*, *gorgio*, *shabane*, *bure*, etc. Gypsy groups are never autonomous, which is why these terms are heavily symbolic. Gajé is 'the other', whom you try to outwit, but also the one upon whom you are economically dependent. 'Man' in a more neutral vocabulary is in Romani called *manush* or *manushi*. Gypsies call themselves *le rom*, *roma*, *rommano*, *kalé*, *sinti*, etc. Finnish Gypsies call themselves *Romane* (pl. *Romanit*) or *Kaalo* (pl. *Kaaleet*), which means 'black'. *Roma* is the term Gypsies prefer in their struggle for recognition as an ethnic group among others in Europe and the world.

Gypsies have for very long, perhaps always, suffered serious persecution. Today ethnic oppression is increasing and public hostility is becoming a major problem in countries around Europe. In Eastern Europe Gypsies are a prime target for ultra-nationalist violence, and are occasionally victims of police brutality. Virtually always they are on the bottom rung of society. This results in severe health problems, illiteracy and often miserable housing.

However, as an ethnic group, Gypsies are normally strong and clever in defending their ethnic identities and often manage to provide for themselves. In Western countries with welfare provisions, they are often quite successful in exploiting social welfare. In the long run this results in new kinds of dependencies on Gajé. Still, there are signs of hope. A new generation of Rom activists is growing and around Europe you find projects that try to increase understanding of Gypsies not as a problematic slum population but as one ethnic minority group among others.

GYPSIES IN SWEDEN

In the records of the Stockholm Municipal Administration from 1512 one can read about a Gypsy encampment: Count Antonius had arrived from 'Little Egypt' with his countess. They were pilgrims and the town presented them with 20 marks. Perhaps these Gypsies truly believed they originated in Egypt, but appearing to be pilgrims was just a trick, which was to their advantage since Europe was witnessing a religious boom at the time.

Swedes were not favourably disposed towards Gypsies for very long. Their life-style and ethics were soon seen as a continuous provocation by a settled, hardworking and God-fearing farming population.

Facing the First World War in 1914, Sweden closed the frontier. Eight Kelderasha Gypsy families, travelling along a northern route, happened to be in Sweden. They decided to stay, regarding being shut out as a worse fate than living permanently in Sweden. These families were mostly nomadic, even during the cold Swedish winter, but they also settled down for shorter periods. They made their living in a traditionally Gypsy way: as tinkers, dealing with horses and various kinds of merchandise – not all business being absolutely honest. They also entertained in the countryside, with music, circuses, fortune-telling and other modest forms of entertainment.

By the beginning of the 1950s it was no longer possible to make a living out of the traditional nomadic Gypsy life-style. A majority of these 'Swedish Kelderasha Gypsies' – approximately 300 – settled down in camps around Stockholm.

Having impoverished Gypsies living around the capital did not exactly please the Swedish authorities. Sweden was then undergoing fast modernisation and the Social Democrats, the hegemonic political party, had great ambitions to build a welfare state, a kind of third way, an alternative to both communism and capitalism. Therefore, in spite of a severe housing shortage, local authorities around Sweden often gave priority to flats to Gypsies over Swedes. In some places they also built small houses specially for Gypsies.

The Swedish Gypsies were, compared with Gypsy groups in other parts of Europe, inclined towards assimilation. Especially after the Second World War they no longer had any strong ties with their kin around Europe.

Another Gypsy group, Finnish Kalé, more numerous than the Swedish Kelderasha Gypsies, also travelled in Sweden. In the middle of the 1950s these Finnish Gypsies, like other northern citizens, obtained the right to move freely in Scandinavia and Finland. Although they were Gypsies, the Kalés were to the Kelderasha just another group with a similar life-style, but they were not kin.

In some respects these small Gypsy groups were advantageous for Sweden, with its growing desire to be a moral example to the rest of the world. If Swedes were able to guide them into modern society – i.e. housing, schools and employment – this would give Sweden political credit internationally.

The Kelderasha (as well as the Kalé) Gypsies responded to the Swedish invitation. They left their camps, moved into modern apartments and adapted to modern life-styles. The traditional Gypsy dress was modified, but not abandoned. Men dressed in good suits, maybe a little too flashy for Swedish taste. Women Westernised, but kept their long skirts and the *dikló* (little scarves in their hair). Different kinds of experts declared that we were now seeing the end of Gypsy life in Sweden; soon they would be absorbed into the Swedish 'folk-home'. The Gypsy life-style was thus understood solely as a result of oppression and stigmatisation, acts of racism. When Gypsies were offered the benefits of modern society, naturally they would want to live the Gypsy life no longer.

However, what seemed to be a process of assimilation was in fact the opposite: a strengthening of the Gypsy minority. Gypsies learnt to live another form of Gypsy life, a modern Gypsy life, which among other things meant that they activated slumbering kin relations with other Kelderasha and Lowara around Europe. They also learnt how to make use of the Swedish welfare system – not that the Swedes were seriously concerned, since the 1950s and 1960s were decades of 'giving'. Gypsies had been Swedish society's failures for a long time, which meant that Swedes had a long-standing obligation to help the oppressed Gypsies.

Gypsy life-style and Gypsy culture, including nomadism and camp life, were never understood as having value in their own right amongst the Swedes.

There were four possible stereotypes that could be applied to the Gypsies:

- good and respectable Gypsies, long oppressed but now more than willing to become Swedes;
- exciting, free and mythical Gypsies, a stereotype favoured by poets, artists, musicians, etc.;
- foreign and dangerous Gypsies, travelling around and for ever being problematic: the traditional political perspective;
- Gypsies deteriorating into a modern slum population: the pessimistic view in social welfare, and a stereotype that motivates responsible political and social action.

Missing from the agenda is Gypsy culture as *counter-culture* – Gypsies as highly competent in defending and rebuilding their ethnic integrity. Also missing is the *ethnically* oppressed Gypsy, later the favourite stereotype among Roma activists.

The first problem to solve was housing. In a cold country like Sweden, living in tents and camping was next to unimaginable. Luckily, these Swedish Gypsies were not too numerous and it is said that in 1963 all Gypsies in Sweden were settled, most of them with housing allowances in rented flats.

Acquiring flats for Gypsies was a new kind of test for the new, non-discriminating Swedish society. At first, some politicians did not understand how fatal it would be to their political career to act or talk in disparaging terms about Gypsies. Some politicians suspected that there would be future conflicts between Gypsies and (other) Swedes. They were proved right, but to air this opinion was becoming taboo. During the 1960s, it was not possible for politicians openly to discuss problems arising from encounters between Gypsies and Gajé (non-Gypsies).

Swedish Gypsies were favoured since they were so few, altogether perhaps fewer than 1,000 persons in the 1950s. This meant that a majority of Swedes had no experience of contact with Gypsies. It was no wonder that most people believed the true but nevertheless one-sided perspective of Gypsies as a severely oppressed minority group. In general, people were aware of Gypsies as having shared the Jews' tragic fate in Nazi concentration camps. Although there was no further systematic oppression of Gypsies in Sweden – sometimes it was even the other way round – there was a national feeling of debt not only to the Jews but also to the Gypsies, a debt that could never be fully repaid.

Gypsies in Sweden, like many other Gypsies, grasped the opportunity and chiselled out a minority status based on their difficult situation. During the 1960s Sweden might well have been the most 'Gypsy-friendly' society in the world.

NAIVE REALISM

When the Gypsies settled down, not able to finance their traditional way of life any more, they met a handful of strongly empathic helpers. Among them one can name Carl-Herman Tillhagen, a folklorist with an interest in Gypsy lore, Sven Andersson, a social inspector in Stockholm, and John Takman, doctor in social medicine and later also a left-wing politician (Andersson 1959; Takman 1976; Tillhagen 1965). They were all eager to help the Gypsies find a better life and they had no doubts about what that involved. Besides decent dwellings, schooling was of great concern – illiteracy would be fought; the Gypsies would first of all be taught how to read and write. They would also be trained in suitable professions, so they could make their own living again in the future. The support was to be clearly defined, extensive and, it was hoped, of limited duration. This was an era of social engineering.

Ivar Lo Johansson, an established and very well-known writer in the field, expressed doubts about this project. In his opinion the Swedish helpers were clipping the wings of the Gypsies and this benevolence was even worse than the former oppression. The chance of the Gypsies surviving this kind of poisoned friendliness was minimal, he wrote. This was understood as hopeless romanticism and a Swedish Gypsy author, Katarina Taikon, criticised his standpoint in her first book about Gypsies in 1963. Ivar Lo Johansson had spent only one summer, many years ago, travelling with Gypsies. He could not possibly understand the problematic modern Gypsy life as Katarina Taikon did. The fact that she had lived with Gypsies only as a child, was married to a Swede and had a Swedish mother, did not matter. She *knew* and Ivar Lo Johansson did not. The Gypsies needed help and the message was that the Swedes should now roll up their sleeves and do what they should have done a long time ago for the Gypsies. There were a lot of good intentions and a will to solve 'the Gypsy question' once and for all. Media supported this project, and suggested that maybe Sweden could even help Gypsies living in other countries. In an editorial in *Dagens Nyheter*, the leading morning paper, one could read on 16 September 1963: 'The Society has reached a realistic perspective on Gypsies too late and because of this the [Swedish] society has certain obligations to this national minority, obligations that should be extended to Gypsies living outside Sweden.'

Three months earlier the same newspaper wrote that the Gypsies in Europe were a group deserving public support. It was believed that there were not too many Gypsies and Sweden now had the opportunity to show that the national concern with racial matters was not just high-flown rhetoric. It was recommended that the Swedish borders should be wide open. This did not only mean that Gypsies were welcome but also that Sweden would give financial support during what was expected to be a short process of assimilation. In fact, around 1970 Sweden even tried to import Gypsies from other countries and refugee camps. A couple of hundred Lowara Gypsies were picked up from a slum district outside Rome and put into ambitious programmes for assimilation. However, it was difficult to find Gypsies in refugee camps. With their experiences in the Second World War, they avoided such places even when the costs were very high. The Swedish idea of organised Gypsy transfer was therefore, not surprisingly, soon aborted.

This was not only a time of *ignorance* about ethnic processes but it was also a time of *realism* in the sense that there was no doubt what would become of the Gypsies and what they were entitled to as Swedish citizens. Official thinking was simplistic, even naïve. It was never seriously asked what the Gypsies themselves wanted and most certainly nobody suspected a hidden 'Gypsy agenda'. The Gypsies were expected to be grateful and play along. In a way they did.

The more aware social welfare workers viewed Gypsies as 'no different from anybody else' and most definitely entitled to a decent life. But this view was only partially held during the 1950s. Behind the scenes, many were still of the opinion that Gypsies were parasites and should be hunted from parish to parish, and best of all would be if they left the country. Therefore, to solve 'the Gypsy question', it was not enough to provide economic support and programmes for assimilation, it was also important to educate Swedish authorities in modern non-discriminatory thinking. The media were interested in this and in the 1960s most of the writing, broadcasting and television was against oppression and strongly in favour of the Gypsies. When it came to conflicts, it was almost never the Gypsies who were in the wrong or mistaken, it was the neighbours, the authorities, the Swedes who were the culprits. The movement in favour of Gypsies was very strong: it was conceded that they were a little different, but if concerned people were patient, they would soon improve, soon become as good neighbours, workers and citizens in the Swedish 'folk-home' as anybody else.

In the 1960s a regular school for Gypsies was set up in the south of Stockholm. The results, however, were not too promising. The Gypsies showed no eagerness to become Swedes. They turned the school into a Gypsy scene, a place where Gypsies could meet each other and do the kinds of things they had done in the old Gypsy camps. The school was not a major interest of theirs: it was regarded as 'Gajé-business'.

A darker picture of Gypsies was emerging, which was new from the Swedish point of view. Gypsies in open conflicts with and routinely insulting neighbours, criminal Gypsies, Gypsies not at all interested in studies or employment, Gypsies exploiting social welfare. How should this be managed? The authorities turned to the social researchers in order to find out what was happening.

AN ANALYSIS OF GYPSY CULTURE

Most social researchers in the 1960s wrote with an ideological bias. Gypsies should and could indeed be studied, but research should be done with maximum participation. Swedes were interpreted as strong and Gypsies as weak and threatened by modern society, an ethnic group in retreat. The idea, however, was not only to help Gypsies as individuals. In spite of what happened around the Gypsies, a loss of Gypsy culture would be a severe loss to the whole world.

At the end of the 1960s this picture was challenged by the psychologist Inga Gustafsson who, with inspiration from the Norwegian social anthropologist Fredrik Barth, painted a picture of Gypsies as ethnically strong and quite successful in defending their autonomy and providing for themselves (Gustafsson 1970). She pointed out that it was not ancient Gypsy customs, beliefs, dressing, etc. that was the heart of Gypsy culture. It was the border between Gypsies and Gajé that should be in focus. How did Gypsies handle interaction across the ethnic divide? The key phrase was 'boundary-maintaining mechanisms'. How did Gypsies encounter Gajé, without becoming assimilated?

Inga Gustafsson's empirical material was collected in the Gypsy school for children and also in educational study groups which were arranged among the Gypsy parents, who were obliged to attend for financial reasons. She was studying what they did and what their view of Gajé was, who put pressure on them and their children to assimilate, and how they responded to all this. Inga Gustafsson pointed out the following Gypsy strategy, as a way of defending Gypsy culture and autonomy:

- Be segregated, live your own life and stay apart as much as possible.
- Social relations with Gajé should have an economic basis.
- Primary relations with Gajé should be economics-based. Whenever possible, personal relations should be transformed into economic relations. The reason for having social relations at all with Gajé is economic gain.
- When Gajé show interest in helping Gypsies, they are to be welcomed, but the role should be similar to fixers or servants. Gypsies should always be in command and Gajé life-style should never be a social model.
- Be mysterious and secretive. Give Gajé as little insight into Gypsy affairs as possible.
- Do not learn too much in Gajé school. To learn how to read and write also means that you have to follow Gajé rules. Then you could not claim ignorance any more. Theory and education are Gajé business.
- In a state of conflict, when relations are getting out of control, leave. Find another place to live in.
- Go back to the beginning again, which means that if a process of assimilation has started, if relations are getting too friendly and close, you had better discontinue in one way or another, and then start all over again.
- Maintain chaos. Gypsy life should not be controlled (and dull). Together with order and control there is risk of Gajé taking over.
- Gypsy vitality is only implicitly treated as a boundary-maintaining mechanism by Inga Gustafsson. Nevertheless, this is of great importance. This means a strong and sometimes also arrogant style of interaction with Swedish authorities. When friendliness and co-operation is not effective you should make strong demands, act in an irritating and even frightening way so that Gajé give you what you want, just in order to get rid of you.

This new picture of Gypsies as very competent in handling Gajé and modern society was most certainly on a collision course with the hegemonic picture of Gypsies as ill-adjusted to and threatened by modern Sweden. It was difficult to see that both pictures were true – that this was a question of perspectives. Today we know it is true to say: of course, Gypsies are threatened by modern society. And, of course, Gypsies are clever at surviving and defending their ethnic autonomy.

SOCIAL WORK AMONG GYPSIES

In the 1950s the Gypsies were understood to be a kind of tribe, a people and a cluster of life-styles not fitting into the modern Swedish project at all. They needed help and were treated *collectively*. Housing, allowances, child care, schools, etc. were directed towards Gypsies as a group. However, when social welfare was well established – at the end of the 1960s – the help became more and more individualised and in practice oriented towards mothers and children. It was economically favourable if there were no fathers providing for their families – so fathers kept out of sight of the social authorities. In theory, there should be no advantage being a Gypsy. Social welfare was intended for individuals with urgent and acute needs. The Gypsies should not benefit solely from being Gypsies. However, in practice the thumbscrews were not squeezed too hard. Social welfare was seen not as charity, but not as a problematic national cost either. Social welfare was part of a system of civil rights, making life safe and secure for everybody living in Sweden.

The Gypsies learned to play by the rules. Amongst other things this meant that they could benefit from being troublesome and disobedient – a paradox in itself. It became a welfare game where Gypsies, through acting out conflicts and demands, were often successful in getting more than basic supplies. It simply was not possible to act in such a way as to be expelled from the system – if misbehaviour did not result in imprisonment, it led in a U-turn right back to the social welfare system. It was no wonder that social welfare became habit-forming; more and more Gypsies showed less and less interest in independent living. They were Swedish citizens, and if they needed help they were entitled to it, without being defiled. They certainly knew this and almost everybody else knew it as well. From the outside Gypsies were not clearly seen as exploitative, as making money out of the welfare system; they were just an unlucky and unsuccessful national minority getting justified help from society.

It was obvious that many Gypsies had no choice other than social welfare, if they were to survive. Whether they were or were not able to make their needs known, these needs were nevertheless real. The list of problems to solve seemed endless.

Inga Gustafsson's research and new perspective, however, never refuted the picture of Gypsies as a needy and discriminated-against ethnic group, but it did change them from being like everybody else into becoming an alien national group, strangers *and* socially disabled.

The logic of the game now demanded bridge-builders, 'hyphen-people'. In the old days Gypsies spoke for themselves in their relations with Gajé. Now, when they needed more than help with acute but clear-cut problems like a camping place for the night, when the questions were complicated and it seemed to take a long time to solve them, the old spokesmen were, in the eyes of Swedish authorities, inadequate or not competent enough. The National

Board of Health and Welfare came up with the idea of family educationists, helpers who could stay close to needy families and be supportive in their contacts with different authorities. The family educationists should have an intimate knowledge of Gypsy culture as well as of Swedish authority regulations and culture, i.e., function as both bridges and bridge-builders. Their job was to:

- be fixers and lubricate contacts across the ethnic borderline;
- inform the Gypsy groups about Swedish rules and regulations;
- inform Swedish authorities about Gypsy culture, life-styles and values;
- be supportive to the Gypsy families;
- build fora, which meant arranging situations where Gypsies and Gajé could meet and co-operate.

In this, family educationists were to be more loyal to the Gypsy families than ordinary social workers. They would not do ordinary social work, i.e., support the authorities when it came to taking charge of children: less professional, more feeling, but nevertheless competent. The goal for this new group of helpers was to make themselves unneeded. In the future, when Gypsies were trained and competent enough, they would (again) be in charge of their own lives.

It goes without saying that family educationists were not a very good idea. The focus on small Gypsy families instead of kin groups was ethnocentric. And what happened to the ethnic and economic survival competence that Inga Gustafsson had exposed? Another problem was that these family educationists were usually young people, who planned to stay in the profession for only a short time. It was hard for the Gypsies to face the fact that well-meaning, but nevertheless quite ignorant, Gajé youngsters exercised power and control over them.

This experiment with family educationists continued for a decade and was also tried with other ethnic groups. Of course, some educationists did good work, but their semi-professional status was difficult to maintain. In Swedish social work nowadays, family educationists are history.

SOCIAL WORK IN THE 1990s

During the late 1960s and early 1970s large-scale housing-construction projects were carried out in Sweden. Today, many of the resulting 'concrete suburbs' appear rigidly segregated and a number of them exhibit many of the traits their critics had warned against. The picture, however, is not totally hopeless and problematic. These suburbs also symbolise a multicultural society, young and rich in human resources.

Rinkeby and Tensta are twin suburbs located in the north of Stockholm, where immigrants to contemporary Sweden live. Among them, approximately 500 call themselves Gypsies: Finnish Kalé, descendants of the Swedish Kelderasha and French and Polish Gypsies, who came to Sweden two or three decades ago. The majority are dependent on social welfare. After the 1980s experiment with family educationists, no special treatment was at first offered to these Gypsies, and at the end of the decade the relations between Gypsies and welfare workers was quite poor in Rinkeby and Tensta. The situation was chaotic and Gypsies who felt discriminated against regularly insulted the welfare workers. In general the Gypsies were regarded as hopeless. They were also strongly disliked – not many social workers wanted to deal with them and wished they would just disappear.

Something had to be done, and the solution was yet another specially designed programme for Gypsies. The ambition was the same as always: to 'domesticate' the Gypsies – this time to integrate them into multicultural suburban life.

A handful of social workers in Rinkeby started to work full-time with the Gypsies and the goals were specified as follows:

- Make the day nurseries and kindergartens work for Gypsy children to the same extent as for other children.
- Give the Gypsies already living in Rinkeby guidelines for peaceful relations with Gajé. Also, equip them with the means of preventing other Gypsies from settling.
- Make it possible for Gypsies to succeed in and intensify their schooling and education.
- Strengthen the motivation to work and support themselves. Be sensitive to traditional Gypsy economics.
- Reduce Gypsies' over-consumption of medical care and be helpful in preventing conflicts between Gypsies and hospital staff.
- Reduce drug abuse among Gypsies.
- Make it impossible to misuse social assistance.
- Develop and give suggestions of practical and useful forms of co-operation between relevant authorities and the different Gypsy groups.
- Make general agreements about limited work objectives. Systematise and document working routines and work plans.

Besides the above-mentioned goals there existed ambitions which were more down to earth:

- Improve relations between social workers and Gypsies.
- Improve relations between the authorities and Gypsy clients.
- Make Gypsies understand how to live in flats; they should not vandalise, or disturb, or in other ways be of a nuisance to their neighbours.
- Make the men/fathers visible to social authorities.

This project started very well. The social workers were enthusiastic and became competent at handling their clients. They had a free hand to form their own work routines, massive professional support and psychological, back-up therapy. It is hard working with Gypsies. In the long run there is considerable risk that social workers will become frustrated, cynical and/or 'burned out'.

The Gypsies were suspicious to begin with, but soon found it advantageous to deal with these specialists. Relations between social workers and Gypsies improved fast and dramatically. One of the main reasons for this was that the social workers were successful in establishing a non-aggressive, 'soft practice'. Amongst other things, this meant that, when addressed in arrogant, shrill tones, they answered in low, kind, friendly ones, implying that 'this is not the way we do business in this place'. The group was also successful in making Gypsies understand that, if they did not pay the rent, mismanaged their apartments or disturbed their neighbours, there was no possibility of being rehoused. They also managed to establish contact with not all, but several, fathers. The specialist group was very successful with their down-to-earth aims.

The social workers managed to gain the confidence of many of the Gypsies. In the reception centre there is still an open and friendly atmosphere and many Gypsies describe their problems quite freely and truthfully.

But when it comes to more complicated questions of assimilation or at least general peaceful integration, this is beyond the reach of social welfare. Most Gypsies still refuse to take ordinary employment, and they do not wish to work for Gajé. Besides, in times of severe unemployment, as is the case for many immigrants in Rinkeby and Tensta, Gypsies without special skills could not get jobs even if they really wanted to. When it comes to their criminal activities there are no signs of positive changes (Arnstberg 1998).

In Rinkeby and Tensta, as elsewhere, Gypsies stick to old habits, loyalties, economic adaptation and Gypsy life-styles. However, in the 1990s another serious problem has emerged – drug abuse of a more serious and widespread sort than before. Alarmingly, many young men from different Gypsy groups have acquired, within the space of two years, heavy drug habits. The older generation of Gypsies were – and still are – deeply troubled. This kind of assimilation was not foreseen and it seems as if the drug-abuse variant of Western culture has a stronger capacity to form identities, habits and networks than Gypsy culture. How to stop the heavy drug abuse among young male Gypsies is difficult to find a solution to.

CULTURAL DISJUNCTION

In Sweden, during the 1950s and 1960s, there was a serious offer to Gypsies to assimilate. However, they did not accept it. Instead they made two simultaneous choices: both to accept generous economic help from Gajé and to strengthen their own culture, the latter inspired by other Gypsy groups around Europe. Today we see the result: Gypsy cultures are probably more effective than ever when it comes to establishing and protecting their identity. At the same time we find the majority of Gypsies in Sweden almost totally dependent on social welfare. Quite a few among them have lost many of their old capacities and talents without gaining new independent ones. Still, many think they are doing well.

It should also be mentioned that churches in Sweden and Scandinavia play a role in shaping a positive Gypsy identity. Groups of gypsies are deeply religious. But this is not an assimilative movement: Gypsy church business is strictly Gypsy concern. In addition to the problems of drug abuse, it is very difficult for Gypsy individuals today to escape the stigma attached to their Gypsy identity. Both Gypsies and social workers are guilty of shaping and upholding the cultural diversion between Gypsies and Gajé. Gypsy culture may be stronger than ever, but the personal costs and the stress put upon individuals is considerable. Being a Gypsy has its advantages. It nevertheless also very often means living a miserable and even tragic life.

SELECTED BIBLIOGRAPHY

Andersson, Sven (1959) *Zigenare i Stockholm. Utredning verkställd av socialförvaltningen och socialvårdens planeringskommittés kansli*. Stockholm.

Arnstberg, K.-O. (1987) *Kulturanalys i praktiken. Svar på 20 frågor som brukar ställas om zigenare*. Norrköping: Statens Invandrarverk.

—— (1998) *Svenskar och zigenare. En etnologisk studie av samspelet över en kulturell gräns*. Stockholm: Carlssons.

Barth, F. (1955) 'The social organization of a pariah group in Norway', *Norveg*, Oslo. Reprinted in F. Refish (ed.) *Gypsies, Tinkers and Others*. London 1975.

—— (1969) 'Introduction', in F. Barth (ed.) *Ethnic Groups and Boundaries. The Social Organization of Culture Difference*. Bergen-Oslo: Universitetsforlaget.

Fonseca, I. (1996) *Bury Me Standing. The Gypsies and their Journey*. New York: Vintage Books.

Gustafsson, I. (1970) 'Studier i en minoritetsgrupps strävan att bevara sin kulturella autonomi'. *Stockholms stads och pedagogiska institutionens försöksprojekt för Stockholms zigenarbefolknings rehabilitering*. Rapport nr 9. Lic.avh. Stockholm University: Samhällsvetarförlaget (2nd edn 1971:4).

Handelman, D. (1983) 'Shaping phenomenal reality: dialectic and disjunction in the bureaucratic synthesis of child-abuse in urban Newfoundland', *Social Analysis. Journal of Cultural and Social Practice* 13, May, Australia.

Heymowski, A. (1969) 'Swedish travelers and their ancestry. A social isolate or an ethnic minority?' Uppsala: Almqvist and Wiksell.

Iverstam Lindblom, I. (1988) *Zigenare. En skrift om möten med zigenare i socialtjänsten*. Norrköping: Statens invandrarverk.

Kaminski, I.-M. (1980) 'The state of ambiguity. Studies of Gypsy refugees', Gothenburg University, dissertation in Social Anthropology.
Marta, C. (1979) *A Group of Lowara Gypsies Settle down in Sweden*. Stockholm University: Imfo-gruppen.
—— (1979) *The Acculturation of the Lowara*. Stockholm University: Imfo-gruppen.
Okely, J. (1983) *The Traveller-Gypsies*. Cambridge: Cambridge University Press.
Takman, John (1976) *The Gypsies in Sweden: A Socio-Medical Study*. Stockholm: Libers förlag.
Tillhagen, Carl-Herman (1965) *Zigenare i Sverigei Natur & Kultur*. Stockholm.

Chapter 11

The 3 Rs in social work

Religion, 'race' and racism in Europe

Naina Patel, Beth Humphries and Don Naik

INTRODUCTION

Human beings occupy a range of identities. How should we consider the service needs of black and minority ethnic groups who have settled in European countries as a result of colonial, economic migration or refugee background? Should we define them by their religion alone or their language and culture or their political and economic position? These things are not straightforward since they assume homogeneity as well as a view that the 'majority' play no part in the determination of minorities' position. A focus on minorities' language, culture, religion or just the experience of racism will produce specific service outcomes. However, the realities of human beings are shaped by several factors and our focus is to look at how religion works in the context of racism for racial minorities.

In section 1 we examine the central concerns of the 3 Rs in our title. This should help the reader establish a general context which is underpinned by our structural perspective on racism. The perspective informs us on how we view and analyse the intersection of religion, 'race' and racism in the European context. Section 2 extends the understanding by looking at the active force of religion through the presence of religious minorities in Europe, through its effect on individuals, and in the provision of services in care and welfare in Europe. Section 3 translates this into a structural framework for direct use by practitioners and teachers of social work. The case study, illustrating the 'new' form of racism in Europe, 'Islamophobia', in this section points to the need to look seriously at the complexity of minority ethnic people's lives as well as to the urgency with which the professionals need to fight against all forms of racism.

As we approach the end of the twentieth century, religion seems to have gained a new lease of life across the world, and particular forms of religious movement (especially fundamentalism) have become a vital force for (and against) social change (Sahgal and Yuval-Davies 1992).

Haynes (1996:1) defines two distinct yet related meanings of 'religion'. It refers first in a material sense to religious establishments (institutions and officials) as well as to religio-political groups and movements whose *raisons d'être* are to be found within both religious and political concerns. It refers also, in a spiritual sense, to models of social and individual behaviour that help believers to organise their everyday lives. In this way religion is to do with the idea of transcendence, related to supernatural realities, a system of language and practice that organises the world in terms of what is deemed holy, and of the ultimate conditions of existence. However, the second of these definitions needs to be placed in the context of the first in order that the impact of personal belief on the practice of social work, or indeed of any human activity may be examined. It is also necessary to examine the ways religion figures in racism and fascism, and the complexities of the notion of equality 'regardless of colour, culture or creed'.

SECTION 1: SOCIAL WORK AND RELIGIOUS MINORITIES IN EUROPE

Religion and European racism

First, in considering religion and religious minorities in Europe, we want to draw attention to fiction and reality in the ways Western civilisation is depicted. Pieterse (1991) quotes the following as a common definition of 'European culture':

> What determines and characterises European culture? . . . Europe is formed by the . . . community of nations which are largely characterised by the inherited civilization whose most important sources are: the Judaeo-Christian religion, the Greek-Hellenistic ideas in the field of government, philosophy, arts and science, and finally, the Roman views concerning law.
>
> (p. 3)

Pieterse argues that this image is wrong because it portrays elite culture as representing culture *tout court*, denying European regional cultures and popular cultures. It defines European culture in terms of the past ('inherited civilization') and totally ignores Europe's contemporary multicultural realities. 'Official European culture, reproduced in declarations, textbooks, media programmes, continues to be the culture of imperial Europe . . . what is being recycled as "European culture" is nineteenth century elite imperial myth-formation' (Pieterse 1991:4–5).

Pieterse offers this challenge to modern Europeans,

> How many of you hail from non-European worlds? Or, to use nineteenth century racist language, how many of you are half-caste? How many of

> you were never represented in this elite European project in the first place – as members of the working class or living in the countryside, or in regional cultures such as the 'Celtic fringe'?

In fact, the great Indian, Chinese and Arab civilisations were in their day more powerful than the European civilisations of the time. India gave birth to Hinduism, which remained largely indigenous to it, and to Buddhism, which died in India but spread through Asia, including China. Arabia gave birth to Islam, which spread through the Middle East and parts of Asia, Africa and Europe (see Siegel 1986).

Moreover, it needs to be said that the ancient Greek philosophy claimed as intrinsic to 'European culture' was heavily influenced by Egyptian and Semitic ideas, what Bernal (1987:1) calls the 'Ancient' model. The version of Greek philosophy which developed during the Enlightenment (the 'Aryan' model) denied any other cultural influences. This denial of any acknowledgement of the African influence on Western philosophy and religion is an example of the impact of racism and chauvinism, and of the ways influential communities construct their own version of 'truth'.

In addition, Webber (1991) describes the reality of cultural and religious influences since the Second World War, when the various countries of Europe looked to different sources of labour, depending on their particular histories and economic relations with the rest of the world. Britain and Holland looked to their colonies and ex-colonies, with Holland also taking workers from southern Europe and North Africa. Belgium and Switzerland looked to southern Europe, to Spain, Portugal and Italy, all countries of emigration. Switzerland's foreign population rose from 90,000 in 1950 to over a million (16 per cent of its population) by 1973. France, West Germany, the Scandinavian countries variously took refugees and other workers from Eastern Europe and North Africa. By the early 1970s there were about 11 million migrant workers in Europe. One-seventh of all manual workers in Germany and the UK had come in as immigrants, and in France, Belgium and Switzerland a quarter of the industrial workforce was immigrant (Webber 1991:12). They brought a dynamic mix of religions and cultures which, meeting and mixing with other cultures, has produced contemporary Europe.

However, what we experience now is not a idyllic multiculturalist, multi-faith community. There has been talk of the 'Islamicisation of France', of 'being rather swamped by people of a different culture' in Britain, and of 'Turk-peoples, the Palestinians, North Africans and others from totally alien cultures. They and only they, are the "foreigner problem" in the Federal Republic' (see Webber 1991). These sentiments have been accompanied by a tightening of European immigration laws, targeted at people from the South, particularly those who are black and whose religion is likely to be Islam. As Sivanandan (1992) puts it:

> A common culture of Euro-racism – which defines all Third World peoples as immigrants and all immigrants and refugees as terrorists and drug runners – cannot tell a citizen from an immigrant or an immigrant from a refugee, let alone one black from another.

The European minority ethnic population is less than 10 per cent (Zakaria 1988), yet is constructed as a threat to the extent that common policies are now in place to exclude ethnic minorities from Fortress Europe.

The persecution of religious groups has a long history in Europe. In different eras, governments in Spain, Poland, France and Germany have acted as a haven for Jewish populations, only then to attack and expel them (Johnson 1987). The 1905 Aliens Act was designed to limit the numbers of Jewish people entering Britain. The Catholic church colluded with fascism during the war of 1939–45, whilst at various times Catholics have been without citizenship rights (Siegel 1986). The spectre of Islam is now seen as the greatest threat to Europe, with the result that European border controls are being tightened, and Muslims are being portrayed as terrorists and illegal immigrants, and thus to be expelled from European countries. Aguirre (1989) writes that NATO (North Atlantic Treaty Organisation) is now looking to the South for the 'new' enemy. He reports that NATO documents identify 'Islamic fundamentalism', poverty and high population growth as the main problems faced by the modern world. This is the background which social workers who deal with religious minorities across Europe need to examine. 'Ethnic-sensitive' or 'anti-racist' practice therefore cannot avoid consideration of the level of internal controls and structured antagonism shown towards black and religious minority groups.

The contradictory role of religion

Not only have people been persecuted for holding to a particular faith, but there have also been internal complexities in terms of the role religion has played. Religion across the world has always had contradictory effects in being drawn in both to oppress people and to support liberation movements. A classic text on this contradictory role is Paul Siegel's *The Meek and the Militant* (Siegel 1986). During decolonisation in India and then in Africa, the churches were initially opposed, then sceptical and finally supported the idea of independence (Haynes 1996). The role of religion has been on the one hand as an ideology of attempted hegemonic control and, on the other, as a vehicle for mobilising community organisation, often to help fend off that control. Both Christianity and Islam are examples of this in sub-Saharan Africa (Haynes 1996). Sometimes the same religious group, at different moments, was involved in both activities.

Haynes identifies the different development of attempts to politicise Christian communities in Africa and Latin America. In Latin America

Christian communities were normally galvanised by radicalised priests. In Africa (except perhaps in South Africa), religious communities generally failed to develop as vehicles of popular power. Haynes documents the development of both Islam and Christianity in Africa, before and after colonisation, along with 'syncretistic' (those which combine a variety of different elements in their spiritual world view) religions. The important thing to note here is the *heterogeneous* nature of both Islam and Christianity (and the other major religions), and that their spread was complex in the ways indicated above. Mbembe (1988) sees the development of modern religions in Africa as the creation of political space in response to the totalitarian ambitions of dictators in some countries. The liberation theologians of Latin America (de Santa Ana 1979) are known worldwide for their mobilisation of poor people against political dictatorship. This is not to say that religious groups are always an emblem of political opposition. Spiritual and community factors are just as important as changes in material circumstances. In addition, religious movements have also been concerned with cultural, regional, ethnic, political and economic tensions which existed before colonialism.

In countries of the North, Christianity has been deeply implicated with power structures for centuries, its bishops at times holding political office and involved in the oppression of the poor. At the same time Christians have been amongst social reformers, as for example in nineteenth-century Britain, worker-priests in France (Edwards 1961), 'Faith in the City' in England (Church of England 1985), the Iona Community and the Gorbals Group in Scotland (Harvey 1987), all radical movements which see the purpose of the church as standing beside and struggling alongside the poor. The stance taken by these groups has at different times brought them into conflict with the governments of the day.

The position of women within religious groups serves as an example of the complex and varied impact of religions. For most African women under colonialism, for example, the prevalence of Victorian attitudes towards women meant that they had no access to education and its associated benefits: 'for most African women . . . the colonial period was characterized by significant losses both in power and authority. . . . Western gender stereotypes . . . assigned women to the domestic domain' (Parpart 1988:210).

In the post-colonial era Mazumdar (1995) describes the oppression of women under Hindu fundamentalism. At the same time, in several countries such as Nigeria and Senegal (Callaway and Creevey 1994) and Sudan (Bernal 1994), religious-based women's organisations have mobilised to create new kinds of political roles for women. Women's Islamic groups are an example of popular religious organisation, especially in countries such as Nigeria and Senegal, where they serve to support women's liberation against male repression. Such groups have skilfully used Islamic precepts to their advantage.

In Britain the dispute over women priests in the Church of England has erupted in recent years, with those in favour having gained an uneasy victory with the admission of women to the priesthood. In the Roman Catholic church the anti-women priests traditionalists still hold the upper hand in this struggle.

In these ways one can see that to speak of religion and religions is to speak of a highly heterogeneous phenomenon which can be used as a weapon against subordinate groups, or can be mobilised in struggles against inequality.

Fundamentalism

Much has been written about religious fundamentalism, and it has become so confused with abusive labelling of Muslims as 'the Barbaric Other', that it has been suggested that the term should be dispensed with altogether. We described above the hysteria and sense of emergency generated in European countries about Islamic fundamentalism. These are orchestrated for the purpose of exclusion. This is not to deny the reality of rise of fundamentalism across different religious groups. Sahgal and Yuval-Davies (1992) show that fundamentalism cuts across religions and cultures and has often been incorporated into and has transformed nationalist movements. Such movements all over the world are basically political movements. They have a religious imperative and seek to harness modern state and media powers to the service of their gospel. They have two features in common: one, they claim their version of religion to be the only true one, and feel threatened by pluralist/secular systems of thought; two, they use political means to impose their version of the truth on all members of their religion, and on others (Sahgal and Yuval-Davies 1992:4). They exist within all the major religions – Christianity, Hinduism, Islam, Judaism, Sikhism:

> [Fundamentalism] can rely heavily on sacred religious texts, but it can also be more experimental and linked to specific charismatic leadership. Fundamentalism can align itself with different political trends in different countries and manifest itself in many forms. It can appear as a form of orthodoxy – a maintenance of 'traditional values' – or as a revivalist radical phenomenon, dismissing impure and corrupt forms of religion to 'return to original sources'.
>
> (p. 4)

There are examples of the rise of fundamentalism globally, operating both in state institutions and legislation, and in the lives of individuals. Some groups make claims to empowerment through fundamentalist beliefs and practices. Sahgal and Yuval-Davies (1992:9) point to a paradox where women, for example, collude with and seek comfort within the spaces allocated to them by fundamentalist movements, whilst at the same time being detrimentally affected by them. Such claims construct constriction as choice (see Humphries 1996), and offer only choice within very narrow parameters, defined and implemented by those in power. As a general rule, fundamentalism equates with intolerance of difference and with extreme moral conservatism.

However, as Sivanandan points out (Institute of Race Relations 1995: 79), there are all sorts of fundamentalisms, some worse than others, some with little organisation and power, some with whole states backing them. He also draws attention to the need to recognise the social processes through which religion passes before it becomes fundamentalist, 'from belief to dogma, from being the "sigh of the oppressed" to becoming the "opiate of the masses"'. Fundamentalism can become fascist, but there is still a point in time when it can be challenged.

Religion and equality

Although it is seldom addressed, not all religions, or rather versions of all religions, assume a goal of equality amongst all people. There exists a potential conflict between notions of equality and religious belief. History bears evidence to this in the subordination and persecution of groups by dominant religions, on the basis of heresy, or ethnicity, or gender, or sexuality, or disability. In each case justification was by reference to divine truth. Modern forms of such persecution range from exclusions of particular groups to 'cleansing' by rape and murder.

Social work education and practice is not immune from these conflicts. For example, some religious-based social work agencies have expressed reservations about treating homosexuals as equal to heterosexuals (see Pilkington 1994). Most people entering social work would not condone the killing of people simply on the grounds of their social identity. However, some see no contradiction between this stance and the social exclusion of groups on similar grounds. Students (and others) who have religious convictions may put limitations on their acceptance of 'equality' where it concerns for instance women, or lesbians and gays. This is not to say that all religious people hold this position, nor is it to say that *only* religious people take this position. The difference seems to be that the prejudice is justified by 'religious convictions' and therefore takes on the aura of the sacred rather than the profane (as in 'blind' prejudice which has no rationale). Some social work courses known to us have admitted students on the grounds that their religious beliefs are sincerely held and therefore excusable, especially if the students are from minority groups themselves.

We also want to point out the problem inherent in many equal opportunities policies which construct a list of people who are disadvantaged without any underlying value base or concept of power. Some equal opportunities statements include 'religious beliefs', ignoring the potential contradiction between this and other parts of the 'litany' of groups identified by the policy. Some religious beliefs legitimate the unequal status of women, or homosexuals, for example, and indeed some exploit vulnerable people for profit and power. This illustrates the problems of formulating a policy which addresses lists which are potentially endless and potentially contradictory.

Another problem with such lists is that they invoke dualistic thinking, a central ideological component of all systems of domination in Western society. This has led to competitiveness for scarce resources, and impossible choices such as whether to affiliate with, say, the black group or the women's group or the disability group. The writer bell hooks (1987) suggests a way of thinking about the issues which centres on the politics of domination. She takes an approach which advocates 'the eradication of domination and elitism in all human relationships' (p. 63). She says,

> it is necessary to struggle to eradicate the ideology of domination that permeates Western culture on various levels as well as a commitment to reorganizing society so that the self-development of people can take precedence over imperialism, economic expansion, and material desires. (p. 69)

This is a position which draws attention to relations of power at interpersonal, institutional and international levels, a useful starting point for understanding present-day Europe. It also acknowledges that groups who have suffered under domination are themselves capable of the oppression of others, that there is nothing in the *essence* of some groups which makes them incapable of dominating others – either inside or external to their communities. Moreover it is a position which engages participants in struggle rather than a passive 'non-discriminatory' stance. And as hooks says, struggle is rarely safe or pleasurable (p. 73). In particular, it demands that domination is resisted, in whatever form it takes, and even where the life-style of those under subordination is personally distasteful. In the next section we look at how relations of power at interpersonal, organisational and international level translates to minority ethnic groups' religious requirements in care and welfare.

SECTION 2: RECOGNISING THE EFFECT OF MINORITIES' RELIGIONS IN SOCIAL WORK

Who are they? What are they?

People's lives cannot be neatly compartmentalised to the exclusion of other factors. 'Minorities', migrants, whatever term we use to signify 'minority' status as a result of being a migrant or a refugee or born of parents who come within this category, occupy a range of identities like those from the majority groups within countries and across Europe. The focus on the 'minorities' is to do with the prevalence of racism and discrimination and the experience of marginalisation as a consequence. This much is at least recognised by the European Parliament since it declared 1997 as the *European Year Against Racism*. The purpose of this section is to consider how 'race', religion and racism are interlinked with reference to demography, in daily living and in service planning and delivery.

The experience of one of this chapter's authors illustrates the intersection of the 3 Rs. In the first week at an inner-city London secondary school having just arrived from India as a Hindu of 12 years of age, a teacher in a Religious Education class remarked: 'in your religion, you could come back as a goat after death', which was met by the laughter of other students. The laughter prompted the teacher to pursue other possibilities of animal reincarnation. This was then extended to 'peculiar' food habits and not eating meat which can 'only stunt your growth' because of 'your strange culture'. Picking on the black and minority ethnic groups' language, culture, religion, their colour is not a new phenomenon, nor is it restricted to one group (see, for example, anti-Semitism in Patel, Naik and Humphries 1998). Racism in our example is the use of professional (teacher) power to devalue the 'other' on an individual basis by virtue of his/her membership of a racial or an ethnic group. The effect of persistent views like the one we have described is well documented: either it leads the young person to reject their culture/religion in the name of 'internalising racism' or creates a reaction which acts as a challenge and salvages self-respect (see various poems in Gambe *et al.* 1992).

Social care and social work

How does the above example translate to the world of social care and social work? Let us consider, for instance, the needs and demands of black and minority ethnic elders in the UK and in parts of Europe: although the current demographic figures suggest a relatively small elderly population from this group (3.22 per cent from Census 1991), the rate of increase will be higher in the next decade because of migration and settlement patterns (e.g. considering age group 45–64 years which stands at 15.18 per cent). This trend is evident across several European countries (Lindblad 1996).

In the UK and Netherlands studies of minority elders (for the UK: Atkin *et al.* (1993), Askham *et al.* (1995) and for the Netherlands, Thomése *et al.* (1995), Nelissen (1997)) have conclusively shown that if sufficient information about welfare services were made available they would be used, but with a qualification. For example, the provision of meals and physical care (male nurses to bathe men) must reflect elders' religious and cultural beliefs since one's identity and dignity are tied to the care of such ordinary matters. And yet we hear of many personal denials and tragedies. In a London borough where one in four of the population is Asian, a 90-year-old Hindu man, a strict vegetarian, was forced to eat meat in a residential home (Moore 1991, cited in Patel 1993). During his employment period, a Turkish elder from Germany commented: 'the food was strange to us. We were often concerned we might be eating pork. At first we mostly ate chicken, we recognised that' (Eberle and Brucker 1998).

Concern has also been expressed in other countries regarding how the death of people from minority groups is treated, from funerals to observance of the rites. This is where various cultural and religious organisations in the UK, Netherlands and France have been critical in making arrangements with mainstream authorities. They have, for example, secured appropriate burials and prayer facilities for their community members.

It is in the absence of mainstream services to respond appropriately to this emerging group of older people that we see a range of self-help organisations or projects developing in the UK, Belgium, France, Germany, Denmark, Sweden or the Netherlands. Often these groups are mindful of the multi-faith nature of their membership in their activities. The Anderston Mel-Milaap Centre in Glasgow, UK, states in its brochure: 'We celebrate: Eid and Vaisakhi; Diwali Festival; International Women's Day; X-mas and New Year.'

Nor are these organisations, often surviving on shoe-string budgets, limited in their vision: the Vietnamese Elderly Community Centre, whose members occupy refugee status in the Netherlands, have their strategy described by Nguyên Xuân Hiên (Amin and Patel 1997) as:

> help yourself first then God will help you.
> . . . Go, See, Listen, Introduce activities and Stimulate the Participation . . .

Similarly, Sarie Adeslam of Alamanar Association in Brussels says:

> there are many questions – how do we defend the moral and material interests of the elderly from the Maghreb without succumbing to the pressures of securing only personal interests? Take safety for example: how do we protect ourselves as elderly and our families against attacks from violence, fascism, racism and xenophobia? What should we do ourselves and what can we expect from the authorities and the wider society? *Almanar* cannot just be satisfied with raising such questions. It has to suggest methods and responses to handle such problems.

We also find demands from minority ethnic elderly women to rethink facilities at places of worship for use by women. The Belgium entry on this aspect states, 'in our mosque there is no . . . room for women . . . to attend lectures . . . or for a meeting place' (Vander Meeren 1998).

The recognition of religion in daily living and care and welfare is also provided at a wider political and potentially policy front. The Council of Europe, the Committee of Experts on Community Relations from fourteen European countries (1991) asserted in their final report:

> For many immigrant and ethnic groups cultural identity is very much bound up with religion. Coping with increasing religious diversity is rapidly becoming a central issue in most European immigration countries. . . . In practical terms, most of the member States are now having to work out what is the proper approach towards the presence in their midst of substantial non-Christian and non-Jewish religious communities, in particular Muslim and, to a lesser extent, also Hindu, Buddhist and Sikh communities. . . . Freedom of religion is a basic characteristic of European society . . . the Committee has noted that, in certain cases, respect for freedom of religion may create practical problems in the following areas:
>
> availability of places of worship;
> funeral customs;
> times of prayer, daily and weekly;
> times of fasting (e.g. Ramadan);
> recognition of religious festivals;
> dress;
> diet (e.g. halal meat);
> availability of appropriate and qualified religious personnel.
>
> . . . The Committee recommends that, as a general rule, such arrangements, which may sometimes include forms of financial support by the State, should also apply to other religions.
>
> (pp. 55–6)

As to training and employment, it recommended:

> Probably the best means of ensuring that public services respond effectively to the varied needs of a multiethnic clientele is to recruit staff who are themselves of immigrant origin. . . . Public services staff should be trained in the need to eliminate unequal and discriminatory treatment and in developing responsiveness to the particular needs of migrants and ethnic groups.
>
> (Council of Europe (1991), Community and Ethnic Relations in Europe, section 274 (final report), p. 66)

Such recommendations, made well before the 1997 European Year Against Racism, give us encouragement not to see the fight against racial inequality in purely cultural/religious terms or to see the inequality in terms of racism, void of minorities' cultural and religious realities and the changing pattern of racisms. Moreover, the link between service provision and employment and training is significant, as well as the fact that the coverage extends across European countries (experts were drawn from fourteen countries). This aspect is important since in debates on racial equality in social work in the European context, expressions like 'such matters are relevant for the UK but not for us' can be heard.

So what does this mean for the social worker working with black and minority ethnic users?

We can make a number of observations: first, religion, religious thoughts, religious practices and spirituality are integral to people's lives, however practised. In working in a multiracial and multi-faith society, social workers face many demands, challenges and possibilities in utilising information. They develop skills and competence which do not necessarily derive from their own cultural and social background. In the trans-European work of *CNEOPSA* Project on dementia / Alzheimer's disease, a manager from an English background running a Jewish residential home said, 'it is important to have staff from the same background because when residents celebrate religious events, staff can share in the *meaning* behind the events' (Patel and Mirza *et al.* 1998).[1]

This is because the 'meaning' involves aspects of celebration, invocation, commemoration and compassion. These aspects can be learnt but require considerable training time. Consequently we often hear requests from professional staff, concerned about their lack of preparation for working with minorities, for a checklist of religious customs and practices. Training programmes in many places have geared themselves to providing such sensitivity through a short burst of 'cultural awareness' programmes. But ask yourself: irrespective of whether you come from a majority or a minority background, how long has it taken you to understand the religious, spiritual and philosophical traditions of your faith? How long has it then taken you to practise social work with users from the same group, displaying diversity of religious practices or otherwise? We often take these for granted and pragmatics take over when we are faced with the 'other'. Its whole complexity we reduce in order to acquire that technical knowledge of 'religious customs and practices' of a minority. Worse still, there is a tendency to lump all minorities together, forgetting the diversity of faiths, their socio-economic status and gender and/or to assume that they are all 'religious'.

Training

A social work training framework at a macro level can reflect the issues we explore in the three sections in this chapter. In the UK such a framework is provided by the Central Council for Education and Training in Social Work (CCETSW). CCETSW is responsible for approving and awarding social work qualifications in the UK. It recognises religion in anti-discriminatory social work as part of the general system of values in social work. On values, CCETSW's Rules and Requirements for the Diploma in Social Work (DipSW) qualification state:

> Social Workers practise in social settings characterised by enormous diversity. This diversity is reflected through religion, ethnicity, culture, language, social status, family structure and life style. . . . They must be self aware and critically reflective, and their practice must be founded on, informed by and capable of being judged against a clear value base.
>
> (p. 18)

To be successful in gaining an award of the DipSW, six value requirements have to be demonstrated in meeting the core competences (communicate and engage; promote and enable; assess and plan; intervene and provide services; work in organisations and develop professional competence). The value requirements are that students must:

- identify and question their own values and prejudices, and their implications for practice;
- respect and value uniqueness and diversity, and recognise and build on strengths;
- promote people's rights to choice, privacy, confidentiality and protection, while recognising and addressing the complexities of competing rights and demands;
- assist people to increase control of and improve the quality of their lives, while recognising that control of behaviour will be required at times in order to protect children and adults from harm;
- identify, analyse and take action to counter discrimination, racism, disadvantage, inequality and injustice, using strategies appropriate to role and context;
- practise in a manner that does not stigmatise or disadvantage either individuals, groups or communities.

(p. 18)

To fulfil the role and values identified above, social workers cannot adequately support people without understanding what it is that they as professionals and their users believe. Religious and spiritual beliefs are critical in the formation of social and cultural values. Not surprisingly, we find references to 'religion, race, language and culture' in legislation concerning children services, adult services and even criminal justice (Children Act 1989;

NHS and Community Care Act 1990 and the Criminal Justice Act 1991 respectively).

At a micro level in a teaching situation in Germany, Professor Hans Walz uses photographs of several religious or cultural monuments in a city like Lisbon to get social work students to consider racial inequality in broad terms. The photographs act as stimuli to express the variation in the meaning of religion and the diversity of population. The physical presence of places of worship can be a focus for racist and fascist attacks (European Race Audit quarterly bulletin produced by the Institute of Race Relations gives factual information on such attacks) or to opposition to the building of mosques, temples; and can also extend social work students' horizons in seeing the multi-faith existence of a city's inhabitants.

In other words a simple tool is needed to begin to look at the 3 Rs which we have been concerned with. This stimulus is made significant by the fact that Walz's survey on social work students and religion in Germany found that students ('who are not even the members of a religious institution or one student who claimed to be a Buddhist') held a common view of religion as 'faith in God or in supernatural forces and church-orientation' (paper given at European seminar IFSW/JCSW 1995 with Graca Andre, Portugal on Religion and Human Rights), reflecting, as we said earlier, a limited view of religion if it omits humanistic and spiritual aspects.

Multi-faith Europe?

We have seen how the 3 Rs interact to produce a range of reactions, practices and effects on the majority and minority groups. At this stage it is worth noting the figures available for selected countries on the extent of their multi-faith societies. The demographic and religion information presented is compiled from Encarta World Atlas (1998) using CIA information. This information is provided in Table 11.1 at the end of this chapter.

We can see in Table 11.1 variations across the countries in the size of minority ethnic groups and their religion. The lack of classification of an 'other' category conceals variations between religions. Therefore Table 11.2 (p. 205) provides a view of the range of variation for one country, the UK. Table 11.2 in turn needs to be supported with further information if we are to look at the Afro-Caribbean community's religious traditions. This is provided in Table 11.3 (p. 205), which looks at Black majority churches. Amin (1998) explains,

> Elaine Foster, as do many others, argues that the churches have given black women and men self-worth, dignity and a positive identity, in contrast to the ways in which 'white British society has alienated, devalued and effectively excluded them from the many forms of legitimate involvement in the wider society'.

In a Comment section in the *Financial Times*, Mortimer entitled his piece a 'tale of two cultures' (1997). He explains that at the 'ideas' stage there may be a difference in the treatment of religious minorities between Britain and France:

> it is true that the idea of a body politic composed of sub-groups or 'communities' with their own leaders sits more comfortably with the British political tradition than with that of Jean-Jacques Rousseau and the 'one and indivisible Republic'.

However, in practice things are not that different. To quote Mortimer again:

> The French *Conseil d'Etat*, consulted by the education minister, decided state school pupils had the right 'to express and display their religious beliefs within educational establishments, while respecting pluralism and the freedom of others, and without prejudicing teaching activities, the curriculum and the duty of diligence'. Subsequent rows have turned on accusations of 'proselytising' within the school, or on whether girls can safely keep their veils on for PE lessons. Such problems are not unknown in British schools. And Britain has so far failed to follow its pluralism to the logical conclusion of allowing 'voluntary-aided' Moslem state schools, alongside the Anglican, Roman Catholic, nonconformist and Jewish ones.

As to the future, Mortimer suggests that

> there is clearly a danger in both countries that Moslems, feeling despised and rejected by the rest of society, will isolate themselves in a hostile and resentful ghetto. French reluctance to recognise a community of any sort is hardly the best way to avoid that outcome.
>
> (Mortimer 1997)

The fact that we see the struggles of several organisations reflected in concrete developments in care and welfare concerning minority ethnic communities provides us with encouragement amid the changing context of the 3 Rs in Europe. In the next section we examine specifically how the 3 Rs operate in social work with reference to one religion. A focus on one religion is designed to illustrate rather than ascribe a particular value of importance. We show how Islam is being accorded a different treatment in the form of Islamophobia, which is explained next.

SECTION 3: ISLAM AND SOCIAL WORK: A STRUCTURAL FRAMEWORK

In this section we consider Islamophobia and its effect on the Muslim community. The practice of Islamophobia excludes the contribution which could be made by Muslims in our pluralist and multi-faith society. The focus on Islam does not imply a 'preoccupation' with one religion. Rather, as Mirza (1992) suggests that in the search for European identity,

> the large Islamic communities in the EC, the geographical proximity of the Islamic world, and the 'demonization' of Islam in the western media and political imagination raise the spectre of 'Europeaness' being defined in contradistinction to 'Islam'. The focus on Islam was not intended to suggest that the consequences of ongoing events in Europe for other minorities were insignificant, but that Islam – being on the front line, as it were – could be treated as a *metaphor* for the serious predicament of all minorities in a changing Europe. [our emphasis]

Consider also the following two quotes:

> If you mention religion and conflict in the same breadth, people assume you are talking about Islam, and usually that the Moslem side is in the wrong.
>
> (Mortimer 1997)

> I fled from Iran because I was not respected as an individual, but it is the same here. Swedes always put me in a category. Nobody asks if I have HIV, but their first question is if I am Muslim. To be a Muslim seems to be more dangerous than AIDS.
>
> (Graham and Khosravi 1997)

Hence the aim of this section is to consider the core features of Islamophobia. A link to social work is made through an outline model of a structural approach to practice as a problem-solving method. This model may have some merit since British Muslims suffer from discrimination in all areas of life, including education, health, housing and employment. They also suffer from acts of violence and harassment (Modood *et al.* 1997).

Islamophobia

The term Islamophobia is of recent origin. It is analogous to xenophobia, implying strange or foreign and phobia meaning dread or horror. Islamophobia has always been present in Western countries and cultures. In the last two decades, it has become accentuated, explicit and extreme. The following is a summary of a consultation paper issued by the Runnymede Trust, entitled 'Islamophobia, its features and dangers' (Runnymede Trust 1997).

When comments are made about Islam, they are invariably accompanied by prejudice and antagonistic statements. Two factors are implied in the use of Islamophobia. 'The object of fear is both out there, beyond natural boundaries, and also here, all too close to home.' Islam is seen as having both these strands of fear and dread. This perception causes many non-Muslims to fear and dislike Islam. The Muslim communities in Britain and Europe are sometimes referred to as 'traitors and the enemy within'. Islamophobia in Britain can be equated with racism. It is based on perceiving the pigmentation of the Muslims as black or brown Muslims. They are regarded as having alien customs, and as being threatening to the British nation.

Although Western countries may be debating religious and theological perspectives regarding freedom of speech, freedom of information, human rights, the place of women and sexual mores, comments made in this area by Muslim religious bodies and organisations are regarded as biased. The avoidance of this form of Islamophobia, which excludes perspectives and insights, could enrich Britain in its multiculturalism and multi-faith dimension.

The features of Islamophobia

1. Differences are drawn between Islam and the non-Islamic world. Such differences tend to cause the 'them–us' syndrome. This then leads to stereotyping. For example, Muslim culture is represented as mistreating women, whereas other religions and cultures have outgrown patriarchy.
2. Islam is seen as hostile to the non-Islamic world. The argument runs that Muslim fundamentalism threatens global peace and security. It also causes national and local disturbance through terrorism.
3. Assertions are made about Muslims using their religion for strategic, political and military advantage.
4. Comments made by Muslims in respect of Western cultures and societies are regarded as inconsequential.

The consequences of Islamophobia

It limits the development of a just, pluralist society and it increases the likelihood of social disorder, with implications for the economy and the justice system; it stifles alternative voices and influences within the Muslim communities; it defeats co-operation between Muslim and non-Muslims in analysing issues and promoting shared solutions to problems; it discourages non-Muslims from appreciating and benefiting from Islam's artistic and intellectual heritage; it damages international relations, diplomacy and trade and renders difficulty for Muslims and non-Muslims to work together (Runnymede Trust 1997).

Islam, social work and the structural model

Islam considers human consciousness as a path to reform and righteousness. It believes it is the best path to a constant, harmonious and happy life (El Sanhoury 1993). These principles and values are also enshrined in Christianity, Hinduism and Judaism.

Islam has a comprehensive order of five values. Briefly they are:

The well-being (welfare) of the community is to be safeguarded.
In Islam, all people are regarded as equal and alike (equality).
There is a relationship between individual freedom and the community's obligations to the individual.
Responsibilities and obligations are intrinsic to the person. An Islamic way of life is therefore more than a matter of conscience and conformity to law.
The principle of consultation in Islam is one of the core principles upon which relationships between people are based.

(Bayoumi *et al.*1988)

These are principles based on the links between the individual, the group and the community. Social support is regarded as co-operation between individuals; equality and justice between people; rendering of social care; sympathy and the concept of consultation as a basis for community affairs and statecraft.

Religious values and principles have played a major role in the development of social welfare as an institution and the emergence of social work as a profession. These values have encouraged people to perform good deeds, to help the needy and the weak in society. Islam, like Christianity, has common characteristics of the welfare concept which can be sensitively incorporated in social work practice. Social workers therefore need to determine their professional position with regard to religious communities. They also need to understand their own personal values as they relate to social work theories and religious beliefs.

We can now describe an outline of a micro-level intervention model in which the ultimate target of change is the social environment. This model aims to improve the quality of the relationship between people and the social environment. It does this by changing social structures which limit human function and aggravate human suffering. It is a structural approach to social work practice which embodies most of the Islamic principles briefly described above. The way in which a problem is formulated places constraints on the range of alternatives from which a solution can be chosen. For example, if a problem such as unemployment is defined as a lack of motivation, then efforts to alleviate the problem will be directed towards motivating the unemployed. On the other hand, if the problem of unemployment is defined as breakdown in the structure of opportunity, then efforts to ameliorate the problems will centre around increasing the number of available jobs and ensuring equal employment opportunity. Definition of a problem, therefore, is a potent force.

This model presupposes that large sections of the population – the poor, the aged, and black and minority groups – are neither the cause of their problems nor the appropriate target for attempts at changes that are directed at alleviating their situation. This does not imply that some people, at times, do not have individual problems.

However, in many instances inadequate social arrangements are chiefly responsible for the problems that are frequently defined as products of those who suffer from them (Ryan 1978). For example, poverty was not created by the poor, nor racism by the blacks. Attempts to change individuals instead of mitigating the social need that causes them to suffer simply perpetuate the existence of such problems.

There are four principles based on the model of structural approach to practice.

1 The worker should be accountable to the service user(s).
2 The worker should follow the demands of the service user's task.
3 The worker should maximise the potential support in the service user's environment.
4 The worker should proceed from an assumption of least contest.

These four general principles shape the approach to social work and also allow for specific strategies to be drawn.

The Structural Model: general and specific strategies for the social worker to follow

General principles	Strategies
Be accountable to service users.	Develop a service contract with the user (verbal or written, whichever is appropriate). Look beyond each user to establish whether there are others facing the same task *Engage in three types of activity:* 1 Work with users on their own behalf

Follow the demands of the user's task	2 Work with users on behalf of others. 3 Work with others on behalf of users. Work with relevant people at different times. Assume roles specific to the strategic action: (a) broker, (b) mediator, (c) advocate.
Maximise support in user's position in the environment.	Avoid occupying the cental helping process (non-egotistic style). Bring to bear change and/or create structures.
Proceed from the position of least contest.	Engage in type 3 activity (as above) before type 2 activity (as above). Assume role of broker before mediator and the role of mediator before that of advocate. The strategy here is gradually to escalate issues unti the required service is provided.

The social worker should take the role of broker prior to the role of advocate, for brokerage is the least threatening role, and advocacy the more threatening role. The social worker can shift from the role of mediator to that of advocate, but he/she cannot reverse the order. That is, once he/she has taken the side of one party in a dispute, he/she loses credibility as a 'neutral person' or as a person equally concerned with both parties. The social worker should establish issues gradually, initiating action at the lowest hierarchical level, proceeding upward until the required service is obtained.

Case example

The social worker may help a Muslim child suffering the consequences of racism at school by talking with his/her teachers about it (type 1 activity described above). In addition, he/she may work with the family and the management board of the school to create an atmosphere congenial to the needs of Muslim children (type 3 activity). If necessary he/she may organise the Muslim children's parents at that school to confront the teachers and the management board (type 3 activity).

In this structural approach to micro-level social work the users are viewed as healthy people, faced by inadequate resources, limited choice, and lack of access to ways of changing their situation. The environmental change, as the goal of intervention, should increase the user's access to resources, thus increasing his/her choices. This structural approach, like any other model, is appropriate in situations that meet the basic assumptions criteria outlined in this section.

Conclusion

We have shown in this chapter the interplay of 3 Rs, religion, 'race' and racism and its implications for social work, social services and training using examples from the UK and/or other European countries. We have located our examination in the context of religion playing a complex role worldwide, at international, national, organisational, group and personal levels. It is a key element in racist constructions in the new Europe. A wide range of groups, sometimes with directly conflicting views, claim religious authority for their beliefs and practices. Humans are able to commit unbelievable atrocities in the name of religion, and to rise to heights of courage and sacrifice for their faith. Any profession which aims to understand what 'makes people tick' should not ignore the place of religion in their lives, in all its contradictory – but very powerful – manifestations.

SECTION 4: SUMMARY

We can summarise the key points which have emerged in this chapter:

- The development of anti-racist/anti-discriminatory social work practice, if it is to be relevant for a multi-faith and multi-ethnic Europe, needs to consider the religious/faith aspects of minorities. Through such consideration, the complexity and challenge of how religion is examined is exposed.
- To plan and provide appropriate care to minority ethnic users, social workers need to appreciate the complex role religion plays in interacting with 'race' and racism. Minorities themselves are in the forefront of developing models of care which incorporate aspects of 3 Rs.
- The role of the social worker as a broker, mediator and advocate in the structural approach to micro-level social work offers the capacity to affect outcomes for users when considering religion and racism (Islamophobia in our example).

Table 11.1 Demography and religion by selected countries in Europe[1]

	Percentages (1995 estimates except where specified)				
Category	*Denmark*	*France*	*Germany*	*Netherlands*	*United Kingdom, 1993 estimate*
Total population	5.2 million	58.0 million	81.6 million	15.5 million	57.2 million
Ethnic divisions	(EUROSTAT 1995) Turks 18.6 Former Yugoslavs 6.3 Norwegians 5.8 Iranians 4.6 Other 42.2	(EUROSTAT 1995) Portuguese 18.1 Algerians 17.1 Moroccans 15.9 Italians 7.0 Tunisians 5.8 Other 24.5	Germans 95.1	Dutch 96.0	English 81.5
			Turks 2.3	Moroccans, Turks, Indonesians, Surinamese and other 4.0	Scots 9.6
			Italians 0.7 Greeks 0.4 Poles 0.4		Irish 2.4 Welsh 0.9 Indians, Caribbean people, Pakistanis and other 2.8
			Other 1.1		

continued . . .

Table 11.1 continued

Category	*Percentages (1995 estimates except where specified)*				
	Denmark	*France*	*Germany*	*Netherlands*	*United Kingdom, 1993 estimate*
Religions	Evangelical Lutheran 91.0	Roman Catholic 90.0	Protestant 45.0	Roman Catholic 34.0	Anglican 47.0
	Other Protestant and Roman Catholic 2.0 Other 7.0	Protestant 2.0	Roman Catholic 37.0	Protestant 25.0	Roman Catholic 16.0
		Jewish 1.0	Unaffiliated or other 18.0	Muslim 3.0	Muslim 2.0
		Muslim 1.0 None 6.0		Other 2.0 Unaffiliated or atheist 36.0	Other Protestant 2.0 Sikh, Hindu, Jewish 2.0 Other or none 31.0

Source: Encarta World Atlas (1998) CD-Rom, Microsoft.

Note
1 Percentages (1995 estimates except where specified).

Table 11.2 Estimates for the main faith communities in the UK

Bahai's	6,000
Buddhists	30,000–130,000
Christians	40,000,000
Hindus	400,000–550,000
Jains	25,000–30,000
Jews	300,000
Muslims	1,000,000–1,500,000
Sikhs	350,000–500,000
Zoroastrians	5,000–10,000

Source: Weller, P. (ed.) (1997) *Religions in the UK: A Multi-Faith Directory*.

Table 11.3 Black majority churches in the UK[1]

	Members	*Congregations*
Church of God of Prophecy	4,938	86
New Testament Church of God	6,665	107
Pentecostal: Afro-Caribbean churches	49,211	605
Of these some of the largest are:		
Four Square Gospel	489	15
Church of Great Britain	1,000	10
New Covenant Church (Pentecostal)	3,500	20
Pentecostal: Oneness Apostolic churches	15,069	212
Of these some of the largest are		
United Pentecostal Church of Great Britain	2,900	17
Christ Apostolic Church, Great Britain	2,000	4
Seventh Day Adventist	18,565	241
African Methodist Episcopal	300	8
Zion Church[2]	450	15
Total	95,198	1,266

Source: Brierley, P. and Wraight, H. (1995), *The UK Christian Handbook* 1996/1997 edition, Marc Europe.

Notes

1 Most have at least some white members.

2 Included here are some of the churches of African origin or some which have a largely African membership although the majority are Afro-Caribbean.

NOTE

1 The CNEOPSA Project consistently found for UK, France and Denmark the importance of religion and spirituality in sustaining the carer and the person with dementia in drawing on deeper long-term memory. The Survey for the UK also found that religion, in the context of faith in God, was used to explain the disease, dementia as 'God's will', while in some cases, the belief in God was doubted or rejected by family carer. This was because of the difficult experience of dementia, particularly when the disease accelerates to 'severe dementia'. If dementia as a degenerative disease is explained away as 'God's will', then there are clear implications for planning, informing and managing care.

REFERENCES

Aguirre, M. (1989) 'Looking Southwards', in D. Smith (ed.) *European Security in the 1990s*, London.

Alison, M. and Edwards, D. (eds) (1990) 'A Speech by the Prime Minister, 21 May 1988', in *Christianity and Conservatism*, p. 338 London: Hodder and Stoughton.

Althusser, L. (1969) *For Marx*, London: Allen Lane.

Amin, K. (1998) 'Ethnic Minorities and Religious Affiliations', in N. Patel, D. Naik and B. Humphries (eds) *Visions of Reality: Religion and Ethnicity in Social Work*, London: CCETSW.

Amin, K. and Patel, N. (eds) (1997) *Our Voices in Europe: The Elderly from Minority Ethnic Groups Speak on Projects in Europe.* Utrecht: NIZW.

Anderson, B. (1983) *Imagined Communities*, London: Verso.

Askham, J. *et al.* (1995) *Social and Health Authority Services for Elderly People from Black and Minority Ethnic Communities*, London: HMSO.

Atkin, K. *et al.* (1993) *Community Care in a Multi-racial Britain: A Critical Review of the Literature*, London: HMSO.

Bayoumi, A.M., El Kordi, D. and Nasr, A.A.S. (1988) *Studies in the Islamic Doctrine and Morals*, Cairo: El Azhar.

Bernal, M. (1987) *Black Athena: The Afroasiatic Roots of Classical Civilisation*, London: Free Association Books.

Bernal, V. (1994) 'Gender, Culture and Capitalism', *Comparative Studies in Society and History*, 36, no.1, pp. 36–67.

Callaway, H. and Creevey, L. (1994) *The Heritage of Islam: Women, Religion and Politics in West Africa*, Boulder, Colo., and London: Lynne Rienner Publishers.

Church of England (1985) *Faith in the City: The Report on the Archbishop of Canterbury's Commission on Urban Priority Areas*, London: Church House Publishing.

Cohen, S. (1996) *Another Brick in the Wall: The 1966 Asylum and Immigration Bill*, Manchester: Greater Manchester Immigration Aid Unit.

Council of Europe (1991) *Community and Ethnic Relations in Europe*, Final Report, Strasburg.

de Santa Ana, J. (1979) *Towards a Church of the Poor*, Geneva: World Council of Churches.

Eberle, B. and Brucker, U. (1998) 'Germany', in N. Patel and H. Mertens (eds) *Living and Ageing in Europe: Profiles and Projects*, Utrecht: NIZW.

Edwards, D.E. (ed.) (1961) *Priests and Workers: An Anglo-French Discussion*, London: SCM Press.

El Sanhoury, A.M. (1993) 'Approach to Social Care', *Report on Islamic Method*, Cairo: Dar El Said Publishers.

El Sherif, O. (1988) 'Notes on the Regime and Administration in the Islamic State', unpublished.

Encarta (1998) *World Atlas*, CD-Rom US: Microsoft.

Gambe, D. *et al.* (1992) *Improving Practice with Children and Families*, Antiracist Social Work Education Series no. 2, London: CCETSW.

Graham, M. and Khosravi, S. (1997) 'Home Is Where You Make It: Repatriation and Diaspora Culture among Iranians in Sweden', *Journal of Refugee Studies* 10 no. 2.

Harvey, J. (1987) *Bridging the Gap: Has the Church Failed the Poor?* Edinburgh: Saint Andrew Press.

Haynes, J. (1996) *Religion and Politics in Africa*, Nairobi: East African Educational Publishers; London and New Jersey: Zed Books.

hooks, b. (1987) 'Feminism: A Movement to End Sexist Oppression', in A. Phillips (ed.) *Feminism and Equality*, Oxford: Blackwell, pp. 62–76.

Humphries, B. (1996) 'Contradictions in the Culture of Empowerment', in B. Humphries (ed.) *Critical Perspectives on Empowerment*, Birmingham: Venture Press, pp. 1–16.

Institute of Race Relations (1995) 'Fighting our Fundamentalisms: An Interview with A. Sivanandan', *Race and Class*, 36, no. 3, pp. 73–88.

—— (1997 series) *European Race Audit*, London: IRR.

Johnson, P. (1987) *A History of the Jews*, New York: Harper and Row.

Lindblad, P. (ed.) (1996) *Elderly People from Minority Groups in Europe: A Review*. Denmark: Gerontologisk Institut.

Mazumdar, S. (1995) 'Women on the March: Right-Wing Mobilization, in Contemporary India', *Feminist Review*, 49, Spring 1995, pp. 1–28.

Mbembe, A. (1988) *Afriques indociles. Christianisme, pouvoir et état en Société post-coloniale*, Paris: Karthala.

Mirza, H. (1992) 'Cultural Identity, Citizenship and Social Policy', Islam in Europe Conference at Bradford University.

Moore, S. (1993) 'Gets Politically Correct', cited in N. Patel 'In Search of the Holy Grail', in R. Hugman and D. Smith (eds) (1995) *Ethical Issues in Social Work*, London: Routledge, p. 41.

Modood, T. *et al.* (1997) *Ethnic Minorities in Britain: Diversity and Disadvantage*, London: Policy Studies Institute.

Mortimer, E. (1997) 'A Comment: Tale of Two Cultures', London: *Financial Times (FT)* 5 March.

Nelissen, H. (1997) *Zonder Pioniers Geen Volgers*, Utrecht: NIZW.

Owen, D. (1996) 'Size, Structure and Growth of the Ethnic Minority Populations', in D. Coleman and J. Salt (eds) *Ethnicity in the Census*, vol. 1, London: HMSO.

Parpart, J. (1988) 'Women and the State in Africa', in D. Rothchild and N. Chazan (eds) *The Precarious Balance. State and Society in Africa*, Boulder, Colo.: Westview, pp. 208–30.

Patel, N. (1993) 'Healthy Margins: Black Elders' Care – Models, Policies and

Prospects', in W.I.U. Ahmed (ed.) *'Race' and Health in Contemporary Britain.* Buckingham: Open University Press.

Patel, N. and Mertens, H. (eds) (1998) *Living and Ageing in Europe: Profiles and Projects*, Utrecht: NIZW.

Patel, N., and Mirza, N. *et al.* (1998) *Dementia and Minority Ethnic Older People: Managing Care in the UK, Denmark and France – CNEOPSA Project*, Russell House Publishing Ltd.

Patel, N., Naik, D. and Humphries, B. (eds) (1998) *Visions of Reality: Religion and Ethnicity in Social Work*, London: CCETSW.

Pieterse, J.N. (1991) 'Fictions of Europe', *Race and Class*, 32, no. 3, pp. 3–10.

Pilkington, E. (1994) 'Anger at Gay Foster Ban', *The Guardian*, 28 October 1994.

Runnymede Trust (1997) *Islamophobia: Its Features and Dangers*, A consultative paper, Runnymede Commission on British Muslims and Islamophobia. London: Runnymede Trust.

Ryan, W. (1978) *Blaming the Victim*, New York: Pantheon Books.

Sahgal, G. and Yuval-Davies, N. (1992) *Refusing Holy Orders: Women and Fundamentalism in Britain*, London: Virago Press.

Siegel, P.N. (1986) *The Meek and the Militant: Religion and Power across the World*, London: Zed Books.

Sivanandan, A. (1992) 'Our Passports on our Faces', *CARF* no. 6, January–February.

Thomése, F. *et al.* (1995) *Het wiel van de buren*, Utrecht: NIZW.

Vander Meeren, P. (1998) 'Belgium', in N. Patel and H. Mertens (eds) *Living and Ageing in Europe: Profiles and Projects*, Utrecht: NIZW.

Walz, H. and Andre, G. (1995) 'Religion and Human Rights', conference paper at IFSW/JCSW, Portugal.

Webber, F. (1991) 'From Ethnocentrism to Euro-racism', *Race and Class*, 32, no. 3, pp. 11–18.

Zakaria, R. (1988) *The Struggle within Islam*, London: Penguin.

Part III

Issues for the structuring of social work's future practice

In the concluding section of our text we return to broader themes and the implications for those teaching, researching, and planning for the future. If the population served by social work is changing, then too the infrastructure that sustains that service must also change. Individuals are not independent of structures, even if they may challenge and reform them: to change the culture of social work requires a re-engineering of its tools. The attention paid in the earlier chapters to questions of terminology and theory, exemplified in the case studies, must be mirrored in the rethinking of the processes of reproduction of the profession through education, research and social policy.

In particular, we believe that social work training must acknowledge in its curriculum the changes that its 'products' will encounter, and prepare them for a world not only of diversity but of continuing evolution. A move from 'pedagogy' to 'andragogy' – a whole-of-life learning strategy – would reflect changes in other professions and might encourage learners to adopt a more equal stance in relation to their clients. In particular this requires attention to the relation of both teachers and learners with people of minority backgrounds. That, however, is only one of the challenges facing the profession in its many guises across Europe.

A second, and possibly deeper, issue is the nature of knowledge itself. Teaching and practice are founded upon the models or stereotypes created through the research process. This activity itself is not immune from change, and the adoption of a partnership strategy whereby users (or clients) and communities are no longer the passive objects of scrutiny can transform the process to the benefit of all concerned. Self-awareness, in research as in teaching and learning, should be a significant part of any study strategy, and the paradigms or categories which are the researcher's tools must be re-examined through the lens of diversity.

In all of this, the role of 'social work' itself and the self-image of the society that such workers construct, reproduce or protect also come in for challenge. There are many myths in a supposedly modern and rational society, including the belief that consensus or stability has ever been achieved. In a Europe that is seeking, ostensibly, to move towards an 'ever closer union', it is important to reflect that this will probably only be achieved by giving greater rather than less rein to diversity. By accepting 'multiple layers' of identity, that all individuals can call upon a variety of repertoires for their support, we may move towards a resolution of the crisis of solidarity and acknowledge that it is possible to serve the individual *and* the groups to which they belong: to see both the wood and the trees.

Chapter 12

Towards an emancipatory pedagogy?

Social work education for a multicultural, multi-ethnic Europe

Charlotte Williams

INTRODUCTION

How should social workers be trained for work in a multi-ethnic, multicultural society? Is there a specific methodology for teaching and practice with minorities? Can social work education as it is constituted serve all students equitably? What is the rationale for such a development across Europe? These big questions lie at the heart of the response of social work education to multicultural, multi-ethnic Europe. This chapter seeks to map some of these concerns and to illustrate some of the tensions that characterise this highly contested terrain.

BACKGROUND

An exploration of trends and issues in relation to social work education for a multicultural society can only be speculative given the dearth of comparative European research relating to this area. Brauns and Kramer's comprehensive review of social work education and professional development across Europe (1986 and 1991) fails to acknowledge this significant development. This does not mean, however, that educational institutions throughout Europe are not at some stage in the development of programmes to promote competency in this area of work. The emerging picture is, however, disappointing. A survey commissioned by the Council of Europe in 1994 of twenty-seven countries across Europe to look at 'the human rights dimension and minority issues' in education and professional practices found a widespread lack of explicit attention to these issues, lack of appropriate study materials, low involvement of minority ethnic people as tutors or students and a social work education that is fundamentally ethnocentric. Despite finding considerable variety in the degree to which social workers were involved in work with ethnic minorities and refugees country by country, the general pattern appears to be one of neglect, of universalist difference, blind practice, or at best of 'special' projects (Council of Europe 1997). Healy's work on the internationalising of social work educational courses world wide comes to a similar conclusion, noting little evidence of a planned coherent strategy to international curriculum development (Healy 1988, 1992 and 1995).

One clear exception to this picture must be Great Britain, where since 1989 the Central Council for Education and Training in Social Work (CCETSW) has prescribed a specific mandate in relation to education and training for work in a multicultural society (CCETSW Paper 30 1989, revised 1995) and developed a range of teaching materials (Northern Curriculum Development Project, CCETSW 1992). Despite this pioneering approach to the institutionalising of this teaching area within social work, developments here have been slow and patchy and lack systematic empirical evaluation. As yet there exists little research to support the tangible effects on practice of this orientation within British social work education.

Comparative analysis is somewhat confounded by the variety of terminology in use to denote this area of work. Work with immigrants (Cheetham 1972), multicultural education, intercultural pedagogy (Hamburger 1994; Friesenhahn 1988), 'cultural animation' (Pollo 1991), human rights education (Satka 1996; EASSW 1997), anti-racist/anti-oppressive social work education (Dominelli 1988, 1996), critical pedagogy (Lorenz 1994; Humphries 1988), international or cross-cultural social work (Healy 1988) are all terms in use. This terminology reflects a diversity of approaches springing from different conceptual paradigms, differences in emphasis and focus given to such work and its perceived location within the curriculum. The only common denominator is some concern to prepare social workers for work with and on behalf of individuals from minority groups and their communities.

The Europe-wide scenario inevitably raises questions as to why educational institutions have been so slow to consider the need to respond to the social and cultural plurality of society; and as to why increased attention is being afforded this issue now. At one level the answer to these questions lies in the different immigration histories of various European countries, in their differing social policy strategies and not least in the nature of and organisation of social work itself within particular contexts. However, deeply embedded in this intransigence may equally lie something of the fundamental ambivalence of Europe to its minorities and an unquestioning approach to the dominant and Eurocentric discourses fostered in liberal visions of Europe. European integration arguably provides an important opportunity for educators in social work collectively to review teaching and learning methodologies for work with minorities, an opportunity to educate for change.

CONTEXTUALISING SOCIAL WORK EDUCATION FOR MULTICULTURAL EUROPE: CONSTRUCTING THE 'PROBLEM OF MINORITIES'

A growing sense of awareness of the 'problem of minorities' and the need for social work education to respond to a changing situation is undoubtedly being felt right across Europe (Satka 1996). What accounts for this increased attention is worthy of exploration because neither migration nor multi-culturality are new phenomena in Europe. Certainly, social work education programmes are increasingly internationalising, opening up new opportunities for cross-cultural encounters. There can be few social work education programmes that have not already participated in exchange schemes such as ERASMUS and now SOCRATES, and a small but significant banking of experience on developing the curriculum towards multicultural learning is emerging (Bradley *et al.* 1995; Hoffman and Reimair 1995; Williams 1996b; Nagy 1996; Kommunaldepartementet 1992; Aluffi-Pentini and Lorenz 1996). What is clear, however, is that European mobility and exchange schemes are largely white, single, able-bodied student preserves in which students from minority groups do not feature (Williams 1996a). This coming together of dominant cultural groupings or the forging of links with more marginalised European countries (TEMPUS, SOCRATES) may well be fruitful in developing some mutual understanding but it neither ensures equality of access to professional mobility (Harris 1990) nor addresses the real issues of 'intercultural' teaching and learning. Neither does it explain the current momentum towards equipping students for multicultural work.

Wider social trends are perhaps more significant in bringing the issues of minorities to the fore. The impact of globalisation of the economy and the massive social movement this entails ensures conspicuous cultural diversity. Ideological changes to welfare systems are transforming the relationship between the individual and the state and producing contexts in which the contraction of state welfarism feeds nationalist agendas of exclusion. The noticeable rise in racial hostility and the regeneration of fascist groupings across Europe is prompting both a growing body of protectionist legislation and policy in relation to minorities and a plethora of organisations aimed at their containment. In addition, an interesting and as yet perhaps embryonic feature of the Europeanising of racism is a developing conscientisation amongst minority groups themselves that is pan-European. Social work education will increasingly be called to respond to what is a new dynamic. In fact, Lorenz (1995) goes as far as to argue that it is not simply a response that is called for but a proactive pedagogy which has an important role to play in the shaping of this New Europe.

This sense of a need for change is being augmented by research evidence firmly establishing that Europe's minorities are not getting an appropriate service from the social work profession. In Britain, for example, there already exists a long and varied critique of social work's response to a multi-ethnic society (Cheetham 1972; Dominelli 1988; Ahmad 1990). Social work in all its varieties is clearly ill equipped to meet these new challenges.

The recognition of the need to change and the appearance of change, however, does not always mean that change is as progressive as it may at first seem. In an analysis of European policy and practice in respect of race and ethnic relations, Mullard (1988) suggests developments and change may often imply progression but be characterised by what he calls 'progressive control' as opposed to true 'transformative change'. Mullard's argument is that policy and practice stemming from dominant definitions of reality will necessarily reflect the object of control. By contrast, transformative policy and practice 'arising from dominated definitions of reality and the nature of the "problem" attempts to transform or structurally change existing racist and ethnicist policy and practice into non-racist policy and practice' (Mullard 1988:360). Closer inspection of the discourses of Europe reflects competing definitions of the 'problem of minorities'.

The majority discourse of Europe presents a construction of the 'problem of minorities' that is littered with double-speak. Policy documents and legislation mirror Europe's ambivalence towards its minorities (Paul 1991). At one and the same time Europe seeks to reconcile its economic imperatives (cheap and available labour) but at the same time to allay fears of swamping by cultural intruders into what is becoming a Fortress Europe (Gordon 1989). Further, it has sought to reject the irrationality of racism and xenophobia (Enlightened Europe) whilst failing to protect the victims adequately (see *Race and Class* vol. 32). Such a Europe cries both: freedom of movement, open borders, integration, solidarity, human rights and yet promotes increasingly rigid immigration control, alien ghettoisation, exclusion and marginalisation. It is these tensions that are negotiated at the front line of social work. (See Lorenz, Chapter 14.)

The minority discourse, by contrast, questions the 'fictions of Europe' (Nederveen Pieterse 1991). From this perspective the 'problem of minorities' is not the plurality of Europe but the homogeneity it attempts to proclaim and defend that is problematic. The minority discourse aspires to negotiated integration, to the retention of identity, individual and collective, and is sceptical of the rhetoric of acceptance and tolerance. The minority discourse is not slow to acknowledge the experience of racism, or afraid to document the open hostility and harassment apparent across Europe. The minority voice asks for acknowledgement of the labourer as well as the labour.

Within social work education the construction of 'the problem of minorities' mirrors these discursive constructions. The rationale for change can become subtly or at times overtly welded to the 'Fortress Europe' objectives. It is not difficult to see how a social work education can be built on the principles of 'progressive control' (Mullard 1988); on the management and containment of the threat of minorities; on the vociferous assimilationism and the whitewashing of diversity in the interests of the 'oneness' of Europe. Too often it is a process of disconnection that is spearheaded within education, whereby the definition of the 'problem of minorities' is separated out from a wider frame of reference of structural relations. In this way the discussion of migrants becomes divorced from a discussion of migrant labour and the moral responsibility and reciprocity this entails, and the response becomes ethnicised. Thus the ethnic and cultural features of the migrant population become the 'problem' for social work and students are trained to operate with sensitivity towards their dietary needs, their custom, language and tradition. Such a 'progression' reflects an implicitly pathological perspective which explains the 'problem' in terms of the social, cultural, economic, linguistic and religious characteristics of minority groups (Mullard 1988:362). This approach can only facilitate a massive distancing between the migrant and the non-migrant population and an elevation of the discourse of cultural influences over structurally informed discourses about power, inequality and exchange. In effect, education therefore aids the process of decontextualising and disconnecting the minority and supports newly emerging forms of social control.

Education does not occur in a vacuum and neither is it neutral to such wider political, social and economic agendas. In fact, it has often been directly harnessed to service national agendas, as in post-war Germany (Lorenz 1994), or conversely has been a vehicle to promote emancipatory movements and social reform. Social work's immediacy to disadvantaged and marginal groups means that it is undeniably implicated in the external and internal controls operated within 'Fortress Europe' strategy (Allen and Macey 1990). Social work education can therefore demonstrate itself to be content with the status quo or committed to transforming it. It cannot stand outside these developments. For this reason social work education should properly embrace a critical and reflective stance to both national and pan-European agendas. Lorenz (1994) argues that such professional autonomy can act as a safeguard against being the instrument of oppressive national agendas.

Yet the emerging literature and practice of social work and minorities appearing across Europe does not indicate such an autonomy (EASSW 1997) and with few exceptions is characterised by an absence of such critical debate on the glaring contradictions of Europe. The focus on liberal visions of European integration acts to shelter critical review of the ways in which the 'problem of minorities' is constructed, and the way in which the salient language of 'race' and racism, power and oppression is diluted. Social workers need to be equipped to reflect critically on the discourses of Europe; to acknowledge the framing and constant reformulation of debates; and to read off the tensions and contradictions of Europe.

A central question therefore becomes not so much 'why' social work education is changing but 'how' it is forging this transition. How can we develop students as critical thinkers, skilled workers and train them for active citizenship?

WHICH WAY FORWARD? DIRECTIONS FOR SOCIAL WORK EDUCATION

The tendency towards largely assimilationist approaches within social work education strongly reflects the liberal traditions of social work thought, i.e. social work as benign, well-meaning and fundamentally embracing 'respect for persons' (see Dominelli, Chapter 3). Such tenets have served to mask gross inequalities and the processes of exclusion and disempowerment. In some European states this may be bolstered by the nation state's refusal specifically to recognise the immigrant status of labour migrants, as in Germany, or rejection of the notion 'ethnic minority' as a significant status as in France. This bedrock of such universalist or 'difference-blind' education has in many countries proved difficult to displace despite a rhetoric of moves towards a distinct intercultural learning and anti-discriminatory practice.

It is possible to identify at least four potential trajectories from such assimilationist mainsprings in relation to teaching and learning for work with minorities that represent a cluster of ideas and command particular criticisms. These can be referred to as *cultural tolerance models*, *conflict models*, *radical models* and a developing *postmodern approach*.

Cultural tolerance models arise largely from functionalist approaches to education and are based on notions of adaptation, adjustment and equilibrium, personal or collective. Varieties of multiculturalism (Switzerland), intercultural education (Germany), anti-discriminatory practice (Great Britain) and human rights teaching all fall within this ambit. This orientation stresses tolerance, understanding and non-discriminatory practice at the interface between cultural groupings. The emphasis is on developing within the individual an appreciation of the culture of others and 'ethnic sensitivity'. Cultural tolerance models differ from abject assimilation in their positive recognition of difference and their concern with prejudice and reducing the barriers of discrimination.

Teaching and learning based on these principles focus on a 'learning to do things together' approach. There will be an emphasis on understanding the culture and traditions of others, and the values of co-operation, solidarity and integration espoused. A characteristic of such an approach may be the development of specialisms, such as 'working with migrant children', 'multicultural work' or 'human rights', with specially earmarked teachers. In some countries, for example Sweden, specialist courses exist for largely white monoculture students to learn about multiculturalism, whilst parallel courses exist for people from minority communities to train for social work. The fundamental basis on which education is organised and delivered remains untouched.

Hamburger's (1994) critique of intercultural education derides the tendency of this approach to ossify cultural groupings, serving to exoticise (or demonise) the supposed incumbent within what is a fixed and static configuration of culture. In addition, such tolerance models assume some notion of equal status between groupings; they fail to question the limits of tolerance and leave social structural arrangements that produce oppressions largely untouched (Essed 1991).

Conflict models, best exemplified by the anti-racist social work education in Great Britain, accept the inevitability of tensions between groups in the struggle for scarce resources. Conflict models pivot on notions of power, domination and subordination and the processes that give rise to these positionings such as class, racism, patriarchy, ageism, etc. In Great Britain the focus on the *anti-racist approach* (Dominelli 1988) presented a far-reaching challenge to the curriculum and the organisation and delivery of social work programmes. '*Altering the social work curriculum in anti-racist/non racist directions means removing its anglocentric basis and arrogance to affirm black people in terms they define and present*' (1988: 60). This approach goes well beyond the inclusion of elements in the curriculum addressing social work with ethnic minority families and argues for changes in the power relations within the academy, critically questions traditional approaches to social work and its knowledge base and argues for greater inclusion of black and ethnic minority people within the academy and social work institutions. In many senses this approach can be seen as radical and gained a lot of ground in terms of pointing to, if not constructing, transformations in educational practice within the UK (see also De Maria 1992).

However, the anti-racist approach has been the subject of considerable criticism, not least for its rapid institutionalisation and deradicalisation within the British context. Strategies which implied the expectation that social workers could resolve the racial ills of society were pilloried and derided in both populist and academic circles. Further, the fundamental essentialism, reductionism and the conceptual difficulties and contradictions the approach embraced have come under increasing criticism (Macey and Moxon 1996). The formulaic and single-issue positioning it fosters suggested the approach as inflexible and unable to accommodate the complexity and dynamic of everyday experiences and rapidly changing realities. Further, the whole notion of category, meta-narrative and universal truths has been increasingly questioned by the emergence of postmodernist thinking.

Radical pedagogical approaches (Humphries 1988; Freire 1972; hooks 1994; Shor 1992) – variously named critical pedagogy, community education, anti-oppressive practice, emancipatory or empowering pedagogy – demand transformation within teaching and learning at the level of practice and the institutional framework in the interests of *all* oppressed groups. There is an understanding within such approaches of the interconnections between oppressions and of notions of oppressed and oppressors as not mutually exclusive entities (Freire 1972; hooks 1994). An understanding of power and powerlessness is fundamental to this approach and it implies an education for emancipation, change and transformation of the power relations within society. It embraces what Humphries (1988) has called 'perspective transformation', i.e., a rigorous examination of world views in use, a rereading of the literature base and the dominant perspectives in the curriculum, a revisiting of the learning environment to ensure the engagement of minority voices, a challenge to dominant modes of assessment and real shifts in power between the community and the academy (Cummings 1986; hooks 1994). The approach is dynamic and seeks to educate towards active citizenship, partnership and change for the benefit of all.

This approach raises questions related to the constraints on social work within a bureaucratic framework: the idea of preparing the 'social revolutionary' for working within and against the state. Concerns arise in relation to the lack of real opportunities to engage in such transformative practice, which will always be circumscribed by institutional and political contexts. The 'dangerousness' and risk of such professional autonomy very easily comes under pressure from standardising processes. Further, as with any emancipatory ideal questions must be asked as to the remit and mandate to change, as to the purpose and moral responsibility of change. Whose change? How far? In whose interests? How best? Simply stated, the issues of conscientisation remain controversial (Banks and Banks 1993).

Postmodernist approaches to social work education reject the totalising tendencies of meta-narratives which produce category as 'everyone is someone else's "Other"' (Gentile 1985 in Solas 1994). Postmodernist approaches differ from critical pedagogy in their shift away from a focus on institutional power and the notion of oppressed groups towards an understanding of power that operates through individual subjectivities and the micropolitics of everyday actions. John Solas (1994) has applied the principles of this approach to social work education. It is worth spelling out what Solas (1994) sees as the core of such a trajectory for social work education:

- The need to attend to and safeguard difference, always and everywhere . . . recognising that the myths embodied in the ideal of the fully conscious, rational, androcentric and Eurocentric person are oppressive to those who are less than ideal.
- A refusal of the terms and assumptions associated with the educator/student and knower/known dualisms as current definitions of educator and knowledge embody powers and privileges which reflect relations of colonialism, sexism, racism, classism, etc. What is required is a reflective cognitive practice, a post colonial mode

of theorisation, which demands that the individual would question the assumptions, conditions and practices they take for granted.

- A need to problematise such powerful structuring practices as expertise, homogenisation, instrumentalism, linearity and reason. This means realising that all voices are not and cannot carry equal legitimacy, safety and power in the classroom.
- The need to politicise social work education; that is, to construct practices in ways that make education and political coalition across differences possible and viable . . . without assimilating to a historically or contextually dominant norm.

(Solas 1994:81–4)

Solas' concern with both an empowering educational process and the development of critical reflectiveness within the individual arguably equips the educational institution for minority students and equips all students for empowering practice. The strategies of such a 'politics of difference' pedagogy include particular techniques of reading, criticism, speaking and writing following Derridean deconstruction (Solas 1994). The approach offers a sophisticated understanding of the ways in which educational processes include and exclude or marginalise, challenging what counts as knowledge, and who counts as speaker. It raises fundamental questions about the ability of a prescriptive social work education to respond to key issues confronting society.

The critique of postmodernism essentially asks to what end such differences are claimed. Where does the endless recognition of the specificity of differences take us? Further, it is argued these deconstructing tendencies are antithetical to the mobilisation of social change as they are fundamentally fragmenting and deradicalising of collective action (Dominelli 1996). The relativistic nature of all social reality purported by this framework ignores fundamental issues of power and it becomes impossible to regard oppression and exploitation as interchangeable.

It is possible to see that all these potential trajectories for social work education contain within them both progressive and regressive elements. The development of the skills of 'ethnic sensitivity' promoted within the cultural tolerance framework are crucial but not to be reified, as are the macro dimensions introduced by more radical perspectives. Postmodernism allows us to recognise small stories that are dynamic and the ever-shifting conceptualisation of what counts as knowledge. All of these areas are important to the progression of minority education and education in minority issues. The question is of emphasis and focus and this in turn reflects particular values. The assumption therefore of a linear shift from assimilationist approaches to postmodern is questionable.

SPECIFIC ISSUES IN MULTICULTURAL EDUCATION

Routes to professional development: 'the competent practitioner' or the 'morally responsible' practitioner?

In the development of social workers for work in a multicultural society a tension exists between those who would argue for the way of 'knowhow' or technique with its focus on standardised prescriptions for skill development and those who would argue for a moral reformative brief or 'the way of emancipation'.

The swift and insidious technocratisation of social work education is well under way in Great Britain, whereby 'the concern with moral responsibility has been neutralised in favour of demonstrating professional competence' (Husband 1995:93). This shift is not solely a British phenomenon and increasingly other European countries are either adopting the 'competency' approach or have developed very much with this orientation, for example Portugal (Anthyade 1986). In this frame intercultural education, or what in Britain is known as anti-discriminatory education, becomes shaped as a technical activity, a set of decontextualised skills/competencies that standardise responses to cultural diversity. Such social work education aims to reproduce the neutral technician who is able and capable in her response to multicultural work and largely 'made safe' within the bureaucratic structures within which she will operate. To this end educational institutions itemise a knowledge base, for example: the customs and traditions of minority groups; cross-cultural communication, policy and legislation in respect of refugees; working with migrant children, etc. The search is on to scientise the response, to standardise and domesticate the project 'working with minorities'. Such extreme instrumentalism strips the practitioner of moral responsibility for the task, divorces the practitioner from the political basis of her work. This is a Fortress Europe strategy which seeks to minimise the risky elements of society (see Lorenz, Chapter 14). Under the guise of developing expertise in working with minorities and the delineation of specialisms such as 'work with refugees' the competency approach upholds newer forms of regulation and control (see Dominelli's critique 1996).

Pitched against this philosophical positioning are those who would argue for a moral and/or political content to education for work with minority groups (Dominelli 1996; Husband 1995). Dominelli (1996), using the term 'anti-oppressive practice', suggests that such an approach 'embodies a person centred philosophy; an egalitarian value system concerned with reducing the deleterious effects of structural inequalities upon people's lives; a methodology focusing on both processes and outcomes' (Dominelli 1996:158). Such an approach implies a worker who is not only appropriately concerned with social justice and equality but who adopts an active role in countering systems of oppression that structure the client's life. Similarly, Husband (1995) suggests a 'moral impulse . . . as a necessary basis for responsible social work intervention' (Husband 1995:99).

The idealism of the moral autonomy protagonists is not without criticism. Moral autonomy as a product of the individual is vulnerable to the generosity of particular commitments at any one time; is vulnerable to obvious conflicts of value systems and is resistant to regulation and standardisation. Further, to confer on social work a political mandate in relation to proscribed cultural categories can be seen as a form of colonialism, for who are the interpreters of change, what is the remit of change and on what basis do they claim this mandate? These fundamental and contested areas are arguably appropriately problematised: *'it is that anguish in the social regulation of caring which must be nurtured and valued, rather than eliminated through professional ethical certitude'* (Husband 1995:99).

It is not difficult to see how these paradigms continue to reflect Western dualist thinking – the reason/emotion, thought/action, theory/practice, theoretician/pragmatist dichotomies, nor to see the problematics of the deductive rather than inductive approaches they deploy. Both positionings grapple with the relationship between theory and practice.

Involvement of minority groups within social work education

The involvement of people from minority groups within social work education as students, teachers and researchers has been advocated by many writers (Freire 1972; Dominelli 1988) and is a growing phenomenon across Europe. Second-generation immigrants in France and the Netherlands, migrant workers in Germany and Sweden and members of minority ethnic communities in Britain are increasingly participating in social work education and training. Arguments for inclusion variously cite the importance of minority representation: as significant to the shift in the power base of institutions; in bringing alternative perspectives to bear; in the need for trained workers from minority communities to work with these communities; and as role models to counteract the inferiorisation of the minority community; in promoting tolerance, harmony and mutual understanding. The involvement of staff members and students from minority communities is therefore generally acknowledged as progressive.

The incorporation of minority workers and students has not, however, been without contention (Stubbs 1988). Minority workers have spoken of tokenistic involvement, rather than real participation, being employed on a casual or part-time basis and particularly employed to teach on courses on minority issues only. Similarly, students from minority groups find themselves restricted to options and career choices that assume they want to practise social work in their own communities. In such ways social work courses effectively marginalise 'multicultural work' to an exotic sideshow in their programme of events. This notion of involvement seeks the co-option of the compliant minority voice whereby alternative perspectives are seen as quaint and interesting but the dominant paradigms remain untouched. It leads to 'dumping' on the ethnic minority community the responsibility for change and to the overloading of workers and students, placing unrealistic expectations on them both to represent and to serve the interests of their community whilst offering no challenge to the dominant framework. Such involvement therefore has the veneer of being progressive but this masks subtle and effective forms of 'progressive control' of minorities.

Cross-cultural assessment

A contentious area both in minority education and in educating for work with minorities is the question of assessment. This raises issues about both the assessment of minority students and the assessment of all students on minority issues.

Educational institutions ultimately are the arbiters of what kind of knowledge and behaviour is legitimated. Cross-cultural assessment is an issue that is at the heart of the challenge to dominant world views and the power base of the academy. Low rates of recruitment from ethnic minority groups and consistently high rates of minority student failure are too often used to pathologise and inferiorise individuals and whole minority communities rather than raise questions about systems of assessment in use. The presence of minority students on social work programmes confronts the dominant paradigms of the educational institution and guarded conceptions of the essence of professionalism. The challenge is therefore far beyond the acknowledgement of linguistic and conceptual competence which is given by far the greater focus.

Brummer (1988) captures the dilemma these latter issues pose for educationalists:

> to fail to apply the same criteria to black students could be racist, because different criteria *might* imply lower expectations. On the other hand to apply rigidly the same criteria can also be racist because the facts of cultural diversity are not taken into account.
>
> (Brummer 1988:30)

The notion of compensatory education and positive discrimination are contentious issues and have been heavily criticised for their stigmatising and ghettoising tendencies. On a straightforward level it should not be too difficult to give students the appropriate language support to open access to mainstream opportunities. An interesting comparison to consider is how the 'myth of bilingualism' can be shattered when an individual is competent in two of the dominant European languages, whereas bilingualism becomes problematic when it involves a minority language. The relationship between language competence and conceptual abilities is complicated, and between language and power (see Chapter 6). It is, however, not simply a matter of language competence.

Cummings' (1986) research on education with minority students focuses the issue clearly with the educational institution:

> it must be emphasised that discriminatory assessment is carried out by well intentioned individuals who rather than challenging a socio-educational system that tends to disable minority students, have accepted a role definition and an educational structure that makes discriminatory assessment virtually inevitable.
>
> (Cummings 1988:30)

Educational institutions are geared to reward those achievements and behaviours that most nearly conform to the conventional and do not challenge fixed power relations (Humphries 1988). Thus educators operate with particular notions of professionalism and the role of the social worker that embrace Eurocentric values, for example on privacy, individualism, confidentiality, normal ageing, relationships within the family, intervention, conduct and even dress. Educators reinforce competitive relationships whereby achievement is defined in particular ways that cannot easily accommodate diversity of experience and the legitimisation of new sources of knowledge. Too often the difficulties of introducing creative forms of assessment are frustrated by the dominant expectations of the academy.

Evaluating learning towards work in a multicultural community

Evaluation of both students' and practitioners' practice in working with minorities is fundamental to the development of good professional practices. One advantage of the competency-based approach is that it offers specific measures for evaluating student and worker competence in this area with its emphasis on specific and measurable criteria. The broader ambitions of emancipatory pedagogy may be much more difficult to evaluate, although some attempt has been made to develop models (Preston Shoot 1995; Cornwell 1992). As yet there is a lack of available substantive research on the outcomes of such multicultural/anti-oppressive teaching on practice. Too much still relies on impressionistic accounts. Soydan's (1995) cross-cultural study of social workers in Great Britain and Sweden used the vignette method to assess workers' decision making in work with 'immigrant' families and found considerable differences between the two countries.

Soydan makes some interesting observations about the bureaucratic, rule-bound and ethnocentric responses of the Swedish cohort of workers as compared with the culturally relativistic and critical questioning approach applied by the British sample. These differences reflect the operating culture of social work organisations and personal dispositions but also perhaps significantly the effects of prior training.

Evaluation studies based on user outcomes, organisational measures of quality assurance and service-based outcomes are, however, a growing feature of European social work practice (Cheetham *et al.* 1998). These are as yet underdeveloped in relation to workers' responses to work with minority clients. Attitude adjustment measures are also available to assess outcomes of specific training regimes. However, the psychological focus of such evaluation, with its emphasis on prejudices, provides only a limited picture of students' development in this area. Studies such as Soydan's raise the profile of the need for education and training for work with ethnic minorities to be a compulsory part of social work training for all students and workers not only in terms of skills for hands-on work but towards broader integrationist and democratic ideals as the responsibility of active citizenship.

Preparing for students' work in combating racism

The rise of xenophobia and overt racism Europe-wide and the harmonisation of policies of exclusion must be of concern to social work educators. Students need not only to be equipped to work with the perpetrators of racism (Lorenz 1994; Aluffi-Pentini and Lorenz 1996) but also to explore their own value base and actions in respect of these issues. Further, the 'Europeanising of racism' will inevitably require a Europe-wide strategy in which the social work profession may have a significant role. Despite the fact that what counts as racism constitutes a major contested area across Europe (see Chapter 1), few would, however, dispute the overt street racism, open hostilities and harassment that are a feature of the lives of many individuals and groups from visible minority communities across Europe (*Race and Class* no. 32, 1991).

These concerns are not marginal to the social work mandate. Anti-racist strategies must be central to the social work task if they are to respond appropriately to the needs of ethnic minorities and promote solidarity and integration in Europe. Opportunities exist within the New Europe to operate in conjunction with other social movements towards the elimination of racism.

There has been considerable focus within the British context to students exploring their own racist attitudes and assumptions and the ways in which these shape their social work interventions (Dominelli 1988 and 1996; Thompson 1997). The European project, however, provides important opportunities for social work to explore on a comparative basis the dimensions of racism and oppression and the processes and structures that give rise to what are many racisms (Aluffi-Pentini and Lorenz 1996). Racism itself is a complex and diverse entity and the responses therefore have to reflect this complexity rather than seek out fixed and inflexible formulations. Students should be given the opportunity to critically debate issues of exclusion Europe-wide and critically review the measures and initiatives taken to protect minority groups. Further, Europe provides an important opportunity to share models and approaches to work with the perpetrators of racism, to develop alliances with social movements pursuing anti-racism and to press for policy changes to ensure the rights of refugees, migrants and minorities.

Towards an emancipatory pedagogy: an emergent methodology?

Social work education clearly must avoid the folly of inflexible prescriptions and formulas for action that very quickly become outdated and unworkable. The Europe project does, however, provide rich opportunities for the sharing of general principles in respect of social work with and on behalf of oppressed minorities. Much of what is emerging is yet to be the subject of rigorous research but nevertheless provides useful descriptive accounts of teaching developments (Friesenhahn 1988; Hamburger 1994; Humphries 1988; Cornwell 1992; Harlow and Hearn 1996; De Maria 1992; Lorenz 1995; Kommunaldepartementet 1992). Teacher education for multiculturalism/ intercultural learning provides an important source of material (Shor 1992; Gagliardi 1995; Banks and Banks 1993; Ray *et al.* 1994; hooks 1994; and Perotti 1994), as do the classic texts such as Freire's (1972) contribution to development of community education. We have still a lot to learn from the connection between social development and social work education models and practice (Midgley 1995) and from those writing with a global perspective (Healy 1992). What is clear is that oppressed minorities will not be appropriately serviced simply by developing students' understanding of cultural needs. A broader approach to education is required, an education that works towards the liberation of oppressed groups. Some very tentative principles might be:

- recognition of the way in which welfare can reproduce and construct major social divisions and perpetuate the minorised position of certain groups and foster exclusion. Students need to be equipped to explore power relations and the processes and dynamics of oppression. Students need to critically debate discourses of Europe and to contextualise these debates against the global context of migration.
- curriculum development that entails a critical rereading of the content and an interrogation of biases in the 'knowledge in use' and the theories, models and approaches of social work, for example in prevailing

conceptions of the norms of family, individualism, privacy, old age, sexuality; a curriculum development that is inductive and can incorporate ways of knowing and doing that are being worked out and constructed by the minority groups themselves. This implies the involvement not only of individual personnel from minority oppressed groups but educational partnerships with minority communities.

- the preparation of students to reflect critically on their own culture as well as learning from the culture of others and to review the project of Europe critically. This could involve the adoption of Freire's (1972) problem-posing approach in which students explore their own internalised cultural myths and test them against alternative meanings.
- teaching and learning strategies that empower *all* students. A liberating pedagogy that transforms teacher/pupil relationships and allows students to learn in ways meaningful to them in both process and content. This will involve opportunities to foster diversity, to promote individual and collective identities but at the same time recognise the complexities of oppressions and their interconnections. It will involve adopting creative and flexible systems of assessment.
- strategies for intercultural education that involve *all* staff and permeate *all* knowledge areas, not a special education for the 'culturally different' or in 'cultural difference' but the development of skills in negotiated diversity and perspective transformation across the curriculum.
- acknowledgement of racism as a pan-European phenomenon that affects the lives of oppressed minorities. Students should be provided with opportunities to explore their own attitudes, prejudices and the nature of discriminatory actions intended and unintended; to consider the nature and processes of racism and critically to review initiatives in respect of the protection of minorities. Students should be equipped for advocacy and action on anti-racism and be empowered to develop skills in forming alliances with wider movements for social change and towards active citizenship.
- the development of systematic research and evaluation of approaches in use and their efficacy in preparing students to meet the needs of oppressed communities and for active citizenship.

The scale of this challenge to the curriculum and the processes of education inevitably produce resistance and fear as this represents real challenges to existing power bases and the status quo. Approaches in use vary from the establishment of elective and specialist courses to attempts towards infusion of all the major learning experiences of the student (Nagy 1996). The processes of transformation can be slow and painful and produce conflicts and at times contradictions. Gains tend to be hard-won. Students need to be supported to acknowledge these fears and overcome them in their education towards critical consciousness. Challenging the dominant paradigms of the academy and of the bureaucracy will produce resistance as powerful interests are protected and those active in promoting change very quickly become labelled as 'radical', 'political', 'subversive', even dangerous in a climate when Europe seeks to 'make safe' the professions. These conflicts will be reproduced both within and outside the profession as opinions vary as to the role of social work and the role of education.

Not all change initiatives within social work education work towards the emancipation of minority oppression or indeed towards the enhancement of sensitive work with minority groups. Clearly an educational approach to cultural plurality is not a short-term remedy. Perotti (1994) argues: 'Multiculturalism is not a transitional situation but a permanent way of thinking associated with a situation of permanent change' (Perotti 1994:25). The development of codes of practice and guidelines to manage what can be ambiguous and changing entities can prove restrictive and unimaginative (Hamburger 1994). It is important therefore continually to problematise our responses to what is a dynamic situation. This may mean that the search for the universalising of specific competencies or the standardisation of responses to multicultural education is misplaced and may fall into the trap of producing a 'European approach' that is Eurocentric, oppressive and mirrors the dominant discourse of Europe.

> Pedagogy or social work which does not examine its contents and aims in a political sense and which relies instead on an assumed 'neutrality', 'objectivity' of its contents and its norms oblivious of their political consequences, is always in danger of becoming the victim of political power games.
>
> (Lorenz 1994:38)

The response of social work education for work with minorities must not be yoked to the 'progressive control' dynamic of European societies but must aim at 'transformative change' in its efforts and its symbolic representations (Mullard 1988). This would be to reclaim a professional identity that transcends national agendas and questions the nation states' prescriptions as to the way in which the professions must manage diversity. Yet without specific organisational frameworks or co-ordinated training initiatives the ideals of such an education might have to be promoted more forcefully within the profession. Arguably, Europe offers a new and potential space for the development of an anti-oppressive education. The challenge is to a European social work education that will either choose to replicate Eurocentrism, protectionism and defensive expediency or seek richer explanations and develop flexible skills in negotiating diversity and coping with the changing faces of Europe. The emancipatory pedagogy offers the possibility of true change and is a flexible instrument that tracks processes as well as outcomes, that is dynamic rather than seeking out ready formulas and that is attuned to the minority discourse of Europe. bell hooks' appeal is to 'teaching to transgress' (hooks 1994).

SUMMARY

- Social work education for work with minorities is characterised by a variety of terminology, approaches and lack of systematic research.
- Social work education reflects particular discourses of Europe. It is not neutral.
- Not all change initiatives within social work education work towards the emancipation of minority group oppression. Education can reproduce new forms of progressive control.
- The development of emancipatory education is an ongoing process associated with a situation of continual change.

REFERENCES

Ahmad, B. (1990) *Black Perspectives in Social Work*. Birmingham: Venture Press.

Allen, S. and Macey, M. (1990) 'Race and Ethnicity in the European Context', *British Journal of Sociology* 41 (3):375–93.

Aluffi-Pentini, A. and Lorenz, W. (1996) *Anti-Racist Work with Young People: European Experiences and Approaches*. Lyme Regis: Russell House Publishing.

Anthyade, F.I.M. (1986) 'Social Work Education in Portugal', in H.J. Brauns and D. Kramer, *Social Work Education in Europe*. Frankfurt: Deutscher Verein.

Banks, J. and Banks, C.A. (eds) (1993) *Multicultural Education: Issues and Perspectives*. Boston: Allyn and Bacon.

Bradley, G., Clark, C. and Kahl, W. (1995) 'Anti-Oppressive Practice and Social Work in Europe', *Journal of Social Work Education* 14 (2):5–10.

Brauns, H.J. and Kramer, D. (1986) *Social Work Education in Europe: A Comprehensive Description of Social Work Education in 21 European Countries*. Frankfurt: Eigenverlag des Deutschen Vereins für öffentliche und privat Fürsorge.

—— and —— (1991) 'Social Work Education and Professional Development', in M. Hill (ed.) *Social Work and the European Community*. London. Jessica Kingsley.

Brummer, N. (1988) 'Cross Cultural Assessment: Issues facing White Teachers and Black Students', *Journal of Social Work Education* 7 (2):12–15.

CCETSW (Central Council for the Education and Training of Social Workers) (1989) *Rules and Regulations for the Diploma in Social Work*. Paper 30. Revised in 1995. London: CCETSW.

—— (1992) Northern Curriculum Development Project. Leeds: CCETSW.

Cheetham, J. (1972) *Social Work with Immigrants*. London: Routledge and Kegan Paul.

Cheetham, J., Mullen, E., Soydan, H. and Teugrald, K. (1998) 'Evaluation as a Tool in the Development of Social Work Discourse: National Diversity or Shared

Preoccupations', *Scandinavian Journal of Social Welfare*, Special Issue: 1998 (forthcoming).

Cornwell, N. (1992) 'From Understanding to Taking Action: Developing and Assessing Anti Racist/Anti Discriminatory Practice', *Issues in Social Work Education* 12 (2):89–110.

Council of Europe (1997) *The Initial and Further Training of Social Workers, Taking into Account their Changing Role. Report on a Co-ordinated Research Programme 1994–1995*. Strasburg: Council of Europe.

Cummings, J. (1986) 'Empowering Minority Students: A Framework for Intervention', *Harvard Educational Review* 56(1):18–36.

De Maria, W. (1992) 'On the Trail of a Radical Pedagogy for Social Work Education', *British Journal of Social Work* 22(3):231–52.

Dominelli, L. (1988) *Anti Racist Social Work*. London: Macmillan (2nd edition 1997).

Dominelli, L. (1996) 'Deprofessionalising Social Work: Anti-Oppressive Practice, Competencies and Post Modernism', *British Journal of Social Work* 26:153–75.

EASSW (European Association of Schools of Social Work) (1997) 'Human Rights and Social Work Education'. Final Report of the EASSW European Seminar, Lisbon 1995.

Essed, P. (1991) *Understanding Everyday Racism: An Inter-disciplinary Theory*. London: Sage.

Freire, P. (1972) *Pedagogy of the Oppressed*. Harmondsworth: Penguin.

Friesenhahn, G. (1988) *Zur Entwicklung interkultureller Pädagogik*. Berlin: Express Edition.

Gagliardi, R. (ed.) (1995) *Teacher Training and Multiculturalism*. Paris: UNESCO International Bureau of Education.

Gordon, P.(1989) *Fortress Europe! The Meaning of 1992*, London: Runnymede Trust.

Gould, N. (1994) 'Anti-Racist Social Work: A Framework for Teaching and Action', *Issues in Social Work Education* 14(1):2–18.

Hamburger, F. (1994) 'Migration and Education in the Federal Republic of Germany'. Paper for the International Scientific Conference 'Interculturality in Multiethnic Societies', Belgrade, 2.6.1994.

Harlow, E. and Hearn, J. (1996) 'Educating for Anti-Oppressive and Anti-Discriminatory Social Work Practice', *Social Work Education* 15 (1):5–17.

Harris, R. (1990) 'Beyond Rhetoric: A Challenge for International Social Work', *International Social Work* 33:203–12.

Healy, L.M. (1988) 'Curriculum Building in International Social Work: Towards Preparing Professionals for the Global Age', *Journal of Social Work Education* 24:221–8.

—— (1992) *Introducing International Development Content in the Social Work Curriculum*. Washington, D.C.: NASW.

—— (1995) 'Comparative and International Overview', in D. Thomas, D. Watts and N. Mayadas (eds) *International Handbook on Social Work Education*. Westport, Conn: Greenwood Press.

hooks, b. (1994) *Teaching to Transgress: Education as the Practice of Freedom*. London: Routledge.

Humphries, B. (1988) 'Adult Learning in Social Work Education: Towards Liberation or Domestication?', *Critical Social Policy* 23:4–21.

Husband, C. (1995) 'The Morally Active Practitioner and the Ethics of Anti Racist

Social Work', in R. Hugman and D. Smith (eds) *Ethical Issues in Social Work*. London: Routledge.

Kommunaldepartementet (1992) *Norge some flerkulturelt samfunn* (Norway as a Multicultural Society). Oslo: Utlendingsdirektoratet.

Lorenz W. (1994) *Social Work in a Changing Europe*. London: Routledge.

—— (1995) 'Nationalism and Racism in Europe: A Challenge for Pedagogy', *Social Work in Europe* 2 (3):34–9.

Macey, M. and Moxon, E. (1996) 'An Examination of Anti-Racist and Anti-Oppressive Theory and Practice in Social Work Education', *British Journal of Social Work* 26: 297–314.

Midgley J. (1995) *Social Development: The Development Perspective in Social Welfare*. London: Sage.

Mullard, C. (1988) 'Racism, Ethnicism and Etharchy or Not?', in T. Skutnabb-Kangas and J. Cummins (eds) *Minority Education: From Shame to Struggle*. Clevedon: Multilingual Matters Ltd.

Nagy, G. (1996) *Pedagogisk Forskning and Fornyelse: Teaching International and Cross Cultural Social Work*. Ostersund: Mitthogskolan.

Nederveen Pieterse, J. (1991) 'Fictions of Europe', *Race and Class* 32 (3):3–10.

Paul, R. (1991) 'Black and Third World People's Citizenship and 1992', *Critical Social Policy* 11(2):52–64.

Perotti, A. (1994) *The Case for Intercultural Education*. Strasburg: Council of Europe Press

Pollo, M. (1991) *Educazione come animazione*. Turin: Libreria Dothrina Cristiana.

Preston Shoot, M. (1995) 'Assessing Anti-Oppressive Practice', *Social Work Education* 14(2):11.

Ray, D. *et al.* (1994) *Education for Human Rights*. Paris: UNESCO International Bureau of Education.

Satka, M. (1996) 'Human Rights: A Challenge for European Social Work Education', *Social Work in Europe* 3 (2):49–50.

Shor, I. (1992) *Empowering Education*. London: University of Chicago Press.

Solas, J. (1994) *The (De)Construction of Educational Practice in Social Work*. Aldershot: Avebury.

Soydan, H. (1995) 'A Cross Cultural Comparison of how Social Workers in Sweden and England Assess a Migrant Family', *Scandinavian Journal of Social Welfare* 4:85–93.

Stubbs, P. (1988) 'The Employment of Black Social Workers: From "Ethnic Sensitivity" to Anti Racism?', *Critical Social Policy* 12:6–27.

Thompson, N. (1993 and 1997) *Anti-Discriminatory Practice*. London: Macmillan

Williams, C. (1996a) 'Erasmus and Socrates in Koblenz: An Alternative View', *Social Work in Europe* 3 (3):29–32.

—— (1996b) 'Sharing Anti-Discriminatory Practice through Erasmus', *Journal of Social Work Education* 16 (1): 54–65.

Chapter 13

Research with ethnic minority groups in health and social welfare

Gurnam Singh and Mark R. D. Johnson

INTRODUCTION

This chapter is not written as a guide for professional researchers on 'how to do' research on ethnic minorities. In adopting a sociopolitical perspective, we aim to engage in a critical discussion of the problems and possibilities in making research relevant to changing, for the better, the situations and contexts of minority ethnic groups in Europe today. These are situations that for many are characterised by high levels of social deprivation and the attendant consequences such as ill health, poverty, unemployment, welfare dependency and violence (SCLRAE 1992). In situations of multiple deprivation, social work is only one of the potential resources or professions which may be relevant to the needs of such populations. Therefore, the issue of research with these groups is also relevant to related professions such as health, justice, and housing. Moreover, under such conditions of powerlessness, minority populations are more likely to come under the gaze of state authorities and professionals and surveillance becomes a normal state of affairs. This itself has implications for the practice of social research by members of these professions, and for the collection and keeping of information relating to minority populations (see Johnson, Chapter 5).

Research activity in such circumstances takes on very specific and conflicting functions. It may become complicit in reinforcing and reproducing oppression by seeking to explain the problems faced by ethnic minority populations in terms of their individual and collective (cultural) pathology. By a process of racialisation one can, for example, see how the vast amount of research on minorities in Britain has been permeated with stereotypical and colonial constructions of Black and Asian people. Whilst the field of epidemiological research is particularly culpable in this respect (Bhopal 1992), there are many examples of the way researchers have legitimised racist oppression by making direct and indirect associations between real or imagined phenotypical characteristics and/or traditional cultural practices.

> This process has a long history and can be witnessed in other areas other than health. Such processes are apparent in the definitions and explanations of, amongst other areas, black people's reproductive capacity, sexuality, intelligence, ability to control the universe, 'rascality', mental breakdown, desire to run away from their slave-masters, lack of political achievements, and so on.
>
> (Ahmad 1993:18)

The other function that can be played by researchers is to counteract the process described above, and focus attention on the social, structural, economic and political domains. At the micro level, this type of what may be termed critical research seeks to understand concepts and phenomena within an understanding of the relationship between language, discourse and power. In developing a critique of various models of social work research, we will advocate a way forward that is based on a genuine partnership between academic researchers, practitioner researchers and research subjects. In doing so, whilst acknowledging the powerful epistemological debates between so-called positivists and phenomenologists (see Hammersley 1993), we will seek to avoid becoming enmeshed in the philosophical nuances. We are more concerned with small-scale local practitioner-based research trying to provide a means for developing welfare services rather than seeking to create 'universal solutions'.

HISTORICAL PERSPECTIVE – MODELS OF RESEARCH

Although the level of interest in ethnic minority and refugee communities across Europe has never been greater, sadly, questions about their welfare have always been subservient to the larger political concerns with the 'problem' of immigration and integration. It is not surprising then that, with few exceptions, much of the research on ethnic minorities has been problematic. Three perspectives have characterised most public policy discussions and research about the provision of welfare services to members of minority ethnic communities in Britain. There is insufficient space to develop a detailed exposition of each perspective; rather, we will indicate some of their problematic aspects.

The dominant and perhaps most enduring perspective is one that has set out to address 'race' from what is essentially an information-gathering exercise. This policy-orientated research paradigm has been born out of both liberal sentiments to help immigrants and refugees to integrate and right-wing fears about maintaining social order and controlling immigration (see Layton-Henry 1984). At both the macro and micro levels, through the use of quantitative methodologies, certain facts about the scale and nature of minority populations coupled with the problems they may be encountering, have been seen as critical to informing the decision-making process. In Britain, for example, we saw throughout the 1960s and '70s huge demographic surveys into race relations that set out to identify empirically both the numbers of minorities in the country and the extent of discrimination and disadvantage they were encountering (see Rose *et al.* 1969; Daniel 1968; Smith 1977; and Brown 1984). The positivist perspective continues to hold the centre stage, as can be seen in the highly influential work of Tariq Modood at the Policy Studies Institute and John Rex at CRER, University of Warwick. At a European level we can see similar examples in the work of Faist (1995), Seifert (1992), Wilpert (1998), and the inexhaustible appetite of such agencies as CEDEFOP (the European Centre for the Development of Vocational Training) and the European Foundation for the Improvement of Living and Working Conditions for documentary statements of the situation, as well as the commissions of the Council of Europe and the European Union!

Whilst one cannot deny the value in having empirical evidence that exposes discrimination and disadvantage, there are many problems with such an approach; mostly, ones which echo the more general critiques of positivism made by feminists (see Roberts 1981 and Harding 1987). Without delving into a detailed critique of the positivist empirical paradigm we would like to point out a number of points of caution about this model:

First, whilst statistics may reveal some interesting features about, for example, the age profile of a particular minority community, they cannot tell us about the particular needs of children and elders in that community which may be influenced by a whole series of factors. Moreover, this type of policy research does little to help one understand more fundamental social and political processes that may result in the production of such issues as higher rates of physical abuse and neglect amongst minority families (Creighton 1992).

Second, the potential consequence of simplistic correlation on the basis of statistical averages can often lead to further reinforcing stereotypical images of minority communities. Sadly, such pathologising tendencies are not restricted to the popular media but can be found amongst academic researchers and professionals. Ahmad (1993) highlights a whole series of instances where, within epidemiological studies on minorities, disproportionate levels of disease or ill-health are routinely attributed to cultural factors. For example, it is observed that:

> Higher rates of consanguinity among Asians, particularly Pakistanis, in Britain has become the ultimate 'explanatory hypothesis' within medicine. This includes serious researchers who wish to disentangle the complex interplay between socio-economic, lifestyle, environmental and health service factors in influencing, for example, birth outcome – perinatal mortality and congenital malformations. A larger group,

> however, is happy to hang anything from poor birth 'outcome' to blood disorders, cancers, diseases of the eye, and much more onto this new found explanatory peg.
>
> (Ahmad 1993: 21)

Of course, not all empirical research is based on statistics – and we are quite sure that there remains a need for descriptive studies. The fact remains that positivism generates narratives which are convincing to policy makers and practitioners. Our concern is that such descriptions should not be uncritical, or informed only by the perspectives and prejudices of the majority or dominant groups.

The second perspective is one which, in attempting to develop a more critical and theoretical dimension to 'race'-related questions, has attempted to understand the features of the lives of minorities from a more phenomenological perspective. Here minorities with particular attributed labels (e.g. immigrants, asylum seekers, etc.) are not reduced to 'social facts', but through the use of qualitative methodologies such as focus groups, participant observation and life-history work researchers have attempted to map out the texture of the day-to-day existence of minority communities. Another important aspect of this paradigm has been rejection of the 'problem'-finding/curing mentality and concentration on describing the concrete interactions of minority communities with one another and with state agencies.

Above all, this approach attempts to subjectify otherwise highly objectified and abstract conceptualisations of minority communities. At its most fundamental, there is a change from enumerating the exotic to describing, with some level of understanding of ethnic minority communities, their needs and aspirations in terms of their new cultural contexts. These inevitably constitute a complex synthesis of past and present. By placing the concepts of culture and ethnicity centrally to the analysis, we saw a whole series of texts written during the late 1970s and '80s that powerfully influenced much of social work practice of the time (see Cashmore 1979; Watson 1977; Khan 1979; Cheetham 1981).

One of the major criticisms of what became known as the ethnic sensitivity approach (Dominelli 1988; Ely and Denny 1987) was the tendency to shift attention away from structural and political issues. Moreover, by focusing too narrowly on the communities themselves – often resulting in promoting a series of misleading constructions of minority cultures' family functioning – explanations tended to reinforce and reproduce the kinds of frameworks emerging out of the black family pathology model evident in much of the social work and health literature of the 1970s and '80s (see Lawrence 1982 for a powerful critique of this approach).

Perhaps unintentionally, what resulted from some of these early attempts by mostly white researchers to address questions of ethnic identity and cultural practices was a series of misleading and stereotypical representations of minority communities. Afro-Caribbean families are very often portrayed as being decadent, culturally deficient, disorganised and disintegrating – the high incidence of single parenthood, offending behaviour and low educational achievement being seen as evidence for this assertion. On the other hand, Asian family life was portrayed as an island of morality in a sea of decadence and immorality. This was an attempt to take a positive view of the Asian community which, in contrast to the broader trends in society of chronic family breakdown (evidenced by high divorce rates and the growth of single parenthood) and the contingent problems of juvenile delinquency, homelessness, etc., has managed to retain a sense of piety, financial independence and social and familial cohesiveness. The problem with such families is seen to lie in their rigid traditional conservative outlook, which may result in narrow repressive 'feudal' regimes within the family!

One of the major obsessions of researchers was the whole question of 'cultural conflict', where minority youth were seen to be trapped between the traditional expectations of their parents and the conflicting social norms associated with the Western culture into which they were being assimilated (Watson 1977). Particularly in relation to what became popularly known as the phenomenon of 'Asian girls running away from home escaping forced marriages', we saw a number of influential social work and other texts presenting such constructions of family life as matters of fact. These highly problematic and simplistic representations of Asian family life were given official credibility by organisations such as the Community Relations Council, which was ironically established to promote a better understanding of the 'ethnic minorities' and their cultures (Lawrence 1982:112). It wasn't until the late 1980s that critiques of this dominant view began to emerge and, somewhat ironically, young Asian women social workers and researchers offered some of the most powerful challenges. Patel, for example, in her research on homelessness amongst young women, found that family conflict was one of many important factors: 'Like many other young women in general, the young black women interviewed were running (away) because of physical violence, emotional and sexual abuse' (1994:35). Where researchers chose to go outside the family or community frame, they tended to focus on interracial conflict or conflict between the minority communities and the state. Legitimate demands for fairer, non-oppressive policing, or equal opportunities in service provision have been reduced to simplistic 'race' relations problems. Of relevance here is a point which Stubbs (1993) makes in his analysis of 'race' and health research:

> Rather than posing fundamental problems of their own making, researchers in 'race' and health tend to operate within a particularly narrow framework of 'policy relevance'. Many studies lack any historical,

> theoretical and political depth. Instead, studies tend to operate within a technical framework in which particular projects are studies relating 'objectives', in a linear way, to outcomes.
>
> (1993:36)

Nevertheless, one can be hardly surprised at a lack of emphasis on the critical questions of racism and the failures of policy makers. After all, they are the ones who have control over the purse strings and/or access to important sources of data (e.g. client case records, daily practices within care institutions) and will determine what research is supported, funded and disseminated (see Barn 1994).

Leaving aside the broader epistemological questions, at the level of research design and execution, one can identify key elements that can characterise the failure of each of the perspectives described above. First, there has been the tendency to present ethnic identification as a given fact and ethnic minority groups as being essentially homogeneous and relatively self-contained. Such an approach, where policy makers and service delivery planners may seek to 'treat all Asian needs as one, or to wish to find a single point of access to the black and minority ethnic population' may be convenient, but it is inappropriate (Johnson 1996:11). A number of critical questions have been ignored. For example, quite apart from the variety of religious affiliations and languages involved, there are questions of gender, class and sexuality and their impact on the ability of members of minority communities to resist oppression and also in relation to determining individual need for the delivery of appropriate social services. Likewise, research has tended to ignore the relationship between white ethnicity as an undefined entity and black ethnicity as something 'other', as has been discussed at length in the introduction to this volume. Indeed, the whole question of identity formation and difference as social and psychological mechanisms has received little or no attention within social policy research until fairly recently.

Second, in failing to acknowledge the many changes, conflicts and struggles that members of ethnic minority community are engaged in, social work research that addresses the question of racial disadvantage, power relations, and questions of culture and identity from a user perspective is almost non-existent. If one believes that research should be 'value-free' and should be devoted to uncovering 'truths', then there is nothing much one can say. However, social work practice does have a clear value base, including amongst other things a requirement to oppose racism and other forms of discrimination (see Dominelli, Chapter 3).

Third, with the exception of feminist researches, the importance of differences between researcher and researched and how these may impact upon the research process – from question formulation right through to dissemination of findings – has tended to be neglected. The failure to take into account the cultural, social and economic position of both the researchers and research subjects has resulted in a 'tendency of research to reinforce and contribute to the plethora of stereotypes and derogatory myths that prevail in the dominant society' (Mama 1990:28).

Towards anti-racist and empowering perspectives

As a direct consequence of the failure of academic and research institutions to develop critical understandings of the politics of research and their own Eurocentric bias (Mama 1990), debates emerged within social work around the need to develop more critical anti-racist and anti-oppressive research. In contrast to all that went before it, this perspective set out make politics its prime concern. Research took on an explicitly political focus whereby the research process and research findings became mobilised to challenge structural inequalities and oppression (Trinder 1996:238).

Drawing on many of the themes of community and radical social work of the 1970s and feminist, anti-racist and more recently anti-disablist social work perspectives in the 1980s and '90s, empowering research takes on very specific modes of operation. Trinder identifies two specific strands which are very much characterised by political rather than 'scientific' concerns, both of which very closely mirror some of the current debates within mainstream social work practice. First, there is the location of the researcher/practitioner, which critically should be 'alongside members of oppressed groups in a non-hierarchical way drawing links between an individual's situation and structural factors' (ibid.:239). In what could be seen as taking a 'postmodern' turn, for Trinder the second strand gets at the very core of the expert/client power dynamic: 'The privileged position and knowledge of the expert is decentred, as the voices of the oppressed and their subjective experiences are moved centre stage' (ibid.:239). In a similar but more specific way, Mama (1990) in her ground-breaking study of professional responses to violence against black women in the home identifies four specific steps that researchers can take to reduce racial inequality in the research process. First, as a means of minimising the possibility of miscommunication and in order to rectify some of the power imbalance, 'ethnic matching of researchers' should be considered. Second, researchers must give credibility to the accounts of research subjects who are best placed to know about their personal circumstances. The third point is closely linked into general critiques of professionals, particularly evident in the work of Foucault (1973), and points out the dangers of viewing their accounts with more credibility than those of the client/research subject. The final point relates to analysing research findings, which according to Mama must be made in the light of the collective histories and cultures of minority groups, paying particular attention to colonial conquests, enslavement and economic exploitation in the Caribbean, Asia and Africa. In other words, in analysing minority experiences in European societies, researchers must never underestimate the continuing legacy of slavery and colonialism that impacts the lives of minority and majority populations in very real (social and economic) and constructed ways (identity formation).

Under the critical anti-racist model a kind of three-way, mutually beneficial partnership between academic researcher, social work practitioner/professional and service user emerges. For academic researchers, one of the obvious benefits of such a partnership is the opportunity of overcoming problems in obtaining access to research sites, subjects and in some instances funding.

For social workers there are a number of very tangible benefits. By engaging in research they can act to enhance and further develop the considerable skills they already possess (e.g. interviewing, observing, recording and analysing). As practitioner researchers, through their proximity to communities and the immediacy of needs, they are required to produce answers as much as to ponder on the unknowable. Therefore there is, for them, a need to engage in critical reflexivity, on their own research as well as on that of others, to ensure that they are not drawn into the sin of the simple solution. And finally, under the growing burden of organisational, legislative and public pressure (as Everitt *et al.* (1992) suggest), as practitioner researchers social workers could reclaim some semblance of professional autonomy, thus providing (as Broad (1994:165) suggests) a mechanism for them once again to be part of a process which is promoting social change.

The clearest benefits for users in the participation model are the possibilities of defining research agendas, gaining self-confidence and raised consciousness and forming support networks. What is more, they are quite likely to be able to access the results of research 'about them', instead of that information becoming the property of others.

Methodological issues

In approaching the research project, a researcher has to make a number of choices. It may be that the resources available to the enquiry dictate the method that will be used – either in terms of the amount of time and money that the practitioner or researcher has available, or because only certain types of records are held in accessible form – and they contain only certain types of information. Equally, the topic of the research will affect the choice of the most suitable research method – whether a quantitative historical approach using data from records, or a qualitative one perhaps involving attitudes – or an experimental approach, seeking to establish what happens when a particular need arises or someone tries to do something. In all cases the *choice* of the method used – that is, questions of methodology – will affect the outcome of the research.

A primary concern is the level of the research – a 'macro-analysis' of patterns of disability across Europe will require approaches very different from a micro-study of an individual's personal history, or the patterns of caring in a family. There is, of course, a middle way as well, and the 'meso-level' study can draw upon both extremes. Indeed, even large-scale studies may benefit from the insight to be gained from including smaller level case studies or examples, as this volume attempts to demonstrate in its structure. Other lessons for the researcher can also be drawn from a reading of the accounts of practitioners – as, for example, can be seen in Segerström's (Chapter 9) description of Somali refugees' responses to community work. It is clear that there was in that situation a difference between the perspectives and techniques of the Aid agencies and the understandings of the people from the Somali community. Such tension (possibly creative) is inherent in all research.

In approaching a question from the research perspective, rather than as a 'politician' or an acknowledged actor in the situation, the researcher must first examine his or her own values, and the degree to which they are conditioned by the very characteristics of the case under review. The child who asked 'Why is the Emperor wearing no clothes?' in the famous story was approaching the scene with no preconceptions, unbiased by the respect and fear which burdened the ruler's courtiers – and not having heard the 'explanation' given by the crafty weavers who had persuaded everyone who was self-conscious that only the most clever and virtuous could see their cloth. However, few of us can approach our research with so light a burden. Equally, few children would possess the breadth of comparative knowledge and technical mastery of statistics, discourse analysis, cartography or other techniques required to back their insights with convincing 'proof'. The researchers too must ask whether they are free from prejudice in examining their own familiar territory but also clear-sighted enough that they do not 'map on' to an unfamiliar society the explanations which would suit their own culture. By culture, incidentally, we must insist that we mean not just Dutch or Scottish or Muslim or refugee culture – every profession and every social work office will have its own norms, technical language and ways of working – its own culture.

There are clear benefits in being an internal researcher – the knowledge of structures, the familiarity with language, the lack of a need to have every irrelevant detail explained just in case it has some significance for the problem. For the qualitative researcher, if the original hypothesis is well founded, access to appropriate informants will be speedy and less time will be wasted in familiarisation. For the quantitative researcher, the availability of data will not be a hurdle, the design of the survey questionnaire and the acceptability of certain forms of question will require little thought, and the computer analysis will ensure that all possible combinations of data will be tried.

And yet – precisely because the researcher is internal – certain questions will not be asked. Certain avenues will be blocked – as anthropologists and ethnographers have found for many years. Social deference, avoidance of extramarital sex, the commercial realism of the housing market, lack of prejudice among professional workers – all of these things are known to be true for (my – your – our) society: and therefore there is no need to ask about them. A degree of *naïveté* permits an unpicking of what is taken for granted, and will ensure that the outsider is given a much fuller explanation of certain aspects of the culture under study. For the quantitative researcher just as much as for the qualitative, the ethnographer and observer, the choice of questions, of what is actually recorded, is critical. In an ideal world, the researcher would question every action, enquire about every motive, and collect information about everything. Most important, therefore, is an awareness of the effect this has on the conclusions that are drawn and the hypotheses that are propounded.

PROCESSES OF RESEARCH

We have raised the question of self-awareness in the researcher – but we have also perhaps to question the whole approach of research. If we are to propose a model of research which is legitimate and transferable across cultures, so that social workers can understand the clients and societies with whom they are to work, we must consider not just the power relationship of the researcher and the researched, and the need to be clear about cultures and 'difference'. We should also think whether the traditional, hypothetico-deductive approach – 'I have an idea of how things might be and then seek to gather data to see if I can prove it is false' – is appropriate or whether this is in fact exploitative and demeaning to those who are subsequently researched. Does the researcher have an obligation to his or her subjects, not to make them simply into objects? Is the exploratory approach the only justifiable method or does this seek to deny the experiences and knowledge of those who already suffer from inequalities and social exclusion? Does the inductive approach, in which the researcher gathers the information and then tries to see what sense it makes, really meet the needs of policy makers and practitioners – or is the increasingly popular 'action research' stance free from bias and different from the processes of 'consultation' that are used to confirm and justify policy decisions which are already in essence formulated and about to be tried?

Many of these questions come into sharpest focus when the research is commissioned by, or is conducted in partnership with, community-based groups. Few of these will be totally disinterested in the outcome. The simple question 'What are the community care needs of the minority population of X?' immediately raises three more difficult and less scientific questions – what resources are available to meet these needs, who will control them, and where else might those resources be used? Because of the history of Western social science, from the origins of modern anthropology as the handmaid of imperial administration to the misuses of eugenics and modern ministries of the interior, many communities settled and living in European cities have at best a mistrust of the researcher and of answering questions asked by anyone remotely connected with the world of officials. However, increasingly too, community leaders and organisations have learned that the only way they can get change brought about, and convince bureaucracies of what they *know* to be true, is to collect 'research evidence'. In the process, community groups and their leaders can be brought together, agree a common agenda, and indeed learn something about their communities and discover issues – such as the contribution of women or another part of the community hitherto excluded from decision making, which take their development forward (Ellis 1991).

In writing for a wider audience than the British, we have also been brought face to face with the fact that there are different traditions and approaches within the European arena. We are conscious that the 'method of sociological intervention' propounded by Touraine (Scott 1991) in France has been little attempted in Britain – and that perhaps its success in France relies upon the esteem with which the academy is regarded there. Similarly, Soydan's (1995) use of vignettes differs in subtle but important ways from the apparently similar testing of psychiatrists (Johnson and Orell 1996) for ethnic bias recently conducted in England. The use of deliberate deception – the 'situation testing' approach used not only by journalists but also the highly respected Policy Studies Institute of London (Brown and Gay 1985) – ran into difficulties in Britain when two doctors sent false credentials to employers to demonstrate racial bias in the medical labour market (Esmail and Everington 1993). In other states, they could have faced prosecution and imprisonment. Even the questions that are taken for granted in Britain and the Netherlands about ethnic and religious affiliation are illegitimate in parts of Scandinavia and the laicised society of France – as discussed in Johnson's chapter on ethnic monitoring. What hope then is there for a 'European model' of social research?

CLASSIFICATION

In nearly any example of social research, and particularly when issues related to social diversity are being explored, it will be necessary to categorise people. The point needs to be reiterated, that such categories are a means to an end, and not the object of the study:

> Studies of different forms of inequality need to differentiate for instance the experiences of black people from the experiences of white people . . . disabled people from those of non-disabled people. However, it is

> neither the *blackness* or *whiteness* nor the *disability* or *non-disability* that forms the focus of the investigation but the differential *experiences* of being black or white . . . that fundamentally reveal how inequalities are maintained.
>
> (Truman and Humphries 1994:3)

Many research texts warn against the dangers of essentialist assumptions, the use of a group label as if it somehow was real and by itself explained difference – and these are not confined to 'race and ethnicity' (Ahmad and Sheldon 1993). Similar dangers can arise in relation to gender (Humphries and Truman 1994), religion (Macourt 1994) or sexual relations and family structures – including the often uncontested nature of 'marriage' and household relationships (Graham 1993). Researchers should not need to be counselled that a person may indeed be 'described' in all of these categories – for example, as a black, female, Buddhist and (lesbian) lone parent; and disadvantaged or advantaged by membership of each group. Equally, one should pay attention to the undefined 'control' category – the 'white' or 'majority'. Very seldom is this group examined or explicitly defined, despite the dangers that this has for scientific explanation (Bonnet 1997). As we would insist that 'racial' or 'ethnic' groups, migrants and other minorities should be seen to contain subdivisions (as above), so does the majority, 'host society', of 'national citizens' – it can be seen that we lack suitable terms to describe this undifferentiated, presumed non-problematic, mass!

The question may be rephrased – it may all be seen to depend upon how we negotiate the notion of difference. We have perhaps argued for a de-essentialised notion of identity, whereby there are no absolutes. However, Spivak (1987) makes an important observation that most people operate and deploy a form of 'strategic essentialism', whereby identity is real and becomes used for specific functions, but cannot be said to be 'real' in any other sense that will determine their entire being. The danger is that the label becomes used in place of the person. As Miles (1989) and others have argued in seeking to avoid the use of the term 'race' (which we and others now tend to place in inverted commas, accordingly), if one argues against racism, then logically one must say that 'race' is an invalid category. However, some things can only be described succinctly if related to 'racialised groupings' – but by using such terms, one 'reifies' (makes real and justifies) their use, and gives succour to those (racists) who argue that 'race' is in fact a real category on which to base one's actions. For communication, it remains true that certain stereotypes and clichés, however dangerous, remain necessary: life is really a series of approximations and simplifications! Researchers must communicate, but at the same time must understand how the terms they use and how identity (the label) work. A person may have several identities, some of which are materially determined (social – such as class, wealth), and others which are symbolic or relational. The researcher should not deny the ability of the person to deploy a repertoire of identities for a variety of functional reasons. The fact that minorities may sing to new tunes and along hitherto undreamed of axes, is part of the excitement. This, in short, is the challenge that diversity raises both for social work and social research.

In sum, we must accept that, as Humphries and Truman insist, there is no such thing as an unproblematic reality – even research is not based solely on objective knowledge, but on (as well as, in the process, making) constructed reality. Therefore, researchers are faced with a number of challenges to their own practice – as well as challenging the assumptions of others. While seeking to (for example) understand and correct the paradoxical use of racial stereotypes by service providers, which may see minority clients described as both pathologically needy but undeserving, incapable but over-claiming, dysfunctional but close-knit and exclusive (Johnson 1986), we are at the same time forced into using the very labels they use – since it is by such labels that their power and explanations operate! Perhaps the best that can be hoped for is that they will be used consciously and with the sort of footnote that Barn feels constrained to add to her challenge to anti-discriminatory research in social work: 'Although the author accepts the concept of race to be a social construction and not a biological entity, the term is being employed here in the absence of other suitable terminology' (Barn 1994:55). Similar points should also be made in respect of other terms used in this volume – such as refugee, 'migrant', and indeed even the label 'minority'. As researchers, it is incumbent upon us to be explicit and aware in our use of such words in our reports.

CONCLUSION

Whether or not one feels that research should be a neutral, dispassionate, fact-finding activity, one cannot escape the historical, political, professional and social contexts in which it takes place. These are contexts in which the distribution of power within society is very much affected by ethnicity, class, gender, age, income, and perhaps other axes of social differentiation as well. Hence the whole process of research, from funding to the types of questions asked, methodologies and dissemination, becomes a political activity which can serve a number of different functions. Since lives and life stories of social work clients are structured by the unequal distribution of power, research can therefore be used to ignore, reinforce or challenge inequalities that may emerge from these dynamics (Trinder 1996:238).

We have in this chapter perhaps asked more questions than we have answered – but then, we too are researchers and it is the function of a researcher to raise questions. To answer one of our own, we do not believe that there is a single answer or a universal model which can be applied to the challenge of conducting social research in an increasingly diverse society of multiple territories, each with its own history and tradition. However, we are also optimists, and do not believe that these difficulties are any reason not to make the attempt. It is clear that there is a need to develop new insights, and to adopt new perspectives. A degree of openness to alternative explanations, and an awareness that diversity brings opportunities as well as threats, will enhance the quality of all social research and may enable the practitioner to see more completely the imperfections in the existing system as it affects all its clients.

In summary, some pointers for future social work research with minority communities:

- With the growth in inter- and multi-disciplinarity social work, health and other welfare fields should draw upon research lessons from each other, remembering that their 'clients' are very often consumers of multiple providers.
- Whilst social exclusion is a reality for all populations, the mechanisms impact differently upon minorities, whose minority status may interact with those processes. There is a need for research to examine the specific impact of social exclusion on minority populations, particularly in relation to determining social care and health status/need.
- Social work research too often ignores the negative effects of professional intervention and the placement of clients into care. For example, the question of 'institutional abuse' is a much neglected subject in need of very thought-out methodologies that can enable the voices of some of the most oppressed members of society to be heard.
- Action research for its emphasis on participation and problem solving has long been favoured by social work researchers. Because of the emphasis on issues, there is little detailed analysis on the methodological considerations, particularly in relation to working with minority communities.

REFERENCES

Ahmad, W.I.U. (1993) 'Making black people sick: "race", ideology and health research' in W.I.U. Ahmad (ed.) *'Race' and Health in Contemporary Britain*, Buckingham: Open University Press.

Ahmad, W.I.U. and Sheldon, T.A. (1993) '"Race" and statistics' in M. Hammersley (ed.) *Social Research, Philosophy, Politics and Practice*. London: Sage 124–30.

Barn, R. (1994) 'Race and ethnicity in social work: some issues for anti-discriminatory research' in Humphries and Truman: 37–58.

Bhopal, R. (1992) 'Future research on health of ethnic minorities' in W.I.U. Ahmad, *The Politics of 'Race' and Health*. Bradford: Bradford University Race Relations Research Unit: 51–4.

Bonnet, A. (1997) 'Geography, "race", and whiteness: invisible traditions and current challenges' *Area* 29, 3:193–9.

Broad, B. (1994) 'Anti-discriminatory practitioner social work research: some basic problems and possible remedies' in Humphries and Truman: 164–84.

Brown, C. (1984) *Black and White Britain: The Third PSI Survey*. London: Heinemann.

Brown, C. and Gay, P. (1985) *Racial Discrimination 17 Years after the Act*. London: Policy Studies Institute.

Cashmore, E. (1979) *Rastaman: the Rastafarian Movement in England*. London: Allen and Unwin.

Cheetham, J. (ed.) (1981) *Social Work and Ethnicity*. London: Allen and Unwin.

Creighton, S.J. (1992) *Child Abuse Trends in England and Wales 1988–1990, and an Overview from 1973–1990*. London: NSPCC.

Daniel, W. (1968) *Racial Discrimination in England*. London: Penguin.

Dominelli, L. (1988) *Anti-Racist Social Work*. BASW, Birmingham: Macmillan.

Ellis, J. (1991) *Meeting Community Needs*. CRER Monograph 2, Coventry: University of Warwick.

Ely, P. and Denny, D. (1987) *Social Work in a Multi-Racial Society*, Aldershot: Gower.

Esmail, A. and Everington, S. (1993) 'Racial discrimination against doctors from ethnic minorities' *British Medical Journal* 306:691–2.

Everitt, A. *et al.* (1992) *Applied Research for Better Practice*. BASW, London: Macmillan.

Faist, T. (1995) *Social Citizenship for Whom?* Aldershot: Avebury.

Foucault, M. (1973) *The Birth of the Clinic: An Archaeology of Medical Perception*. Translated from the French by A.M. Sheridan, London: Routledge.

Graham, H. (1993) *Hardship and Health in Women's Lives*. Brighton: Harvester.

Hammersley, M. (ed.) (1993) *Social Research: Philosophy, Politics and Practice*. London: Sage/Open University.

Harding, S. (ed.) (1987) *Feminist Methodology*. Bloomington: Indiana University Press.

Humphries, B. and Truman, C. (1994) *Rethinking Social Research* Aldershot: Avebury.

Johnson, M.R.D. (1986) 'Citizenship, social work and ethnic minorities' in S. Etherington (ed.) *Social Work and Citizenship*. Birmingham: British Association of Social Workers.

—— (1996) *Good Practice and Quality Indicators in Primary Health Care*. Leeds: NHS Ethnic Health Unit, in association with NAHAT and KCW Health Authority.

Johnson, S. and Orell, M. (1996) 'Insight psychosis and ethnicity – a case note study' *Psychological Medicine* 26, 5:1081–4.

Khan, V. (ed.) (1979) *Minority Families in Britain: Support and Stress*. Basingstoke: Macmillan.

Lawrence, E. (1982) 'In the abundance of water the fool is thirsty: sociology and black "pathology"', in *The Empire Strikes Back, Race and Racism in the '70s* CCCS, University of Birmingham: London: Hutchinson: 95–142.

Layton-Henry, Z. (1984) *The Politics of Race in Britain*. London: Allen and Unwin.

Macourt, M. (1994) 'Using census data: religion as a key variable in studies of Northern Ireland' *Environment and Planning Series A* 27:593–614.

Mama, A. (1990) *The Hidden Struggle: Statutory and Voluntary Responses to Violence against Black Women in the Home*. London: London Race and Housing Research.

Miles, R. (1989) *Racism*. London: Routledge.

Patel, G. (1994) *The Porth Project: A Study of Homelessness and Running Away amongst Young Black People in Newport, Gwent*. London: The Children's Society.

Roberts, H. (1981) *Doing Feminist Research*. London: Routledge.

Rose, E. *et al.* (1969) *Colour and Citizenship: A Report on British Race Relations*, Institute of Race Relations. London: Oxford University Press.

SCLRAE (1992) *Europe 1990–2000: Multiculturalism in the City – the Integration of Immigrants*. Strasburg: Council of Europe – Standing Conference of Local and Regional Authorities of Europe (Studies and Texts 25).

Scott, A. (1991) 'Action, movement and intervention: reflections on the sociology of Alain Touraine' *Canadian Review of Sociology and Anthropology* 28:30–45.

Seifert, W. (1992) *Ausländer in der Bundesrepublic Deutschland: soziale und ökonomische Mobilitat*. Berlin: Wissenschaftzentrum Berlin für Sozialforschung.

Smith, D. (1977) *Racial Disadvantage in Britain*. London: Penguin.

Soydan, H. (1995) 'A cross-cultural comparison of how social workers in Sweden and England assess a migrant family' *Scandinavian Journal of Social Work* 4:85–93.

Soydan, H. and Stål, R. (1994) 'How to use the vignette technique in cross-cultural social work research' *Scandinavian Journal of Social Welfare* 3:75–80.

Spivak, G. (1987) *In Other Worlds: Essays in Cultural Politics*. London: Methuen.

Stubbs, P. (1993) '"Ethnic sensitive" or "anti-racist"? Models for health research and service delivery' in W.I.U. Ahmad (ed.) *'Race' and Health in Contemporary Britain*, Buckingham: Open University Press: 35–47.

Trinder, L. (1996) 'Social work research: state of the art (or science) in child and family social work' *Child and Family*: 1 (4):233–42.

Truman, C. and Humphries, B. (1994) 'Rethinking social research in an unequal world' in Humphries and Truman, *Rethinking Social Research*. Aldershot: Avebury: 1–20.

Watson, J.L. (ed.) (1977) *Between Two Cultures: Migrants and Minorities in Britain*. Oxford: Blackwell.

Wilpert, C. (1988) *Entering the Working World: Following the Descendants of Europe's Immigrant Labour Force*. Aldershot: Gower.

Chapter 14

Social work, social policies and minorities in Europe

Walter Lorenz

This chapter places the phenomenon of migration in the context of globalisation and argues that the increasing cultural diversity, particularly in urban European locations, heralds a world-wide process through which space and time get redistributed. Migrants share many characteristics with 'indigenous' dispossessed people who are being subjected to new and well-established forms of displacement and exclusion. The chapter attempts to show that for social work to respond to the challenge of finding appropriate methods for the work with dispossessed migrant populations it needs to place less emphasis on the special requirements of such groups and give greater attention to the mechanisms of exclusion as such, not least because social workers themselves can easily become unwitting instruments of exclusion. The close and uncritical relationship of social services with the nation state is evidence for this and care needs to be taken that this dependence on a nationalist agenda is not repeated at European level.

> In 1990 21.2% of the population of Greater London were black, 'foreigners' (excluding foreign-born citizens) constituted 16% of the resident population of greater Paris . . . in Amsterdam at the beginning of the 1990s 22% of the population were 'foreigners' – and half of the primary school population – in Frankfurt about 25%, and in Brussels some 28%.
>
> (Therborn 1995:50)

Cultural diversity had certainly arrived in the urban centres of Europe by the last decade of the twentieth century, at levels comparable to those prevailing in New York. Europeans find this astonishing, sometimes alarming; they got used to considering their territories as ethnically homogeneous and regard the rising number of ethnically distinct groupings as a disturbance of this 'established' pattern – oblivious, on the whole, to the fact that the pattern of homogeneity was of quite recent origin. Only by 'around 1950 had the states of Europe achieved an unprecedented ethnic homogenization of their populations' (Therborn 1995:47), and this came about largely as the indirect or direct result of the impact of Nazism on Europe and the world, its racist policy of the extermination of whole populations, its aggression against countries near and far, and an armistice settlement that, while not repeating the Wilsonian doctrines of the Versailles peace treaty, nevertheless gave renewed impetus to the identification and political utilisation of cultural and political boundaries. This homogenisation was achieved through the deliberate, politically motivated displacement of minority populations, most notably by Nazi Germany in the territories it occupied, and after the war of the German population of Eastern Europe, creating among them some 10.7 million refugees (Niethammer 1991). Austria and Finland received 6 per cent and 10 per cent of their populations respectively in refugees, Italians were expelled from Dalmatia and Istria (Therborn 1995:46). With the exception of the Soviet Union, Yugoslavia and Switzerland, the European nation states came to consider themselves as mono-ethnic, though mostly allied to political blocks that superseded and 'dampened down' their nationalism.

The political recipe that was to ensure peace in Europe after the devastation of the Second World War was in this sense strangely reminiscent of the formula of appeasement which had produced the welfare state consensus: it, too, regarded society as basically homogeneous, and solidarity as something that had been achieved through the coalition of former adversaries. Any deviation from the rational norm of 'good citizen behaviour' was treated as a matter of individual pathology. The refugees who arrived and had to be 'integrated' counted as 'indigenous', at least in a political sense (not just Germans who had escaped an alien, i.e. communist, regime, but also refugees from the uprisings of Hungary and Czechoslovakia belonged to 'our side'), even if at a cultural level mistrust and conflict were all too apparent. These political refugees stood in contrast to the economic migrants who started to appear in Western (and to some extent in Eastern) Europe a decade or so later, who were not regarded as refugees and instead, in countries like Germany and Switzerland, were made to retain their status as foreigners over several generations.

Historically speaking, cultural homogeneity of major cities in Europe certainly was an anomaly. Therborn calculates the proportion of the population of capitals which by today's criteria would have represented the typical national ethnicity in Central and Eastern European countries in the decades before the First World War as ranging from 36 per cent (Prague), 38 per cent (Bratislava), 40 per cent (Bucharest), 46 per cent (Helsinki) to 62 per cent (Warsaw), 75 per cent (Zagreb), 85 per cent (Vienna) and 89 per cent for St Petersburg (the highest 'indigenous' proportion for those capitals, Therborn 1995:44). The 1950s therefore completed a process of social homogenisation constructed around ethnic concepts. This tendency had set in with the political transformations of Europe in the post-Napoleonic era, had been fuelled by the patriotic movements which gave rise for instance to German and Italian unification in the latter half of the nineteenth century, had spread into global rivalry in the period of aggressive colonialism, had resulted in the break-up of the remaining multi-ethnic empires at the end of the First World War, flared up again in nationalism, fascism and Nazism in the inter-war period and plunged the world into cataclysmic destruction in the Second World War.

Ethnic diversity and rivalry in the recent post-war era of (assumed) homogeneity had by no means disappeared, but it was not made thematic. The Cold War confrontation saw to that in East and West, as did the determination behind the Western European integration efforts not to let nationalist rivalry become ever again the fuse that set the world ablaze. The Franco-German accord between de Gaulle and Adenauer was symbolic of this – the new generation of French and Germans youth had offers of exchange programmes heaped on them. Europe suggested itself to the immediate post-war generation as 'the solution' to old rivalries, a quasi-country with which young Germans could identify without shame, without the tyranny of a domineering culture and of stuffy traditions.

A similar political agenda contributed to the integration of the refugees in West Germany, officially called 'out-settlers' (*Aussiedler*), 'German nationals' from beyond the Iron Curtain who came to constitute 16.4 per cent of the population of the Federal Republic of Germany (Castles and Miller 1993). In popular perceptions their official title differed little from the customary 'refugee' (*Flüchtlinge*), which was often a means of referring not only to East Germans, Poles and Sudeten-Czech, but in southern Germany also to everybody who spoke with a 'posh' northern-German accent. The cultural diversity they created was notable: language patterns shifted, the difference between Protestant and Catholic regions levelled, culinary traditions changed, folk customs from far-away places occasionally became visible. But the diversity was framed in such a way that it was 'neutralised', subsumed under the much more important 'greater identity' of being German, or rather, of being Western, being an inhabitant of 'the free world'.

During the first two decades after the Second World War, two types of population movements coincided in Western Europe: the displacement and reception of refugees, mainly from Central and Eastern Europe, whose arrival had deep symbolic significance in that it served as a constant reminder of the repressive nature of the socialist regimes, and the recruitment of workers from Mediterranean countries and the Caribbean to fill vacancies in the labour market in the context of the reconstruction of the European economies. Both were considered transient, despite the fact that the fall of communism seemed ever more utopian and despite the rhetoric emanating from annual gatherings of ethnic groups (*Volksgruppen*) and 'people displaced from their homeland' (*Heimatvertriebene*); the refugee-settlers from East Germany, Poland, Hungary and Czechoslovakia were quietly regarded as permanent members of Western societies. By contrast, the permanency of recruited migrant workers was never accepted. Their relationship as 'guest-workers' with the 'host society' was considered as purely instrumental, a contractual arrangement with few implications for political integration and the acquisition of residency and citizenship rights.

It is against this historical background that the role of the social professions in relation to migrants, refugees and ethnic minorities in Europe has to be evaluated. Social services and social work methods of intervention are not in the nature of private arrangements between individual service users and independent service providers who seek to resolve crises over resource shortages and personal adjustment. Rather, such interactions are framed by this historical background and affected by the various political agendas at every stage and in every detail. Ultimately the traditional mandate of social service staff is to legitimate the boundaries of solidarity of a society, to ensure that solidarity is being extended only to 'the right kind of people' and that as many as possible of those remaining on the margins of society are being transformed into 'the right kind of people'. The assumed ethnic and cultural homogeneity of post-Second World War European societies made this task appear to be soluble largely with reference to psychological methods. The excluded were distinguished by behavioural or cognitive deficits, which prevented them from fully taking part in that solidarity. They had to be helped to adjust or they could not be helped and were left to the care (and control) of institutions. Behind the principle of 'client self-determination' stood a whole range of measures, which ensured conformity and assimilation, but they were seen as outside the domain of social work. Social workers were keen to 'treat people as people', to do justice to their professionalism by disregarding cultural and ethnic diversity and thereby to remain 'politically neutral', without questioning the very specific political assumptions and interests behind this neutrality and assumed universalism.

It is not surprising, therefore, that the articulation of ethnic diversity in European societies which occurred during the 1980s and '90s raised fundamental questions not only about social work methods but also about the role of social work in society. It is with this in mind that the more detailed look at social work in relation to migration can serve as an opportunity for the comprehensive assessment of social work's position in such societies' becoming more aware of their cultural diversity and the diminishing significance of the nation state.

As the immediate experience of the Second World War fades and the 'block-thinking' of global confrontation disintegrates, the nature of political crises in Europe and in the wider world changes fundamentally. They can no longer be subsumed under established patterns of lines of confrontation. The boundaries between 'them' and 'us' have become uncertain and unpredictable. Since the fall of the Iron Curtain and the visible permeability of borders more generally which it heralded, boundaries have to be re-established both on a global scale and at the community level. An immediate response to this uncertainty is the reference to the earlier experience with migration, which had set a pattern of distinction between political and economic migrants. This is being invoked as a regulatory principle for the treatment of refugees at both national and European level even though the distinction has become totally blurred (Castles and Miller 1993).

This results in an escalation and a short-circuiting of measures between national and European policy decisions which amount to a much tighter restriction on entry to the EU for political refugees and a relative openness to migration suited to or demanded by changes in the economy. The latter applies not only to the active encouragement of the mobility of labour, which is one of the central tenets of the European economic integration process, but also a relative toleration of illegal immigration in parts of Italy (Vasta 1993) and Spain and the persistent recruitment drive in response to labour shortages in Germany in certain parts of industry, notably the building and construction sectors and increasingly now also the personal and care services sector.

Migration highlights not only the existing diversity of every society; it also tests the boundaries of solidarity. All responses to the arrival of refugees are politically sensitive because they expose the prevailing rationale for the existence of boundaries of belonging, social responsibility and the conditions of citizenship and all their inconsistencies and weaknesses. In the context of the globalisation not just of the economy but of social relations generally (Waters 1995), national boundaries assume an ever more arbitrary character and become irrelevant for the purpose of defining the limits of social responsibility. This is reminiscent of the upheaval at the beginning of capitalist industrialisation when the system of parish responsibility for the poor and destitute became totally abstract and untenable in an industrialised nation state that required labour mobility. But while that marked the transition between, in Durkheim's terminology, mechanical and organic solidarity for which the state was *de facto* the new organising principle, today's transition from the national to the global scale has no new institutional framework (Beck 1994). It is open and therefore constantly prone to premature closure. Individual consciences are implicated in world events. The media present wars and disasters in far-away places with unprecedented immediacy. People respond personally to crises like famines or the plight of orphans in other countries or continents by becoming emotionally and often very practically drawn into giving direct help. The spread of ecological awareness illustrates further the connectedness of all world systems. And yet there are no longer any agreed guiding principles with which to limit this infinite burden of responsibility and to legitimate limits of responsibility and solidarity, let alone effective systems of governance to deal with global issues. The arrival of the new refugees on the Western doorsteps is inescapable evidence of the fact that economic and political problems can no longer be externalised, that no society can isolate itself from world events or deal with them from a distance. Their arrival is so uncomfortable because it highlights the sliding loss of control by First World societies over the process of boundary drawing, a form of control which they have come to take for granted.

The crisis of the limits of solidarity also represents a crisis of collective and individual identity and this leads to a new preoccupation with ethnicity (Bastenier 1994). The (re-)ethnification of social relations in Europe has two fundamental aspects. On the one hand it helped minority groups to articulate their cultural identity in a political arena which had become sensitised to cultural differences. This allowed them to recognise and utilise the collective assertions of power invested in claims to distinct ethnicities, particularly where they were associated with claims to national independence (Rex 1996). Alternatively, it gave those groups at least the possibility of offering effective resistance against the pressure to assimilate through positively revalidating the labels that had been used by the majority society to exclude them. On the other hand, using ethnicities as markers of the boundaries of community and solidarity reactivates nationalist mechanisms which had been so powerful (and disastrous) in the history of European nation states. Ethnicity in this sense always implies hierarchical orders of superiority and inferiority (Wieviorka 1994).

The re-emergence of nationalism and neo-fascism directed in aggressive forms against foreign and minority populations, as for instance in France, Austria and Germany, has the effect of ethnifying social and political conflicts further. Neo-fascist ideologies suggest 'simple solutions' which ultimately amount to the 'choice' between assimilation (on the terms dictated and controlled by the dominant group) and ethnic separation, expulsion or the redrawing of political boundaries (Radtke 1994). But ethnicity cannot be treated as a 'natural category' to be recovered and retrieved from historical oblivion; these conflicts show that it is a means of social classification and as such the product of very specific historical conditions and political interests.

The ambivalence of the ethnic argument exposes the contradictory premises on which solidarity as national solidarity is predicated. It suggests nationality as a taken-for-granted reference point that distinguishes nationals from foreigners with reference to some intrinsic qualities. In European history it has come to imply an ethnified concept of the nation (Hobsbawm 1990) and thereby places the qualities and prerequisites of 'belonging' beyond the reach of political discourse while at the same time being unable to substantiate the assumed equivalence of ethnic and national boundaries (Gellner 1983). There are strong indications that European identity and thereby solidarity is being fashioned according to the recipe of the nation state, through closure constructed on ethnic lines which confirms a Fortress Europe mentality, and not just in relation to asylum seekers (Pieterse 1995). The fundamental changes in the nature of the welfare states and the selective manner in which a European social policy agenda is being developed point in that direction. It no longer suffices to be born into the community of a nation to be entitled to a minimum of support. This support has to be 'earned', not necessarily financially but in terms of loyalty to the nation and conformity with its standards. Fortress Europe is being erected not just against foreigners, but also against homeless people, single mothers, people who seemingly brought about their own hardship. For economic reasons the 'contract between the generations' which had ensured the payment of old age pensions from contributions paid by those earning a wage is being questioned. Solidarity no longer extends automatically between the economically active and those in retirement, who get constructed as a separate group on lines akin to those of ethnicity. Both on the inside of nation states and on their external boundaries, fortified by the European unification process, boundaries of solidarity are being mapped out anew, but the criteria by which these boundaries are being determined have long lost their universal validity and legitimacy. Solidarity reveals itself as whimsical, fashion-driven, media-dependent, ultimately arbitrary. The encounter with migrants and refugees activates those very uncertainties in localised, everyday, inescapable contexts and interactions.

What is more, the ambiguity of national boundaries is indicative of a fundamental reordering of the command over time and space in the course of globalisation. In the analysis of Giddens and Harvey, accelerating trends in late modernity or postmodernity have completed the distanciation of time and space, which resulted from the formation of international sets of relations by the nation states and was supported by the emerging national economies of the nineteenth century and the concomitant technological advances (Giddens 1984, 1991, 1994; Harvey 1989). Time and space have not only separated from each other and have become independent of a locality, but the technology to 'shrink' space and to create virtual simultaneous encounters across the globe is having the effect of a dramatically increasing time–space compression. This is not an inevitable linear development of history; it is the direct result of the power to command the use of time and space accumulating in the hands of an elite. In other words, globalisation is about the redistribution of time and space, about their very unequal redistribution. The rich and powerful occupy space, which they claim as their own (while running out of time in the process, which has to be utilised ever more efficiently as the global stock market never closes), whereas the dispossessed have 'time to kill' and are being squeezed out of economically usable space and become ghettoised in wastelands (Bauman 1997). This is the motor for global, end of twentieth-century migration patterns which puts jobseekers from declining national rural regions in the same contested metropolitan arena as migrants and asylum seekers from distant places. Globalisation is about a forceful and rapid rupture within space and time. Additionally, it reduces the migrant population and the 'indigenous' excluded to an over-reliance on time: they are being eliminated from the present and relegated to the past, made to carry around with them an oversized baggage of history of which they are being constantly reminded. They are being identified with traditional forms of behaviour as former peasants, as left-overs of a working-class culture, as settled nomads who have never left behind their habits. In a similar vein, one of the mechanisms of excluding women is their identification with traditional values and roles as bearers not only of children but also of historical continuity and a particular type of social order. This prevents these groups from ever fully arriving in the present and laying claim to a piece of contemporary territory. It also sets them in competition with each other as different groups of dispossessed populations and reveals another insidious aspect of the sporadic popularity of neo-fascist ideas among disaffected youth and insecure sections of the working class: by clinging to their ethnic identity they can easily become hooked on a selective, tendentious version of history and thereby remove themselves from the economic battleground of the present. Consequently, they can only make their presence felt in violence and provocative disruptions.

It is therefore not surprising that conflicts over the unequal distribution of resources erupt with increasing frequency in open violent conflicts over territories. Seen from this perspective, conflicts ranging from inner-city riots to neo-fascist agitation and certain forms of violent crime share with the wars in former Yugoslavia, in different parts of the former Soviet Union and Northern Ireland the same underlying connection to the redistribution of time and space under globalisation. They are extreme means of settling the boundaries and conditions of belonging. Their appearance as untimely relicts from the past belies the logic of their acute contemporary role as manifestations of globalisation. The distinction between political and civil conflicts becomes as tenuous as the distinction between economic and political refugees. Populations can become a 'threat' to each other without being physically on the move, at least not at the moment of the conflict. Once the right of one part of the population to 'belong' fully has become contested, references to past migrations and displacements become moral justifications on the dominant side of such conflicts for claims of having 'been here first', no matter how arbitrarily such historical data are chosen. These conflicts represent desperate attempts to reconnect time and space, territory and culture, with reference to a reified past unity. Ethnic cleansing is evidence of a fundamental contemporary conflict over the disappearance and the symbolic reconstruction of criteria for social and political solidarity (Brubaker 1996). The message of 'simple, self-evident' and thereby deeply racist solutions it contains is bound to set the scene for endless future conflicts because it localises a problem that is in fact global. The exclusion from territory and the denial of contemporary time go hand in hand.

What is now the significance of this analysis for social work? Direct social work with refugees and asylum seekers is of marginal importance to the whole field of the social services. Although the work with these minority groups shares many characteristics with general social work, helping people to come to terms with the experience of a crisis, with the trauma of displacement, with the financial insecurities, it has become in most countries a highly specialised field and usually not one that is exclusively the responsibility of the social work profession. Nevertheless, seen against the background of this analysis and in the context of a general crisis of social solidarity, social work with refugees and migrants assumes a paradigmatic significance. It challenges the profession ethically and methodologically to clarify its reference points for intervention. The work with migrants, with people whose citizenship status is in doubt, tests the relationship of social work with the project of the nation state and its possible over-dependence on it. Was it ultimately the national agenda that gave it a mandate to ensure national solidarity, to contribute towards the creation of a national identity at the breaks and fault-lines of modern societies? Has the distinction between the 'deserving' and the 'undeserving' cases, which was always part of the profession's patriotic legacy, really disappeared and given way to a universal, critical, scientifically based approach to diagnosis and intervention? Or does social work, having ostensibly adjusted to the realities of multicultural societies, operate with notions of solidarity which are ultimately infused with a categorical concept of diversity (see Soydan, Chapter 2) and which make it inherently prone to misuses for racist purposes?

Social work with refugees is therefore basically not at all a specialist area, which requires a separate set of methods and principles. Instead, it may be more conducive to regard this area of work in line with 'mainstream social work', notwithstanding the necessity to develop 'special techniques' and even the occasional suspension of 'normal practice' in war conditions, as described in the chapter by Hessle and Hessle in this volume (Chapter 8). Under the impact of globalisation all users of social services are in danger of being displaced from the present, of losing a foothold in the imaginary territory of solidarity, of being reinvented as 'strangers among us' whose lack of self-reliance testifies to their existence beyond the pale. Or seen the other way round, the specialised forms of knowledge and skills developed in the area of work with refugees, in war zones and with people trying to 'settle' have far-reaching, critical implications for general social work which is grappling with fundamental transformations in society everywhere.

These methodologies will not emerge as straightforward prescriptions, which resolve dilemmas in a one-dimensional way. The contradictory effects of national (and indeed European) social policies in relation to migrant populations are indicative here. These policies oscillate broadly between attempts at 'integration through dispersal', through the avoidance of ghetto formations and the ensuing stigmatisation and discrimination (e.g. in France and to some extent the UK), and strategies directed explicitly at special needs and the acknowledgement of separate ethnic, cultural identities (e.g. the Netherlands and Sweden) (Castles and Miller 1993:210). Both are aimed at integration and the avoidance of conflict, but the experience has been quite universally one of 'unintended consequences': dispersal encounters the resistance by the migrant or ethnic groups concerned against the implied disregard for their collective identities, while special attention creates grounds for new inequalities in comparison with other marginalised groups.

These political dilemmas apply equally at the level of direct interaction. Social work methods that have been developed in relation to ethnic minorities, refugees and migrants are subject to the same ambiguities. Approaches that ultimately supported assimilation were often applied by social workers in the belief that this was the most effective way of preventing or eliminating discrimination. In the process they disregarded the importance of cultural continuity for identity formation and reinforced the perception of non-native life-styles as inferior or deviant. Similarly, a superficial multiculturalism that tries to give 'special attention' to cultural differences either reduces inequalities to a matter of culture and life-style or it 'essentialises' socially constructed differences. It thereby renders intercultural dialogue and critique of values and standards impossible (for instance with the 'safe' formula of same-race fostering and adoption). The reproduction of discrimination and exclusion as a result of such interventions is not a consequence of the methods or strategies as such but of their being 'overtaken' by structural inequalities and the prevailing racism in societies which constitute the problem in the first place.

It has now been recognised in most European countries that developing social work methods for work with migrant groups and ethnic minorities is therefore not primarily a matter of concentrating on migration or cultural differences as the specific causes of the social problems to be dealt with; nor can such methods be designed by way of ignoring those specific conditions and reverting to 'treating people as people'. Rather, the tension between the specific forms of exclusion encountered by those groups and the general nature of exclusion as encountered by all users of social services has to be explored in both directions. As Dominelli states in Chapter 3, all forms of social work are in danger of either bringing pressures to bear on people to assimilate to prevailing norms or of 'othering' clients, of arresting them in their categorical otherness and thereby confirming, even legitimating, their being excluded.

The reflection on the impact of racism on social work practice helped to bring out these connections in the discourse on social work methods. But it does not therefore follow that such methods can simply be exported to other countries. Seeing methodological developments as linear would imply a monocultural bias, as if, for instance, other European countries would have to wake up, sooner or later, to the necessity of applying the anti-racism approaches that have become a feature of some aspects of British social work. In the case study of Yemen (see Segerström in Chapter 9) culture-specific responses had room to assert themselves which had not initially been apparent to the Western aid workers instigating the project. The engagement with racism and exclusion needs to recognise the multifaceted and constantly changing manifestation of contemporary racism and the historical dynamics of exclusion. In particular, the discourses over methods need to take account of three reference points in the formulation of these specific responses, as becomes evident in the literature review by Hummrich, Sander and Wöbcke (1998):

(a) The different academic and disciplinary traditions prevalent in the social professions: social work in the form of community work is not inherently more political than that in the form of social pedagogy or counselling, and yet each discipline makes visible different mechanisms and consequences of exclusion.
(b) The differences in political culture that exist in different countries, particularly in relation to the degree and kind of mobilisation of civil society: there is no formula as to whether state or non-state services and agencies are less discriminatory, but what is important is the way the relationship between citizens and the state is mediated by associations and self-help movements. This is of special significance for the development of social services in former communist countries.
(c) The different legal conceptions regulating 'citizenship' as the manifestation of national solidarity, for instance the principle of *ius sanguinis* in Germany as against the *ius solis* and the emphasis on cultural integration as an expression of citizenship in France.

The encounter with users of social services whose basis of 'belonging' to a given society and nation is in question on psychological, cultural and legal grounds gives occasion to reflect on the need for a 'multilayered' approach to methods generally. This confirms the analysis central to Soydan's chapter that social work responses, particularly in the area of dealing with ethnic and cultural diversity, need to acknowledge explicitly the interplay between personal and political factors.

It is through this combination of perspectives and skills that social work has an important contribution to make to the development of a critical social policy perspective in Europe which is being shaped by new programmes and directives, but also by the way those affected by them can participate in their shaping. At European level the treatment of refugees and asylum seekers in comparison to that of migrant workers is highly contradictory and indicative of the fact that principles of selective exclusion, which had prevailed in the formation of nation states, are being reproduced rather uncritically at European level. Social workers know that it will not be possible simply to 'manage' those tensions except by force. In any case the policy of defining 'Europeanness' by means of exclusion will not produce a sense of European social solidarity or European citizenship unless there is a broad consensus on the principles by which to construct such solidarity positively. The convergence of European immigration policies from the Schengen Agreement to the Dublin Convention and their ratification in the Amsterdam Treaty of 1997 was intended to strengthen the perimeter fence around Europe while allowing greater mobility between EU countries. Measures taken concentrated on negative aspects, on keeping out 'undesirables', and it is very significant that refugees and immigrants from outside the EU are regarded in line with drug traffickers and terrorists for the purposes of controls and surveillance. The intergovernmental committees dealing with such questions operate under a cloak of secrecy and are not subject to effective democratic controls.

This 'Fortress Europe' mentality is antagonistic to the attempts to define positively a European sense of belonging and solidarity. A defensive, excluding fortress mentality is also becoming the hallmark of national social policies in the wake of the advance of the neo-liberal critique of the welfare state. The better off in society feel under siege from welfare claimants; their property rights appear threatened by high levels of taxation and redistributive policies. This amounts to a serious erosion of social citizenship, just as migrants are denied political and often civil citizenship. But formal and legal arrangements by which citizenship rights will be established or secured are one important dimension of the political process. Equally important is the actual practice of citizenship in everyday contexts, particularly between citizens and state officials, between clients and professionals, between claimants and service providers. In other words, the political dimension of social work is brought to bear not only on campaigning, on social workers contributing to the debate on social rights and submitting evidence to social policy committees, but also on the form of the actual practice of delivering a service to users of social services. It is at this level that 'substantial' citizenship in the distinction of Bottomore (1992; see Chapter 1 by Soydan and Williams) is either established or denied.

What is suggested here is the equivalence between the political 'framing' of actions around consistent sets of anti-racist principles (see Dominelli, Chapter 3) and the extension of those principles and their 'substantive' interpretation and application in all direct personal interactions. The physical arrival of minority groups among the ranks of social service users raises the question of citizenship in a highly acute form. It highlights the deep ambivalence contained in European practices around citizenship by triggering well-established mechanisms of ethnic closure and thereby exclusion. Of these the most prominent and the most insidious is the inversion of cause and effect: the arrival of migrants can be construed as 'causing' xenophobia and racism, just as the appearance of homeless people in the streets 'causes' aggressive reactions from the public, or the establishment of a hostel for people with schizophrenia in a respectable neighbourhood 'causes' social tensions. Social workers themselves, on account of the attention they direct to those problem areas and their failure to make them invisible, also become implicated in having caused or contributed to them. Underlying this ideology concerning the formation of social problems is always the assumption that a community is essentially homogeneous, that standards of normality are something akin to a natural phenomenon that a society then strives to 'preserve', and that homogeneity is a guarantee against the emergence of social problems. Citizenship status is then only bestowed on those who already possess the assumed qualities of that community (Parekh 1995). This detracts from the realisation that such normality is not a natural state but a social construct and a means of legitimating the boundaries of society, externally as well as internally.

Minorities do not need to migrate at all to become entangled in these mechanisms; they can also encounter them by finding themselves on the wrong side of the border (and in most parts of Europe there are examples of ethnic conflicts arising not over the moving of people but over the moving of national boundaries). As far as social work is concerned, the underlying pattern is the same: social workers invariably deal with people who find themselves on the wrong side of a border or who are being shunted back and forth between agencies or departments who contest their claims for support. The difference between political and social boundaries becomes further relativised when one recognises that boundaries are always social constructs and as such manifestations of power interests: rivers, mountains and other markers on the physical landscape, like skin colour, appearance, language and habit on the social landscape, are merely the symbols that serve to legitimate, however spuriously, the planting of a border post and the operation of sentinels or of special rules.

'The migrant' is therefore a paradigmatic test case for social work. Displaced, dislocated people challenge social work to declare whether its values are rooted in (an ideology of) a place, in nationalism or even in racist assumptions about the given, innate qualities of those who deserve to belong or whether it succeeds in transcending the securities of territory and nation to realise its universal potential. 'Migrants', non-citizens, hold up a mirror to our societies, which have come to expect seeing a picture of themselves as enlightened, rational, well-ordered modern entities. But seeing themselves reflected in the expectations and claims of those 'others' shatters the mirror image into the fragments of postmodernity. The insecurity, relativity and arbitrariness not just of national boundaries but of the prevailing principles of order and cohesion emerge with uncomfortable clarity. The problems the others 'cause' are evidence that we are not in control of our circumstances, that fundamental issues of order and cohesion lie unresolved at the core of the rationalisation project of Western civilisation, that our social and political organisations are incapable of facing up to the complexity of situations to which they have all contributed. Social work has been an intricate, small but important part of this civilising project. It now sees itself questioned in that role and plunged into the uncertainties associated with globalisation.

Globalisation brings with it individualisation and fragmentation of social relations, the redistribution of time and space referred to above, and social workers have to examine critically what functions they are called upon to fulfil in this new scenario. Globalisation transforms social problems and issues into risks, into something that has to be and therefore will be eliminated by technical means (Beck 1992). The technical management of such risks has the function of securing the new distribution of space and time, of protecting private spaces which occupy more and more what was formerly public space, from leisure amenities which now exist for private profit to hospital beds and places in educational institutions. The elimination of risk, the exclusion of ambivalence, of free spaces in which the unpredictable may happen, very often involves the exclusion of those who are seen as causing the risk. This leads to

> attempts to burn out the uncertainty in effigy – to focus the abhorrence of indetermination on a selected category of strangers (immigrants, the ethnically different, vagrants, travellers or the homeless, devotees of bizarre and thus conspicuous subcultures) while hoping against hope that their elimination or confinement would provide the sought-after solution to the problem of contingency as such and install the dreamt of routine.
>
> (Bauman 1995:128)

Indiscriminate deportations of refugees originating in countries that have been declared 'safe' is an institutional solution parallel to the indiscriminate reception into care of all 'at risk' children.

Paradoxically, globalisation itself teaches that it is impossible to externalise risks, that there is a global, systemic nexus between all human activities, most vividly demonstrated in ecological matters. But this awareness and the skills required to act accordingly are by no means automatic consequences of the suspension of national boundaries and the arrival of satellite media conveying global cultural influences in even the remotest corners. On the contrary, as the treatment of migrants shows, first reactions mobilise defensive ideological responses, both at the personal and at the political level. In Beck's analysis (Beck 1994) societies find themselves on the threshold of a second phase of modernity which has direct and very specific implications for social work. The reflexivity, core characteristic of modern societies (Giddens 1991), becomes conscious of its own insecurities, of the unreliability of the norms of rationality in which modernity had invested so much. Overburdened by this need for constant reflexiveness and unable to gain from it, many sections of modern society retreat into constructions of 'counter-modernity', into 'fabricated, manipulable self-evidence' (Beck 1994:473). Territorial ideas of identity abound and with them the fallacy that identity could be something simple, unequivocal, a product of simplified dualisms. The ethnification of social relations is therefore part of this counter-modern backlash. The warning references to the consequences of such simplifications under Nazism and its 'final solution' are not sufficient to avert the dangers of neo-nationalism and neo-fascism in Europe. The 'ethnification of social work methods' would be equally inappropriate as it reduces all differences, all problems encountered to fixed, undifferentiated categories.

What is required instead, and this becomes clear in practically all social work situations, is a dual strategy around which social work methods capable of engaging with 'Europeanisation' and globalisation need to be constructed. This applies not just to the work with migrants and refugees but must become a feature of all social work in multicultural, diverse societies. One requirement is that it fosters psychological security through competence in reflexivity, allowing individuals to accept fully their multilayered identities in the context of 'fluid' communities. The other is that these identities and the conflicting demands on others that arise from them are negotiated with regard to civil and political rights. Differentiated social groups and communities require rules, not in the form of externally imposed rules, but as frameworks of rights and obligations, which those affected by them can shape collectively. This means, for instance, that in the work with offenders or perpetrators of violence their human rights get established, the ties of mutual obligations with various sectors of the population get re-established, that institutional segregation, where it becomes necessary, does not mean the end of regarding inmates as members of society and of distinct communities of interest. The uncertainties and anxieties not just on the part of the excluded but also on the part of those benefiting from globalisation and the expansion of their space can only be met effectively by the development of new social and political structures. Globalisation challenges social work to contribute imaginatively to this reconstruction of 'the social' which neo-liberalism had declared all but obsolete.

This reconstruction is above all a moral question, 'since it is only the *full* relationship, a relationship between spatially and temporarily *whole* selves, that may be "moral", that is embrace the issue of responsibility for the other' (Bauman 1995:134). But as a moral question it becomes an immensely practical question, a matter of action not of attitude. The reconstruction of what constitutes a social self begins with daring to show social responsibility in non-routine ways, in ways that build trust, mutual obligations, sets of agreed rules, negotiated structures and hence communities, in ways that allow criticism of other life-styles and cultural traditions and make reference to universal principles. The approach does not start with regarding communities as given entities with fixed rules and linear continuities. Continuity is desperately important, particularly for those who experienced forceful disruptions and dislocations, for children caught in the cross-currents of incompatible demands and from societies in transition. Language can be a crucial factor in ensuring such continuity, as the reference by Drakeford and Morris to the use of the Welsh language in social work shows (Chapter 6). But this continuity cannot come from references to ontological qualities like race and culture, nation or blood or soil, which are products of deception and will always render those putting their faith in them powerless and disoriented once they experienced their unreliability. Continuity can only be secured in the interplay between personal freedom and social responsibilities which has found its diverse manifestations in modern notions of citizenship. Taking citizenship as a lived experience, as moral practice among people who recognise each other's multilayered, dynamic identities, could provide a reference point for social work not just with migrant groups, but for social work in the age of globalisation *per se*.

Within the prevailing politics of recognition where ethnic identities and other 'expressions of self-interest' have currency, where political correctness conjures up notions of moral righteousness, social workers are ill advised to choose the road of 'ethnified approaches' as a means of refuting the suspicion of racism and other inherent biases. Such 'partiality' alters nothing about the nature of discrimination in society and ultimately plays into the hands of power interests that utilise ethnic boundaries as markers for discrimination and exclusion. Furthermore, from an ethical point of view it locks social work into a fundamentalist framework which Giddens warns against:

> A Nietzschean view is sometimes lauded these days as allowing for that recognition of the 'other' – that necessary cosmopolitanism – which makes possible a multi-national world. It does nothing of the sort. What it leads to, in fact, is precisely a world of multiple fundamentalisms; and this is a world in danger of disintegration through the clash of rival world-views.
>
> (Giddens 1994:252)

His proposal of a 'generative equality', negotiated through 'generative politics', is very much the domain of social work because such equality needs to be worked out primarily 'at the basis', at community level, as the condition of tangible, substantive, experienced, lived citizenship.

To summarise the main arguments of this chapter:

- Ethnic and cultural diversity of societies is a constituent problem for most European nation states that built their national identity on the 'ideal' of homogeneity. Homogeneity, to the extent to which it was achieved at all, was largely a result of massive population displacements and of enforced 'border corrections'.
- The ideology of homogeneity places migrants under pressure to assimilate or, if they resist, to remain deprived of citizenship status.
- Social work's mandate implies a policing of the internal boundaries of solidarity in a society. In a professional context this was usually

interpreted as meaning that criteria of individual suitability, willingness and ability to be integrated into society were applied without regard to ethnic and cultural differences.

- In the light of cultural diversification and under the impact of globalisation, the criteria of social solidarity become disputed. They either get redefined along lines of ethnicity (and nationalism) or arbitrary and inconsistent parameters come to promote extreme forms of individualism.
- Social work appears to face a stark choice between allying itself to this process of ethnification of social relations on the one hand and a retreat to a project of uncritical support for the nation state on the other, which latter could also mean supporting a unified Europe characterised by a 'fortress mentality'.
- However, the analysis of this polarisation could clear the way for a third choice in which social work methods are geared towards creating the conditions for citizenship as a means of establishing mutually negotiated rights and obligations as the 'non-essentialist' basis for solidarity.
- These methods and competencies are not technical matters but call for a firm grounding of social work in ethical discourses and for a differentiated engagement in political processes.

REFERENCES

Bastenier, A. (1994), Immigration and the ethnic differentiation of social relations in Europe, in J. Rex and B. Drury (eds), *Ethnic mobilisation in a multi-cultural Europe*, Aldershot: Avebury.

Bauman, Z. (1995), *Life in fragments, essays in postmodern morality*, Oxford: Blackwell.

—— (1997), Schwache Staaten; Globalisierung und die Spaltung der Weltgesellschaft, in U. Beck (ed.), *Kinder der Freiheit*, Frankfurt: Suhrkamp.

Beck, U. (1992), *Risk society*, London: Sage.

—— (1994), Nationalismus oder das Europa der Individuen, in U. Beck and E. Beck-Gernsheim, *Riskante Freiheiten*, Frankfurt: Suhrkamp.

Benz, W. (1992), Fremde in der Heimat: Flucht – Vertreibung – Integration, in K. Bade (ed.), *Deutsche im Ausland – Fremde in Deutschland*, Munich: C.H. Beck.

Bottomore, T. (1992), Citizenship and social class, forty years on, in T.H. Marshall and T. Bottomore (eds), *Citizenship and social class*, London: Pluto Press.

Brubaker, R. (1996), *Nationalism reframed, nationhood and the national question in the New Europe*, Cambridge: Cambridge University Press.

Castles, S. and Miller, M.J. (1993), *The age of migration – international population movements in the modern world*, London: Macmillan.

Gellner, E. (1983), *Nations and nationalism*, Oxford: Blackwell.

Giddens, A. (1984), *The constitution of society*, Cambridge: Polity Press.

—— (1991), *Modernity and self-identity*, Cambridge: Polity Press.

—— (1994), *Beyond Left and Right – the future of radical politics*, Cambridge: Polity Press.

Harvey, D. (1989), *The condition of postmodernity: an enquiry into the conditions of cultural change*, Cambridge: Cambridge University Press.

Hobsbawm, E.J. (1990), *Nations and nationalism since 1780: programme, myth, reality*, Cambridge: Cambridge University Press.

Hummrich, M., Sander, G. and Wöbcke, M. (1998), Practice and research literature about social work methods with immigrant clients, in H. Soydan *et al.*, *Socialt arbete, invandrare och etniska minoriteter. Litteraturöversikt* (forthcoming).

Niethammer, L. (1991), *Die volkseigene Erfahrung*, Berlin: Rowohlt.

Parekh, B. (1995), Politics of nationhood, in K. van Benda-Beckmann and M. Verkuyten (eds), *Nationalism, ethnicity and cultural identity in Europe*, Utrecht: ERCOMER.

Pieterse, J.N. (1995), Europe among other things: closure, culture, identity, in K. van Benda-Beckmann and M. Verkuyten (eds), *Nationalism, ethnicity and cultural identity in Europe*, Utrecht: ERCOMER.

Radtke, F.-O. (1994), The formation of ethnic minorities and the transformation of social into ethnic conflicts in a so-called multi-cultural society: the case of Germany, in J. Rex and B. Drury (eds), *Ethnic mobilisation in a multi-cultural Europe*, Aldershot: Avebury.

Rex, J. (1996), Ethnic and class conflict in Europe, in J. Rex, *Ethnic minorities in the modern nation state, working papers in the theory of multiculturalism and political integration*, London: Macmillan.

Therborn, G. (1995), *European modernity and beyond – the trajectory of European societies 1945–2000*, London: Sage.

Vasta, E. (1993), Rights and racism in a new country of immigration: the Italian case, in J. Wrech and J. Solomos (eds), *Racism and migration in Western Europe*, Oxford: Berg.

Waters, M. (1995), *Globalization*, London: Routledge.

Wieviorka, M. (1994), Ethnicity as action, in J. Rex and B. Drury (eds), *Ethnic mobilisation in a multi-cultural Europe*, Aldershot: Avebury.

Index